Comprehensive Nursing Care
for Parkinson's Disease

Lisette Bunting-Perry, MScN, RN, is the assistant clinical director of the Parkinson's Disease Research Education and Clinical Center (PADRECC) at the Veterans Affairs Medical Center in Philadelphia, Pennsylvania. Ms. Bunting-Perry earned her undergraduate degree in nursing from the University of Maryland and her master of science in chronic care and management from The Johns Hopkins University, School of Nursing. She currently is a doctoral student at the University of Pennsylvania, School of Nursing, where she is focusing her work on palliative care in elders with Parkinson's disease. Ms. Bunting-Perry is a John A. Hartford Foundation Building Academic Geriatric Nursing Capacity Predoctoral Scholar and has received funding from the Mayday Fund for the study of pain in older adults with Parkinson's disease. Ms. Bunting-Perry has been active in numerous clinical trials, both as a clinical coordinator and principle investigator, and she has earned a certificate in the science of clinical investigation from The Johns Hopkins University School of Medicine. Through her publications and presentations, Ms. Bunting-Perry has received international recognition as a nurse expert in Parkinson's disease.

Gwyn M. Vernon, MSN, CRNP, is a certified registered nurse practitioner (CRNP), and has been caring for those with Parkinson's disease and their families for over 20 years. She has functioned in the capacity of coordinator for an American Parkinson Disease Information and Referral Center, a National Parkinson Disease Center of Excellence, a clinical research coordinator, and a direct provider of patient care and services. Gwyn has authored or coauthored over 25 articles or chapters on Parkinson's disease and related topics and has lectured nationwide. She is on the faculty of the School of Nursing at the University of Pennsylvania and is currently in private practice.

Comprehensive Nursing Care for Parkinson's Disease

Lisette K. Bunting-Perry, MScN, RN
Gwyn M. Vernon, MSN, CRNP

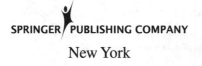
SPRINGER PUBLISHING COMPANY
New York

Springer Publishing Company, LLC
11 West 42nd Street
New York, NY 10036
www.springerpub.com

Acquisitions Editor: James Costello
Managing Editor: Mary Ann McLaughlin
Production Editor: Carol Cain
Cover design: Joanne E. Honigman
Composition: Apex Publishing, LLC

07 08 09 10/ 5 4 3 2 1

Library of Congress Cataloging-in-Publication Data

Bunting-Perry, Lisette K.
   Comprehensive nursing care for Parkinson's disease / Lisette K.
Bunting-Perry, Gwyn M. Vernon.
       p. ; cm.
   Includes index.
   ISBN-13: 978-0-8261-0237-9 (alk. paper)
   ISBN-10: 0-8261-0237-9 (alk. paper)
   1. Parkinson's disease—Nursing.   I. Vernon, Gwyn M.   II. Title.
   [DNLM: 1. Parkinson Disease—nursing. WY 160.5 B942c 2007]
   RC382.B95 2007
   616.8'33—dc22   2007008216

Printed in the United States of America by Bang Printing.

To nurses and other health care providers who seek to improve the quality of life of people living with Parkinson's disease. May you continue to inquire and find the knowledge needed to serve our patients and their families.

Contents

List of Contributing Authors

Heather J. Cianci, PT, MS, GCS
Geriatric Clinical Specialist
Dan Aaron Parkinson's Rehabilitation Center
Pennsylvania Hospital
Philadelphia, Pennsylvania

Barbara Fitzsimmons, RN, MS, CNRN
Nurse Educator
Department of Neuroscience Nursing
The Johns Hopkins Hospital
Baltimore, Maryland

Gretchen L. Glenn, LSW
Social Worker
Parkinson's Disease Research Education and Clinical Center (PADRECC)
Department of Veterans Affairs
Philadelphia Veterans Affairs Medical Center
Philadelphia, Pennsylvania

Susan Heath, MS, RN, CNRN
Movement Disorders Clinical Nurse Specialist
Associate Director for Clinical Care
Parkinson's Disease Research, Education, and Clinical Center (PADRECC)
Department of Veterans Affairs
San Francisco Veterans Affairs Medical Center
San Francisco, California

Julia E. Howard MS, CCC-SLP
Speech Language Pathologist
Philadelphia Veterans Affairs Medical Center
Philadelphia, Pennsylvania

Rebecca Martine, APRN, CS, BC
Associate Director of Education
Clinical Nurse Coordinator
Parkinson's Disease Research, Education, and Clinical Center (PADRECC)
Department of Veterans Affairs
Philadelphia Veterans Affairs Medical Center
Philadelphia, Pennsylvania

Jacqueline H. Rick, PhD
Department of Psychiatry
University of Pennsylvania School of Medicine and
Parkinson's Disease Research, Education, and Clinical Center (PADRECC)
Department of Veterans Affairs
Philadelphia Veterans Affairs Medical Center
Philadelphia, Pennsylvania

Amy M. Sawyer, Ph.D.(c), R.N.
Clinical Nurse Specialist, Sleep Disorders
VISN 4 Eastern Regional Sleep Center
Philadelphia VA Medical Center
Doctoral Candidate, University of Pennsylvania School of Nursing
Philadelphia, Pennsylvania

Constance (Connie) Ward, MSN, RN, BC, CNRN
Clinical Nurse Coordinator
Department of Veterans Affairs
Parkinson's Disease Research, Education, and Clinical Center (PADRECC)
Michael E. DeBakey VA Medical Center
Houston, Texas

Heidi C. Watson, BSN
Clinical Nurse Coordinator
Parkinson's Disease Research, Education, and Clinical Center (PADRECC)
Department of Veterans Affairs
Philadelphia Veterans Affairs Medical Center
Philadelphia, Pennsylvania

Preface

The nursing profession has provided us with the opportunity to be an integral part of interdisciplinary teams serving people with Parkinson's disease (PD) and related movement disorders. We have chosen this time to collaborate with friends and colleagues to bring *Comprehensive Nursing Care for Parkinson's Disease* to the nursing community and disseminate our collective clinical knowledge in hope of improving care for patients and families living with PD.

The international specialty of PD Nurse Specialists is in early development. We were fortunate to have met, as an international group of highly trained clinicians, at the First World Parkinson Congress in Washington, DC, in February 2006. Our shared training, vision, and passion for nursing brought us together to evaluate our mission, goals, and vision for the future. PD Nurse Specialists from Israel, the United Kingdom, Sweden, the Netherlands, Canada, Australia, and the United States attended a special session to discuss the creation of a global organizational structure. During the course of the evening we considered the following questions: Where have we been? Where are we now? Where are we going? What are our roles? And who do we serve?

WHERE HAVE WE BEEN?

In addressing the first question—where have we been?—we should look back at the landscape of movement disorder nursing as it has evolved over the past 25 years. At the World Parkinson Congress, Mary Baker, MBE, president of the European Parkinson's Disease Association, and Linda Caie, PD Nurse Specialist in Scotland, eloquently presented the development of the PD Nurse Specialist's role in the United Kingdom. In February 2006, there were 218 PD Nurse Specialists in the United Kingdom, with a goal of reaching 240 PD Nurse Specialists by 2008. The model of care for PD in the United Kingdom includes community health, hospital-based programs, and prescriptive authority for PD Nurse Specialists. Privileging as a PD Nurse Specialist in the United Kingdom is achieved through certification supported by a program of clinical and didactic education. In the United Kingdom, certified PD Nurse Specialists work closely with regional general practitioners and are highly valued members of the interdisciplinary team.

Undeniably, the United Kingdom has the most developed nursing organization for the training and development of nurse specialists for PD. How can we learn from their success? Mary Baker spoke of the importance of approaching the development of PD Nurse Specialists through building partnerships with physicians and by evaluating the "economic evidence" to support the role of the nurse in the interdisciplinary team. Funding in the United Kingdom for PD Nurse Specialists is supported through public and private partnerships. Additionally, pharmaceutical companies have generously supported the development of the PD Nurse Specialist's role in the United Kingdom.

Furthermore, the commitment of the United Kingdom to developing PD Nurse Specialists globally is evident in the establishment of PD Nurse Specialists' roles in Australia. Two nurses, Janet Doherty and Jo Chadwick, serve a diverse population of Parkinson's patients in remote areas of western Australia. Thus the training and dissemination of knowledge between the United Kingdom and Australia is enhanced through this partnership.

In the United States, movement disorder nurses were the first to form a special focus group within the American Association of Neuroscience Nurses (AANN; 1989), paving the way for the development of many special focus groups. Limited in scope, the movement disorder nurses' special focus group provides educational symposia at the national American Association of Neuroscience Nurses annual conference, a mechanism for networking and sharing of resources and information. The specialty of movement disorder nursing has benefited from the generosity of nonprofit organizations such as the National Parkinson Foundation (NPF) and the American Parkinson Disease Association (APDA). Both the NPF and APDA have funded PD Centers of Excellence and information and referral centers. In addition, the U.S. Congress allocated funds in 2001 to fund six Parkinson's Disease Research, Education, and Clinical Centers (PADRECC) with a mission to conduct research, provide clinical care, and present education programs in the Department of Veterans Affairs. Each PADRECC is paired with a large university-based medical center with a world-class movement disorder practice. Nursing is central to the model of patient care delivery in each PADRECC.

Through these federal, private, and nonprofit entities, enlightened neurologists have hired, trained, and mentored registered nurses in the care and treatment of patients with PD and related movement disorders. The mission of these nurses has been to provide patient care, disseminate knowledge, and support clinical and basic science research. Nurses working in specialty centers have also been trained in the conduct of clinical trials, case management, and community outreach. Through clinically based training within interdisciplinary teams, movement disorder nurses in the United States have evolved into highly skilled researchers, educators, and clinical specialists. This skill set contributes to the unique and valuable nature of nursing in movement disorder centers and has been used as a model in other chronic disease states.

In contrast to the UK model, there is no current certification for PD Nurse Specialists in the United States. Nurses in the United States have the opportunity to sit for certification through a variety of credentialing agencies, depending on level of education and licensure. The AANN provides advanced certification in neuroscience nursing for those meeting requirements and passing a rigorous examination. Nurses having completed graduate course work as nurse practitioners or as clinical specialists may sit for certification through the American Nurses' Association–approved American Nurses' Credentialing Center.

Globally, nurses working in movement disorder centers have recently become involved in the care and coordination of patients undergoing deep brain stimulation surgery. The advancement of deep brain stimulation technology is providing new hope for patients with PD, essential tremor, dystonia, and Tourette's syndrome. The advent of deep brain stimulation technology has dramatically changed the role of movement disorder nursing by opening opportunities for collaboration with neurosurgery and developing skills as deep brain stimulation programmers.

WHERE ARE WE NOW?

The World Parkinson Congress (2006) provided us with an exciting opportunity for nurses to come together at an international conference. As we examined our collective history, it was imperative that we assessed where we were at that juncture in time. We are bound together by our shared nursing education, training, and commitment to patients with PD. We are a service profession, composed primarily of women who are reaching middle age. We have few male nurses in our specialty and a sparse representation of people of color. By virtue of our being in the clinical setting, we have brought nursing to the treatment team and have influenced the history of care of Parkinson's patients and their families. Moreover, nursing is now recognized as an essential part of the interdisciplinary movement disorder team internationally.

In numbers, where are we now? There are approximately 500 nurses internationally focusing their practices on the care of patients and families living with PD. While we are proud of our growth, we realize that in the United States alone we have 1,500,000 people with PD to serve. Thus we must be creative in our work and generate a certain contagious enthusiasm for our passion to attract nurses into the caring of those with PD and their families.

WHO DO WE SERVE?

As nurses who specialize in the care of patients with movement disorders, it is important to recognize that we serve primarily older adults in developed nations. PD and other movement disorders are primarily a focus of countries with advanced medical care and fiscal resources to devote to specialized neurological services.

The aging of the U.S. and European populations positions our specialty at a point in time where we are now witnessing a dramatic increase in the reporting of the prevalence and incidence of PD globally. Older adults have higher rates of comorbid conditions, affecting the role of the PD nurse through the need to managing populations with multiple chronic conditions. The emerging economies of China, India, South Africa, and other nations will eventually develop a need for nurses to provide care and join interdisciplinary teams to meet the challenges of clinical services for people with PD globally.

WHERE ARE WE GOING?

Although we are young as an organized group of clinical experts, we have a rich history. The struggles ahead will challenge us to examine our mission and goals. Our future is shaped by who we serve. We serve our patients and their families.

As we evaluate the future, we need to ask, What are the needs of people with PD, and do our current models of care meet their needs? Are there other nursing organizations that can assist us in the development of our specialty? What portion of our work should be devoted to the various roles we play, and where is the benefit greatest for our patients?

To guide us in the development of our specialty, we need to understand the demographics and symptom profiles of the patients we serve. Two nurses have provided excellent examples for us. Janet Doherty, PD Nurse Specialist, presented data at the World Parkinson Congress on the population of PD patients she serves in Australia. Ms. Doherty reported the following symptom profile: cognitive decline (28%), depression (45%), and hallucinations (36%). Through understanding symptoms and illness, Ms. Doherty can design models of care to best meet her patients' needs. Julie Carter, Adult Nurse Practitioner in the United States, has contributed to the medical and nursing literature on the burdens faced by caregiving PD spouses as they travel through their loved ones' stages of illness. This research helps us, as nurses, to anticipate and offer appropriate care suggestions for the caregivers of our patients.

How will our role change to meet the needs of our patients and their families? Do we have the skills to develop new models of care and evaluate care effectiveness? Through global collaboration we can move interdisciplinary care to new levels of effective care for people with PD. To accomplish our goals, we need to attract, educate, and retain young nurses to the nursing profession. In identifying candidates to the specialty, we should examine the opportunity to recruit males and people of color to reflect the population we serve. Currently, only the United Kingdom has a strategic plan to address the need to educate, certify, and retain young nurses to the specialty of PD nursing. We need to advocate for modules on Parkinson's education in undergraduate training. We need to mentor student nurses at all levels of their education. We need to continually publish, speak, and educate practicing nurses on the care and treatment of patients with PD. Furthermore, the emerging needs of PD patients in developing countries will challenge us to reach out and collaborate with neurologists, generalists, and nurses in underserved areas of the world.

WHAT IS OUR ROLE? WHAT AREAS OF ROLE DEVELOPMENT ARE NEEDED?

Our current roles include research coordinator, deep brain stimulation management/programmer, case management, neurosurgery nurse, educator, advocate, direct patient care provider, and coordinator of community outreach activities. Our future will be influenced by the science of discovery in laboratories and clinical settings. We will need to gain skills in genetic counseling to support the needs of patients and families as the genetics and risk of developing PD become more defined.

Our current representation as researchers is limited. Negotiating a place with physician researchers to bring nursing into the interdisciplinary research agenda should be a focus in addressing the needs of people with PD from a uniquely nursing perspective. Collaborating with basic scientists and clinical researchers to translate their work into development of new models of care for PD should be a priority. In addition, disseminating nursing knowledge should be a focus for nurses in setting standards of care and treatment. Currently, we have little evidence-based practice to support our models of care. This paucity of literature should be considered as we move ahead in defining our specialty.

ORGANIZATIONAL NEEDS

The consensus of nurses attending the World Parkinson Congress suggests that we work toward an organizational structure. Mary Baker suggested that this may be possible through collaboration with the International Council of Nurses, based in Geneva, Switzerland. The European Parkinson Nurse Network, based in the United Kingdom, is another organization with the infrastructure to support the need for developing a cohesive specialty for PD Nurse Specialists globally. Yet another model, disease-specific, is that of the International Society of Multiple Sclerosis Nurses.

To move forward, we should consider recording our living history. Thus we can review where we have been and learn from our past. A new international organization could support nurses as care providers, researchers, educators, and mentors by documenting the work of PD Nurse Specialists around the globe. We should celebrate our success and support each other in our professional development through the dissemination of knowledge.

In summary, we must not forget to preserve what is distinctly nursing within the interdisciplinary team, and we must not be consumed by tasks that are extensions of physician practice. We often walk a thin line between the role of physician extender and professional nurse. We should be mindful of the important and unique role we bring to the treatment team. Furthermore, we should be aware of how the team perceives our role and how nursing is valued by the team, patient, and family.

By discussing our past, present, and future, we can develop a successful road map for the development of PD Nurse Specialists on a global scale. In looking forward, our mission is to evaluate the needs of the people we serve and to develop models of care to meet the complex clinical profile of people with PD and their families.

Lisette K. Bunting-Perry
Gwyn M. Vernon

November 8, 2006

Foreword

As any expert neurologist in the treatment of Parkinson's disease (PD) will attest, comprehensive nursing care is a critical component of PD management. Indeed, nurses have been key in developing most of the major PD and movement disorder centers. The editors themselves have a long track record of achievement in PD. Gwyn Vernon cofounded the Parkinson's Disease Center at the University of Pennsylvania and was instrumental in helping the center evolve into a worldwide Center of Excellence, providing care and innovative medical and surgical therapies to thousands of patients annually. Lisette Bunting-Perry started her career helping to build the PD program at The Johns Hopkins University before becoming one of the founders and developers of the Parkinson's Disease Research, Education, and Clinical Center at the VA Medical Center in Philadelphia, a key component of the center at the University of Pennsylvania.

In this text the editors have assembled an array of ancillary health care providers who specialize in the management of PD. Each has broad experience in clinical care and provides invaluable information for those interested in the comprehensive treatment of PD. While basic aspects of diagnosis and medical and surgical therapies are included, it is particularly noteworthy that significant attention is paid to aspects of PD often overlooked in medical texts and yet crucial to understanding how best to treat our patients and how wellness is really defined. Chapters on psychiatric problems, nonmotor complications, caregiving and psychosocial issues, and rehabilitation underscore the importance of a comprehensive approach to patient care and how quality of life is defined by more than motor abilities. A chapter on alternative therapies addresses a subject most of our patients pursue but often fail to discuss with their physicians. Finally, the role of palliative care as it applies to PD is addressed as a novel and useful paradigm for the management of patients and families dealing with advancing PD.

The chapter on the role of the nurse in PD management understates how important nursing care is to patients with PD. Not only do patients with a chronic illness need to communicate readily with health care providers, but nurses often are the key therapeutic partners to patients and families dealing with chronic illness. This text is an important resource for nurses and ancillary health care providers treating PD patients. Physicians treating PD and other neurodegenerative diseases will also find that its contents have broad applicability and value. Finally, patients and families dealing with PD will derive invaluable information that will assist them in adjusting to living with PD, finding the right blend of professional assistance and comprehensive care, and discovering that quality of life and a sense of well-being are well within their grasp.

Matthew B. Stern, MD

Parker Family Professor of Neurology
Director, Parkinson's Disease and Movement Disorders Center
University of Pennsylvania

Acknowledgments

We recognize the extraordinary commitment made by the contributors of *Comprehensive Nursing Care for Parkinson's Disease*. Each chapter is presented by dedicated, passionate, and skilled professionals who have years of expertise working with patients with Parkinson's disease and related movement disorders. We are fortunate to know many of the contributing authors and consider them not just colleagues, but friends. We could not have published the text without the support and mentorship of family, co-workers, and friends. Our husbands, Jim Perry and Mark Vernon, have gone the extra mile in providing encouragement, technical support, patience, and oceans of love. Special thanks go to Christine Bunting in providing remarkable editorial work. We recognize the leadership of the Philadelphia, Houston, and San Francisco Veterans Affairs Parkinson Disease Research, Education, and Clinical Centers in supporting contributors in the development of manuscripts and expert content review. Dan Weintraub, MD, an international expert on depression in PD, was generous in his review of our chapter on psychiatric symptoms associated with PD. Our ongoing relationship with the University of Pennsylvania Schools of Medicine and Nursing continues to provide us with mentors and inspiration to improve the quality of life of people living with Parkinson's disease. Finally, we acknowledge Matthew B. Stern, MD, Howard I. Hurtig, MD, and John Duda, MD, three enlightened neurologists who provide us with opportunities to change the landscape of movement disorder nursing.Comprehensive Nursing Care for Parkinson's Disease

Comprehensive Nursing Care
for Parkinson's Disease

1

Parkinson's Disease — Then, Now, and in the Future

Gwyn M. Vernon, MSN, CRNP

Movement disorders are neurological syndromes in which there is either an excess of movement or a paucity of voluntary and autonomic movements, unrelated to weakness or spasticity.

(Fahn, 2003, p. xix)

Parkinson's disease (PD) is often called the prototype or most common of the hypokinetic movement disorders. Characterized by a paucity of movement, PD is the movement disorder for which we have the best neuropathological and neurophysiological understanding. Yet this body of knowledge is growing by such leaps and bounds that one must wonder if we only truly understand a fragment of the disease. Just over four decades ago, scientists considered PD symptoms to be caused simply by a shortage of dopamine-producing cells in the substantia nigra. While this is true, this fact is now known to be just a piece of a very complex and evolving puzzle. While early scientists classified PD as a so-called movement disorder, we now appreciate the disease as having motor, nonmotor, and even neuropsychiatric symptoms.

This chapter will introduce PD—the evolution of findings, as we understand them now, and where we are headed in the future. The history of the early recognition of the disease and a journey through almost two centuries of discoveries will be discussed with the relationships they have had to treatment development. Epidemiology will include a brief introduction to the exploding world of the exploration of environmental and genetic factors. An introduction to the neuropathology, symptomatology, disease presentation, progression, and prognosis will be discussed. Differentiating PD from those conditions that resemble PD, the *parkinsonisms* or *atypical*

PD, will be presented. This introductory chapter will prepare the reader for the chapters to follow. The text as a whole will prepare nurses in a variety of settings to care for those with PD and their families along the continuum of the disorder.

THE EARLY RECOGNITION OF PARKINSON'S DISEASE (PD)

Every book on PD begins with the very interesting story of Dr. James Parkinson. Dr. Parkinson, a British physician, eloquently described people he observed on the streets of London. He described a phenomenon he called the "shaking palsy," or *paralysis agitans* (Parkinson, 1817). He described people with tremor at rest, stooped posture, and a shuffling gait, with a tendency to pass from a walking to running pace. He also wrote in his essay that the "intellect and senses were spared" (p. 1). Dr. Parkinson's first three cases were ages 50, 62, and 65. One he attributed to alcohol consumption and another to sleeping on the cold, bare earth for several months while aboard ship. Although Dr. Parkinson's original description of PD comprised narrative case reports, it continues to be the foundation for this common disease that bears his name today. His *An Essay on the Shaking Palsy* (1817) was published by Neely and Jones in London and contains six case histories of the disorder. Dr. Parkinson was a prolific writer, and in the British style of the 18th century his essay reads like a novel. It can be found in many medical library museums around the world. Dr. Parkinson worked and lived within 5 minutes of St. Leonard's Church, Shoreditch, London, where a plaque bearing his name and the dates of his birth and death (1755–1824) can be found.

Dr. Jean Marie Charcot, a famous French physician, is said to have elaborated on Dr. Parkinson's original description of the features of the disease and to have named the disorder after Dr. Parkinson; hence, today, we call it PD, not the shaking palsy or paralysis agitans (Duvoisin, 1987). Dr. Charcot's theory on the etiology of PD was that it was due to stress on the body, a theory with which Dr. Gowers, another prominent physician of the late 19th century, concurred. Many other early scientists believed that PD was a phenomenon of aging. Perspectives on the cause of PD expanded in the 20th century after the 1918 worldwide influenza epidemic and an outbreak of encephalitis, which became an interest due to an unusual form of parkinsonism that followed.

The influenza epidemic of 1918 was legendary. By its end, the death toll exceeded in 1 year that of World War I, World War II, the Korean War, and the Vietnam War combined (Kolata, 1999). Shortly before the influenza epidemic, Baron Constantin von Economo (1917) published a paper describing a "sleeping sickness," originally given the name *encephalitis lethargica* and later called *von Economo's encephalitis.* This illness caused patients to sleep continuously. However, they could be aroused and would answer questions and follow commands. Left to their own, the patients would resort to a somnolent state (Kolata, 1999). Encephalitis lethargica killed 5,000,000 people, and of those remaining, 5,000,000 developed a form of parkinsonism characterized by a frozen look, being unable to respond or speak, and eye movement abnormalities. Although initially thought to be linked to influenza, von Economo's postencephalitic parkinsonism could develop even years after the illness, with or without one experiencing the influenza of 1918. Neuropathological findings revealed inflammatory changes in the midbrain and degeneration in the substantia nigra (Dickman, 2001).

Naturally, the events of encephalitis lethargica and the influenza epidemic of 1918 led to etiologies other than aging and stress as causative agents of PD to be considered, such as infectious and viral causes. By the 1950s, concern regarding industrialization and increasing interest in environmental issues as causes for PD were being entertained. In the late 1950s and into the early 1960s, it was noted that the drug reserpine, an antihypertensive medication, and some neuroleptics in common use at that time could deplete or block dopamine in the brain and cause a Parkinson-like picture. As the middle of the 20th century approached, a variety of theories were being considered as causes of PD: stress, aging, infectious agents, industrialization (i.e., possibly environmental), and the effects of certain drugs. However, the answer was, and continues to be, elusive.

EXPANSION OF KNOWLEDGE IN THE SECOND HALF OF THE 20TH CENTURY: LEARNING MORE ABOUT THE ANATOMY AND PHYSIOLOGY OF PD AND EARLY TREATMENT INITIATIVES

Brissaud (1895) may have first suggested that there was a neuronal loss responsible for the symptoms of PD, but it was approximately 150 years after Dr. Parkinson's original description in 1817 that modern technology allowed the discovery of the rudimentary neurochemical basis of PD. Using analytical chemistry techniques and radioisotopes, a neurotransmitter, dopamine, was noted in the substantia nigra. *Substantia nigra* is Latin for "black substance," a part of the midbrain. In approximately 1963, Dr. Oleh Hornykiewicz, of the University of Vienna, and Dr. Ehringer identified degeneration of the nigrostriatal pathway and dopamine depletion in autopsied brains of those with symptoms of PD. This led to the introduction of the use of levodopa (L-dopa), a precursor of dopamine, in 1967, with Dr. George Cotzias leading the team of investigators. L-dopa did significantly treat the symptoms of PD, making the disease the first to respond to neurotransmitter replacement therapy. L-dopa remains the mainstay for many patients even today in the 21st century.

Neurotransmitters are chemicals that serve as messengers to modulate signals between neurons. Within cells, they are packaged and are ready to release in a process called *exocytosis*. They then diffuse across the synapse, where they have an effect at the postsynaptic receptor. Neurotransmitters are receptor-specific and action-specific. There are excitatory and inhibitory potentials. Dopamine is an inhibitory neurotransmitter and is released from the substantia nigra to the striatum, the input nuclei of the basal ganglia. Together with the substantia nigra, the subthalamic nucleus, and the motor neurons of the spine, the basal ganglia make up a larger system called the *extrapyramidal motor system* (a functional concept rather than a true anatomic entity). This motor system is responsible for the initiation of movement, starting and stopping, posture, and balance. Along with the cerebellum, the extrapyramidal system maintains muscle tone, equilibrium, and coordination. Dopamine's complementary excitatory neurotransmitter partner is acetylcholine. With dopamine in short supply the effect of acetylcholine becomes prominent, tilting the balance. In the mid-20th century the neuropathology of PD was thought to be quite simple, a balance between dopamine and acetylcholine, and treatment options were quite simple—replace dopamine with levodopa, or calm the excitatory neurotransmitter acetylcholine with anticholinergics. Both, however, were limited in controlling symptoms and caused many side effects.

It was noted shortly after the development of levodopa that each dose lasted for a shorter period of time. Often, in the process, patients began to experience excessive abnormal treatment responses in the way of jerky or writhing movements, which are called *dyskinesias*. This sensitizing effect of levodopa, called *priming*, has now been found to modify subsequent levodopa responses and therefore dyskinetic severity (Brotchie, 2005). It also appeared early on that treatment responses could take the opposite effect—that of an insufficient or even total lack of response. This variability in response soon became labeled the *on–off phenomenon,* as if the brain receptors were indeed turning on and off to an individual dose of levodopa. The movie *Awakenings* (1990), based on the book written by Oliver Sacks, MD, tells the most unusual story of the on–off phenomenon and the striking response experienced by PD patients new to levodopa. The movie won three Oscar awards. It is certainly a must-see for all those caring for people with PD.

The on–off phenomenon is due to pulsatile or erratic firing of dopaminergic presynaptic neurons. Recognizing this led to the development of a new class of agents for the treatment of PD in the early 1980s: the dopamine agonists. These chemicals directly stimulate the postsynaptic dopamine receptor, smoothing out the response. As you will read in subsequent chapters, these agents are now used in early and advanced PD. Two studies, REAL and CALM-PD, suggested that using dopamine agonists in early PD slows down the loss of dopaminergic terminal function, as documented by positron emission tomographic (PET) scan in the former and single photon emission computed topography (SPECT) in the latter (Brooks, 2004). Whether this is truly a neuroprotective effect in the long term remains the question. Data to date do show that dopamine agonists have a good symptomatic benefit and can delay and spare the use of levodopa and therefore the priming effect that is thought to lead to dyskinesias.

One of the most historic breakthroughs in PD was the discovery of the toxin MPTP (1-methyl-4-phenyl-1,2,3,6-tetrahydropyridine) as a causative agent in PD. The first human case was noted in 1979, however, it was not until 1982 when multiple cases appeared in drug addicts in California who were manufacturing heroin. An error in the heroin manufacturing process occurred, and these individuals injected themselves with a narcotic-like drug, suddenly developing a severe form of drug-induced PD. These cases were identified by Dr. William Langston. Together with Dr. Stanley Burns, he showed that MPTP directly and selectively destroyed dopamine-producing cells in the substantia nigra. The idiopathic form of PD may take years to develop, and it is estimated that 80% of the dopaminergic cells have degenerated by the time symptoms become evident. In the MPTP cases the presentation was of advanced, end-stage PD within 2 weeks of injection of the tainted heroin. *The Case of the Frozen Addict,* written by Dr. William Langston (1995), tells in graphic detail the story of these unfortunate individuals. As a consequence of discovering MPTP-induced PD, new animal models of PD were developed that have been extremely beneficial in providing an improved understanding of disease onset, progression, and basic science research to advance novel therapeutics.

An early research innovation, related to the discovery of MPTP, was the first neuroprotective study in PD: the Deprenyl and Tocopherol Antioxidatiave Therapy of Parkinsonism study. On the basis of the hypothesis that monoamine oxidase (MAO) breaks down dopamine, thereby releasing toxic byproducts, or oxidants, research was designed to study the role of antioxidants in PD. To study the question of whether antioxidants may slow or halt PD, the first trial included two antioxidative strategies, a MAO-B inhibitor, selegiline (l-deprenyl), and a-tocopherol (vitamin E). A consortium was formed, the Parkinson Study Group (PSG), funding from the National Institutes of Health was obtained, and enthusiasm was high. The study began in 1987 with 800 patients from 28 U.S. states and Canadian sites. No evidence for neuroprotection was found in the vitamin E group. Interestingly, the blinded portion of the study (the time period during which the investigator and patient did not know which compound, or if a placebo, was being administered) was concluded early as it appeared the selegiline group showed statistically significant improvement. However, when the study was continued for a few more months, this analysis did not hold. Investigators concluded that selegiline has a symptomatic benefit, not a neuroprotective benefit.

With the MPTP model, research momentum escalated. Scientists who for so long had few leads to follow now had new avenues to explore. Other possible triggers of pathogenesis of PD have been under study. Some of the areas that have become important to understanding the keys to PD development include mitochondrial dysfunction, glutamate excitotoxcitity, failure of neurotrophins, and cell necrosis or *apoptosis* (another term for self-programmed cell death).

Mitochondria are the energy or power of the body. They are membrane cytoplasmic particles with many functions, including involvement in the citric acid cycle and fatty acid oxidation pathways. They play a role in adenosine triphosphate production and oxygen and calcium regulation. They are involved in apoptosis. An increase in glutamate activity has been shown to increase the inhibitory action of the pallidus to the motor thalamus and may therefore have a role in PD, particularly in bradykinesia or akinesia. Glutamate receptor agonists, a new class of PD medications, are currently under study. Neurotrophy refers to the nutrition and maintenance of tissue in the nervous system. Neurotropic factors have been found to be decreased in postmortem studies of those with PD. Therefore research has been stimulated by the model of MPTP, basic research has gained strides, and we are moving toward experimental trials and hopefully marketable agents that will address these issues in PD pathogenesis.

The second half of the 20th century also raised awareness of further complexities of the neuroanatomy and neurophysiology of the disease process and exploration for triggers of PD. The presence and location of Lewy bodies, which were once thought to be just a hallmark finding in PD, have changed dramatically their role to a more active one in the pathogenesis of PD.[1] Alpha-synuclein, a protein, is the major component of the Lewy body, and studying this protein has proved the pathology to be more extensive than just within the confines of the "black substance" (substantia nigra) due to dopaminergic cell loss, as once thought. Alpha-synuclein is a protein unique to central nervous system (CNS) neurons, but it has wide distribution among neurons within the CNS. A change is thought to take place in this protein, allowing it to misfold or change its binding capacities. Within the Lewy bodies this misfolding results in clumping and aggregating and initiates a cascade of events that may lead to neuronal death.

Dr. Heiko Braak (2005), from the Institute of Clinical Neuroanatomy, Germany, stated during the papers presented at the Ninth International Congress of Parkinson's Disease and Movement Disorders that "idiopathic PD is a multi-system disorder in which predisposed nerve cells in specific regions of the brain become progressively involved." He found that the process begins and advances predictably and involves cortical and subcortical structures. He describes six stages of the idiopathic PD neuropathological process: Stages 1 and 2 are presymptomatic stages, whereby the pathology is confined to the brainstem; Stage 3 and 4 patients begin to be symptomatic, and the pathology is traveling its course to the midbrain and beyond; Stages 5 and 6, the final stages, find the pathological process involving the cortex of the brain, causing further impairments in the physical being, cognition, and behavioral and emotional domains. Braak further described clinical correlates to the neuropathological stages, which will be discussed in the clinical presentation of PD segment later in this chapter.

The view of PD as a more complex central nervous system disorder spreading from the brain stem to the cortex, and the extension of Lewy body understanding from hallmark to perhaps involvement with pathogenesis underlines that PD is no longer a disease simplistically caused by dopamine deficiency. Likewise, the effect of levodopa as a priming agent for long-term complications has changed our thinking about simple dopamine replacement therapy. The elusive cause and myriad of suggested avenues continues to expand into the 21st century as we add the unfolding genome to the list of paths to explore. Clearly momentum is strong past the decade of the brain (1990–2000) into the 21st century in seeking knowledge about PD.

SEARCHING FOR THE CAUSE: ARE THERE CLUES IN GENOME RESEARCH OR EPIDEMIOLOGY?

Today, we know that PD is a common neurodegenerative disorder. It is progressive, results in disability for many patients, and is costly. Yet we do not know the cause or causes of PD. Many theories continue to be postulated, and while it remains elusive, many consider that the cause must be multifactorial. As mentioned, stress, aging, infectious, industrialization, environmental, and drug-induced etiologies have certainly been entertained. Pesticide use as an environmental factor came into focus about 20 years ago and again recently. Genetic clues are expanding yearly.

Genetics and PD

Interest in PD as a genetic disorder can be traced back to Gowers's (1903) text *A Manual of the Diseases of the Nervous System.* However, up until one decade ago, PD was considered spontaneous, idiopathic, and purely nonhereditary. Today, it is considered a "complex disorder with a well established genetic component in a considerable subset of patients" (Klein & Schlossmacher, 2006, p. 136). This subset may be 5% to 10% of cases. The first genetic clue was reported in 1990 and was further confirmed in 1997. The presence of a gene mutation in an Italian–Greek American family was noted in a gene coded for the protein, alpha synuclein. An overabundance of alpha synuclein was observed. This protein is a large part of the Lewy body (Vila & Przedburski, 2004). Now we know that there are over 10 regions in the human genome linked to PD, with over 500 locations that may contribute—there may be even more yet to be identified or, of course, possibly some will be eliminated with time. Many of these genetic mishaps involve mitochondrial dysfunction or aggregation of abnormal proteins that cannot be eliminated properly. While this chapter does not allow for an in-depth discussion of genetics and would most likely be out-of-date when published, there are several general concepts regarding genetics and PD worth mentioning in this nursing text.

The literature separates familiar types of parkinsonism into two subgroups, which are called the PD phenotype (Type I) and the PPS phenotype (Type II). Basically, PD phenotype (Type I) refers to what is considered clinically consistent with typical idiopathic PD and a positive response to levodopa therapy. PPS phenotype (Type II) is more atypical in presentation—occurring in younger patients with a more aggressive course, little or no improvement with levodopa therapy, and additional clinical as well as neuropathological features supporting more widespread neurodegenerative disease.

Genetic susceptibility factors, gene expression, and penetrance are also important concepts when considering the role of genetics in the development of PD. Does it take an environmental trigger to turn the gene off or on, to cause the gene to express itself, or to mobilize the gene to mutate? If we consider that PD has a long preclinical phase and that an estimated 80% of the dopaminergic neurons degenerate before the symptoms appear in the individual, this implies that physiologically, a process is taking place for a very long time before symptoms become noticeable. We must consider also that some of the identified genetic mutations have been found in people who do not express clinical symptoms of PD.

Yet another concept to consider is that of known patterns of genetic transmission. To date, autosomal dominant and autosomal recessive patterns have been connected to PD. Some studies have found families where multiple areas of the genome and patterns of transmission seem to be present. Monozygotic twin studies have at best shown us that we need better methods to identify preclinical disease and years of long-term follow-up and autopsy confirmations. These considerations make the role of genetics in PD much more complex than other genetic neurological disorders, such as Huntington's disease, where the pattern is clearly, and only, autosomal dominant. Table 1.1 presents highlights of the genome work being performed.

TABLE 1.1   Genetic Overview of Parkinson's Findings

Designation	Mutation noted	Comments	Pattern	Chromosome localization
PARK 1	a-synuclein protein[a]	Discovery of a-synuclein mutation led to understanding it as a component of Lewy bodies; gene triplication and duplication.	**AD**	4 Q
PARK 2	Ubiquitin-protein ligase[a]	Younger, juvenile, and/or dystonia at onset. Ubiquitin important to cell's normal self-protective functions, eliminating abnormal proteins.	**AR**	6 Q
PARK 7	DJ-1	Mutations destabilize or reduce the protection from oxidative stress. Rare, early-onset PD.	**AR**	1 Q
PARK 6	PINK 1,[a] mitochondrial associated protein kinase	Mitochondrial protein kinase may prevent cells from stress, mutations lead to instability.		1 P
PARK 8	LRRK2/ Dardarin[a]	Perhaps most common cause of genetic late-onset PD; mixture of neuropathological changes noted, including those seen in Parkinson's disease, diffuse Lewy body disease, and Alzheimer's disease.	**AD**	

Note. AR = autosomal recessive; AD = autosomal dominant. This is an overview of genes with clear links to PD, not an extensive list of genetic findings or research underway. [a]Commercial genetic testing now available for research studies.

Epidemiology of PD

Kurland (1958) published the first community-based estimates of PD. Incidence and prevalence rates as well as disease distribution patterns were at that time, and continue to be, imprecise at best. There are a multitude of reasons why incidence and prevalence studies of PD are difficult to conduct. PD is not a reportable disorder in the United States. There is no county, state, or national mandate, nor a Centers for Disease Control and Prevention tracking system. The diagnosis is based on a clinical exam. This leads to human interpretation and error. Issues of standardizing diagnostic criteria and patient classification are superimposed on an evolving, progressing disorder. For example, to point out the range in crude incidence rates of idiopathic PD, 4.5–19 per 100,000 people per year have been cited. Prevalence ranges from 100 to 200 per 100,000 people (Marras & Tanner, 2004).

Worldwide, epidemiological studies likewise vary and have been biased by case ascertainment, identification difficulties, and study design. Attempts to improve accuracy, by utilizing a racially diverse population in a tightly controlled study in a focused geographical location, would also be flawed as this may exclude certain environmental influences and lifestyle factors in the individual before or after relocating to the new culture. In today's mobile world it is not unusual for individuals to live in several culturally diverse environments, further complicating epidemiological studies in a disorder like PD, which has a long preclinical phase and is progressive over time.

The National Parkinson Foundation states that approximately 60,000 new cases are diagnosed each year, joining the 1,500,000 currently diagnosed in the United States. Many are over the age of 65, however, 15% are diagnosed under the age of 50. Men, women, and all socioeconomic and ethnic as well as geographical groups in the United States are affected (National Parkinson Foundation, 2006). Lifetime risk of developing PD is 2% for men and 1.3% for women (Lang, 2005).

Despite the frustrations of understanding the pure numbers of those affected, which undoubtedly will continue, epidemiological studies offer perhaps more value and pursuable information about trends that may lead to clues into the causes of PD, risk factors, populations at higher risk, environmental toxins, and genetics. The *American Journal of Epidemiology* published "A Retrospective Study of Smoking and Parkinson's Disease"

(Nefzinger, Quadfasel, & Karl, 1968), paving the way for most subsequent case-controlled studies to report an inverse relationship between PD and cigarette smoking. More recently, a similar but not as well established inverse relationship has been suggested between coffee consumption and PD in several studies (Ascherio et al., 2001; Beneditti et al., 2000; Ross et al., 2000).

As discussed earlier, the toxin MPTP has been proven to cause PD by selective destruction of dopaminergic neurons. Otherwise, perhaps the most consistent positive association with PD found in epidemiological studies is pesticide exposure. Meta-analysis studies from North America, Europe, and Asia first supported this in 1999 (Priyadarshi, Khuder, Schaub, & Shrivastava, 2000). Ascherio (2006) further contributed to this research in the July issue of the *Annals of Neurology* with a review of 143,000 participants in the U.S. Cancer Prevention Study II Nutrition Cohort (1982–2001 group). He found that the long-term risk of developing PD increased by 70% if exposed to pesticides, without regard to occupational exposure or amount or duration of exposure. On the contrary, a study done in western Washington found that pesticides did not play a role in the development of PD in that population (Firestone et al., 2005). Further work must be done on the etiological role of pesticides in PD and to determine which chemicals within pesticides may be the most toxic.

While pesticides appear to have a strong association with PD, environmental and other risk factors have demonstrated relationships, albeit inconsistently. These include other metals, such as manganese; chemicals; carbon monoxide; dietary fat intake; head trauma; and occupational type, to name just a few. None of these factors to date have shown a consistent positive association with the development of PD, although some individual studies have suggested a correlation.

CLINICAL PRESENTATION OF PD

The onset of PD is slow and insidious. Many patients experience a prodrome of just not feeling like themselves. They may have an internal tremor, or a sense of apathy or depression. A resting tremor of the extremities may come infrequently or not at all. Family members may note that the individual is slower in activities of daily living but consider age or arthritis the cause. A masked facies may develop, but again, this may be considered aging or disinterest, when in reality, the "thief of expression" may have arrived (Christensen, 2006). A loss of olfaction is frequently noticed in early PD (Stern, 1994; Ward, Hess, & Calne, 1983).

As the symptoms evolve and become more obvious, patients most often develop the characteristic signs asymmetrically. Hughes, Ben-Shlomo, Daniel, & Lees (1992) stated that 72% to 75% of patients have asymmetric onset. The clinical triad of resting tremor and cogwheel rigidity found on examination and bradykinesia (slowness of movement) is seen in PD, and its elements may appear in no particular order.

As the diagnosis of PD is a clinical diagnosis that can only be confirmed upon autopsy, the rate of misdiagnosis is quite high. In fact, only about 75% of clinical cases are confirmed at autopsy (Hughes, Daniel, Kilford, & Lees, 1992). This rate is largely due to the varied presentation of PD and the lack of a specific diagnostic test during life for confirmation. Clinical diagnosis correlation can be enhanced to concur with postmortem evidence to approximately 98% if patients are evaluated by an experienced movement disorder neurologist and team (Hughes, Daniel, Ben-Shlomo, & Lees, 2002). Neuroimaging has not yet become readily available, perfected, or U.S. Food and Drug Administration approved for diagnosis. Research with PET scans shows promise as a diagnostic tool in PD but is not yet readily available or reimbursable by insurers for PD.

Most experts agree that patients must have two of the three cardinal signs to meet diagnostic criteria (Stern, 1993). While some patients meet all three criteria, not all patients with PD develop tremor. In fact, only about 70% develop tremor as a feature of the disease. As the disease progresses, a fourth sign, postural instability, appears, as do many secondary symptoms. It is important for nurses to be comfortable with understanding each of these classic or primary symptoms individually so as to recognize typical PD from atypical parkinsonism and also to be aware of functional issues, limitations, and the need for nursing support and patient education.

Tremor in PD

The tremor of PD is a tremor at rest. It is present when the patient has the arm or leg still, frequently while sitting still or walking with arms at the side. Initially, it is intermittent and quite mild, perhaps involving only a finger or two. Most often, it begins unilaterally, with no relationship to the dominant side. The resting tremor oscillates at a frequency of 4–5 hertz (Hz, a unit of frequency equal to one cycle per second). Some patients may develop an action tremor or a postural or kinetic component, but by far, these qualities should be outweighed by the resting tremor. Most patients will report that the resting tremor gets worse with excitement (good or bad), stress, cold, anxiety, pain, and concurrent illness.

Cogwheel Rigidity

Cogwheel rigidity may not be apparent to the patient but is found by the examiner on range of motion of the limb. This increase in tone, a "ratchety" rigidity, can often be brought out by distracting maneuvers in the contralateral limb, for example, asking the patient to make a fist with the opposite hand. The rigidity is not smooth, but irregular, such as "cogs in a wheel," and is thought to reflect a superimposed tremor. It is found on flexion and extension in the limbs and can also affect the neck and trunk. Cogwheel rigidity is specific to PD and has a very different character compared to other types of muscle rigidity, such as spasticity, lead pipe/smooth, and gegenhalten tone.

Bradykinesia

Bradykinesia in early PD is not specific; it can be seen in the psychomotor slowing of depression, Alzheimer's disease, and other neurodegenerative disorders. It is, perhaps, the most disabling of symptoms for most PD patients. Early in the course of PD, and perhaps even before the diagnosis, it may appear as normal slowing of aging. With time it is noted to be out of proportion for normal aging. Distal signs may appear first, such as finger and hand movements, micrographia, and loss of dexterity. With time, symptoms progress to more generalized bradykinesia and axial signs (Paulson & Stern, 2004). One of the most difficult diagnostic challenges when confronted with a patient with severe bradykinesia and no tremor is differentiating between PD and the psychomotor slowing of severe psychiatric depression. Bradykinesia affects all activities of daily living, walking, talking, swallowing, speaking, and even thinking. The slowness of thought described by individuals with PD is termed *bradyphrenia*.

Postural Instability

Postural instability, the loss of postural reflexes, results in falling and injuries in the PD patient. It should not appear early in the disorder, and if so, one should suspect an atypical process. Many patients will note that they will tend to *retropulse,* or continue stepping back rapidly and uncontrollably. Other patients may *festinate,* or take quick short steps forward uncontrollably. Both retropulsion and festination can lead to falls. Yet other patients suffer from postural tilts and imbalance combined with such severe truncal rigidity that they simply fall over when attempting to turn, change their weight, or even look in another direction. Falls lead to further disability in PD. At the very least, they create problems with confidence and contribute to a fear of falling. With significant injury, such as fractured hips, rotator cuff injuries, or head trauma, falls result in tremendous morbidity and mortality.

Secondary Symptoms

While the presence of two of the three classical signs of PD (resting tremor, cogwheel rigidity, and bradykinesia) are necessary for clinical diagnosis, patients experience a myriad of other bothersome symptoms. These symptoms may reflect a primary sign, for example, a patient experiencing bradykinesia and muscle (cogwheel) rigidity may complain of difficulty getting out of a chair. However, the complaint may actually be considered a secondary manifestation of PD, such as a painful dystonic cramping of the toes. Other secondary manifestations may include cognitive and mood changes, visual changes, decreased olfactory function, edema, compression neuropathies, sensory symptoms, autonomic dysfunction, seborrhea, and sleep disorders.

In a study by Malecki, Vaughan, and Anderson (2004) that was presented at the American Academy of Neurology in San Francisco, CA, patients ranked the symptoms that were most troubling. Loss of balance; trouble speaking; loss of memory; unpredictable periods when symptoms worsen; and involuntary, uncontrollable movements were the top five concerns noted in this report. It is important for nurses to recognize and differentiate those classic signs associated with diagnostic criteria from those concerns most bothersome to patients when planning nursing care. Please refer to chapters 4 and 5 for a comprehensive presentation of these secondary and neuropsychiatric symptoms and their management.

STAGES OF PD, PROGRESSION, AND PROGNOSIS

Practitioners frequently use a staging system for communicating the PD state. There are several commonly used staging scales. The Hoehn and Yahr scale (Table 1.2), published in 1967, continues to be widely used as a quick description of the patient's disease state (Hoehn & Yahr, 1967).

It is important when counseling families to emphasize that this staging system is not related to any prognostic factor regarding progression of disease. Progression is variable, and the Hoehn and Yahr scale does not implicate any time frame for progression; it is only a statement as to where the patient is at the current time. Another important point for family counseling is to note that while patients frequently reached Stage V in the pre-levodopa era, with the currently available treatments, patients are often spared this devastating debilitation.

The Unified Parkinson Disease Rating Scale (UPDRS) is a six-section scale that was developed in the 1980s and is currently being revised. This scale documents the patient's functional status, level of activities of daily living, motor function, mood, cognition, and treatment-related manifestations (Fahn, Elton, & Members of the UPDRS Development Committee, 1987). This scale is presented in Table 1.3. The UPDRS incorporates the Schwab and England Capacity for Daily Living Scale, which is a very helpful tool for nurses to gain an understanding of the daily needs of the patient and caregivers.

Another staging system has recently been proposed by Braak to correlate clinical features with his six stages of pathological progression. Braak's staging recognizes the nonmotor, motor, cognitive, and treatment-related intolerances as the disease progresses. Interestingly, Braak's staging makes one take note of the long preclinical phase, wherein pathological and nonmotor symptoms are beginning to occur prediagnostically. Braak's staging of PD is presented in Table 1.4 (Braak, Ghebredmedhin, Rub, & Del Tredici, 2004).

Braak's staging of PD and the UPDRS, like the Hoehn and Yahr scale, do not imply any time frame of progression. They are a mark in time at

TABLE 1.2   Hoehn and Yahr Stages of Parkinson's Disease

Stage	Clinical findings
I	Unilateral
II	Bilateral mild disease with or without axial involvement
III	Mild to moderate bilateral disease with deteriorating balance
IV	Severe disease requiring considerable assistance
V	Confinement to wheelchair or bed unless aided; with feeding tube or tracheostomy

Adapted from Hoehn, M. M., & Yahr, M. D. (1967). Parkinsonism: Onset, progression and mortality. *Neurology, 17*(5), 427.

the point the patient is rated. While the UPDRS and Hoehn and Yahr scale have been shown to have interrater reliability and validity, there is a significant portion in the UPDRS that is subjective information the provider asks of the patient. It is very common in clinical practice to note the caregiver disagreeing with the patient on the subjective portion, either verbally or with hidden gestures or head shakes. Medications being utilized and timing within the dosing schedule can greatly alter the rating scales. Many PD research centers attempt to rate the patient at the same time within a medication schedule or in both the on and off medication states for comparison and to attempt to measure disease progression over time.

Idiopathic PD has wide variation in the rate of disease progression. Until the 1990s, most clinicians divided PD into three subgroups when speaking of progression based on clinical observations of the apparent natural history of the disease. One-third of observed cases progressed rapidly. Often, these patients developed signs of atypical PD or other forms of parkinsonism with more extensive neurodegenerative changes, such as progressive supranuclear palsy (PSP), multiple system atrophy (MSA), or Shy-Drager syndrome (SDS), to name just a few. One-third progressed slowly and insidiously. The final one-third were said to progress very slowly, often remaining quite functional for decades.

In the mid-1980s and into the 1990s, Jankovic and others began to describe the heterogeneity of PD and prognostic implications (Jankovic et al., 1990; Zetusky, Jankovic, & Pirozzolo, 1985). Experts were gaining skill at earlier recognition of the atypical forms of parkinsonism.

TABLE 1.3   Unified Parkinson's Disease Rating Scale

I. Mentation, behavior, and mood

1. Intellectual impairment

0 = None.

1 = Mild. Consistent forgetfulness with partial recollection of events and no other difficulties.

2 = Moderate memory loss, with disorientation and moderate difficulty handling complex problems. Mild but definite impairment of function at home with need of occasional prompting.

3 = Severe memory loss with disorientation for time and often to place. Severe impairment in handling problems.

4 = Severe memory loss with orientation preserved to person only. Unable to make judgments or solve problems. Requires much help with personal care. Cannot be left alone at all.

2. Thought disorder (due to dementia or drug intoxication)

0 = None.

1 = Vivid dreaming.

2 = "Benign" hallucinations with insight retained.

3 = Occasional to frequent hallucinations or delusions; without insight; could interfere with daily activities.

4 = Persistent hallucinations, delusions, or florid psychosis. Not able to care for self.

3. Depression

1 = Periods of sadness or guilt greater than normal, never sustained for days or weeks.

2 = Sustained depression (1 week or more).

3 = Sustained depression with vegetative symptoms (insomnia, anorexia, weight loss, loss of interest).

4 = Sustained depression with vegetative symptoms and suicidal thoughts or intent.

4. Motivation/initiative

0 = Normal.

1 = Less assertive than usual; more passive.

2 = Loss of initiative or disinterest in elective (nonroutine) activities.

3 = Loss of initiative or disinterest in day-to-day (routine) activities.

4 = Withdrawn, complete loss of motivation.

(continued)

TABLE 1.3 *(continued)*

II. Activities of daily living (for both "on" and "off")

5. Speech

0 = Normal.

1 = Mildly affected. No difficulty being understood.

2 = Moderately affected. Sometimes asked to repeat statements.

3 = Severely affected. Frequently asked to repeat statements.

4 = Unintelligible most of the time.

6. Salivation

0 = Normal.

1 = Slight but definite excess of saliva in mouth; may have nighttime drooling.

2 = Moderately excessive saliva; may have minimal drooling.

3 = Marked excess of saliva with some drooling.

4 = Marked drooling, requires constant tissue or handkerchief.

7. Swallowing

0 = Normal.

1 = Rare choking.

2 = Occasional choking.

3 = Requires soft food.

4 = Requires NG tube or gastrotomy feeding.

8. Handwriting

0 = Normal.

1 = Slightly slow or small.

2 = Moderately slow or small; all words are legible.

3 = Severely affected; not all words are legible.

4 = The majority of words are not legible.

9. Cutting food and handling utensils

0 = Normal.

1 = Somewhat slow and clumsy, but no help needed.

2 = Can cut most foods, although clumsy and slow; some help needed.

3 = Food must be cut by someone, but can still feed slowly.

4 = Needs to be fed.

(continued)

TABLE 1.3   Unified Parkinson's Disease Rating Scale
(continued)

---

10. Dressing

0 = Normal.

1 = Somewhat slow, but no help needed.

2 = Occasional assistance with buttoning, getting arms in sleeves.

3 = Considerable help required, but can do some things alone.

4 = Helpless.

11. Hygiene

0 = Normal.

1 = Somewhat slow, but no help needed.

2 = Needs help to shower or bathe, or very slow in hygienic care.

3 = Requires assistance for washing, brushing teeth, combing hair, going to bathroom.

4 = Foley catheter or other mechanical aids.

12. Turning in bed and adjusting bed clothes

0 = Normal.

1 = Somewhat slow and clumsy, but no help needed.

2 = Can turn alone or adjust sheets, but with great difficulty.

3 = Can initiate, but not turn or adjust sheets alone.

4 = Helpless.

13. Falling (unrelated to freezing)

0 = None.

1 = Rare falling.

2 = Occasionally falls, less than once per day.

3 = Falls an average of once daily.

4 = Falls more than once daily.

14. Freezing when walking

0 = None.

1 = Rare freezing when walking; may have starthesitation.

2 = Occasional freezing when walking.

3 = Frequent freezing. Occasionally falls from freezing.

4 = Frequent falls from freezing.

(continued)

TABLE 1.3 *(continued)*

15. Walking

0 = Normal.

1 = Mild difficulty. May not swing arms or may tend to drag leg.

2 = Moderate difficulty, but requires little or no assistance.

3 = Severe disturbance of walking, requiring assistance.

4 = Cannot walk at all, even with assistance.

16. Tremor (symptomatic complaint of tremor in any part of body)

0 = Absent.

1 = Slight and infrequently present.

2 = Moderate; bothersome to patient.

3 = Severe; interferes with many activities.

4 = Marked; interferes with most activities.

17. Sensory complaints related to parkinsonism

0 = None.

1 = Occasionally has numbness, tingling, or mild aching.

2 = Frequently has numbness, tingling, or aching; not distressing.

3 = Frequent painful sensations.

4 = Excruciating pain.

III. Motor examination

18. Speech

0 = Normal.

1 = Slight loss of expression, diction, and/or volume.

2 = Monotone, slurred but understandable; moderately impaired.

3 = Marked impairment, difficult to understand.

4 = Unintelligible.

19. Facial expression

0 = Normal.

1 = Minimal hypomimia, could be normal "poker face."

2 = Slight but definitely abnormal diminution of facial expression.

3 = Moderate hypomimia; lips parted some of the time.

4 = Masked or fixed facies with severe or complete loss of facial expression; lips parted 0.25 in or more.

(continued)

TABLE 1.3   Unified Parkinson's Disease Rating Scale
(continued)

20. Tremor at rest (head, upper and lower extremities)

0 = Absent.

1 = Slight and infrequently present.

2 = Mild in amplitude and persistent, or moderate in amplitude but only intermittently present.

3 = Moderate in amplitude and present most of the time.

4 = Marked in amplitude and present most of the time.

21. Action or postural tremor of hands

0 = Absent.

1 = Slight; present with action.

2 = Moderate in amplitude, present with action.

3 = Moderate in amplitude with posture holding as well as action.

4 = Marked in amplitude; interferes with feeding.

22. Rigidity (judged on passive movement of major joints, with patient relaxed in sitting position. Cogwheeling to be ignored.)

0 = Absent.

1 = Slight or detectable only when activated by mirror or other movements.

2 = Mild to moderate.

3 = Marked, but full range of motion easily achieved.

4 = Severe, range of motion achieved with difficulty.

23. Finger taps (patient taps thumb with index finger in rapid succession)

0 = Normal.

1 = Mild slowing and/or reduction in amplitude.

2 = Moderately impaired. Definite and early fatiguing. May have occasional arrests in movement.

3 = Severely impaired. Frequent hesitation in initiating movements or arrests in ongoing movement.

4 = Can barely perform the task.

(continued)

TABLE 1.3 *(continued)*

24. Hand movements (patient opens and closes hands in rapid succesion)

0 = Normal.

1 = Mild slowing and/or reduction in amplitude.

2 = Moderately impaired. Definite and early fatiguing. May have occasional arrests in movement.

3 = Severely impaired. Frequent hesitation in initiating movements or arrests in ongoing movement.

4 = Can barely perform the task.

25. Rapid alternating movements of hands (pronation-supination movements of hands, vertically and horizontally, with as large an amplitude as possible, both hands simultaneously)

0 = Normal.

1 = Mild slowing and/or reduction in amplitude.

2 = Moderately impaired. Definite and early fatiguing. May have occasional arrests in movement.

3 = Severely impaired. Frequent hesitation in initiating movements or arrests in ongoing movement.

4 = Can barely perform the task.

26. Leg agility (patient taps heel on the ground in rapid succession, picking up entire leg. Amplitude should be at least 3 in.)

0 = Normal.

1 = Mild slowing and/or reduction in amplitude.

2 = Moderately impaired. Definite and early fatiguing. May have occasional arrests in movement.

3 = Severely impaired. Frequent hesitation in initiating movements or arrests in ongoing movement.

4 = Can barely perform the task.

27. Arising from chair (patient attempts to rise from a straight-backed chair, with arms folded across chest)

0 = Normal.

1 = Slow, or may need more than one attempt.

2 = Pushes self up from arms of seat.

3 = Tends to fall back and may have to try more than one time, but can get up without help.

4 = Unable to arise without help.

(continued)

TABLE 1.3 Unified Parkinson's Disease Rating Scale
(continued)

28. Posture

0 = Normal erect.

1 = Not quite erect, slightly stooped posture; could be normal for older person.

2 = Moderately stooped posture, definitely abnormal; can be slightly leaning to one side.

3 = Severely stooped posture with kyphosis; can be moderately leaning to one side.

4 = Marked flexion with extreme abnormality of posture.

29. Gait

0 = Normal.

1 = Walks slowly, may shuffle with short steps, but no festination (hastening steps) or propulsion.

2 = Walks with difficulty, but requires little or no assistance; may have some festination, short steps, or propulsion.

3 = Severe disturbance of gait, requiring assistance.

4 = Cannot walk at all, even with assistance.

30. Postural stability (response to sudden, strong posterior displacement produced by pull on shoulders while patient erect with eyes open and feet slightly apart. Patient is prepared.)

0 = Normal.

1 = Retropulsion, but recovers unaided.

2 = Absence of postural response; would fall if not caught by examiner.

3 = Very unstable, tends to lose balance spontaneously.

4 = Unable to stand without assistance.

31. Body bradykinesia and hypokinesia (combining slowness, hesitancy, decreased arm swing, small amplitude, and poverty of movement in general)

0 = None.

1 = Minimal slowness, giving movement a deliberate character; could be normal for some persons. Possibly reduced amplitude.

2 = Mild degree of slowness and poverty of movement that is definitely abnormal. Alternatively, some reduced amplitude.

3 = Moderate slowness, poverty, or small amplitude of movement.

4 = Marked slowness, poverty, or small amplitude of movement.

(continued)

TABLE 1.3 *(continued)*

IV. Complications of therapy (in the past week)

A. Dyskinesias

32. **Duration: What proportion of the waking day are dyskinesias present?** (historical information)

0 = None.

1 = 1–25% of day.

2 = 26–50% of day.

3 = 51–75% of day.

4 = 76–100% of day.

33. **Disability: How disabling are the dyskinesias?** (historical information; may be modified by office examination)

0 = Not disabling.

1 = Mildly disabling.

2 = Moderately disabling.

3 = Severely disabling.

4 = Completely disabled.

34. **Painful dyskinesias: How painful are the dyskinesias?**

0 = No painful dyskinesias.

1 = Slight.

2 = Moderate.

3 = Severe.

4 = Marked.

35. **Presence of early morning dystonia** (historical information)

0 = No.

1 = Yes.

B. Clinical fluctuations

36. **Are "off" periods predictable?**

0 = No.

1 = Yes.

37. **Are "off" periods unpredictable?**

0 = No.

1 = Yes.

(continued)

TABLE 1.3 Unified Parkinson's Disease Rating Scale
(continued)

38. Do "off" periods come on suddenly, within a few seconds?

0 = No.

1 = Yes.

39. What proportion of the waking day is the patient "off" on average?

0 = None.

1 = 1–25% of day.

2 = 26–50% of day.

3 = 51–75% of day.

4 = 76–100% of day.

C. Other complications

40. Does the patient have anorexia, nausea, or vomiting?

0 = No.

1 = Yes.

41. Any sleep disturbances, such as insomnia or hypersomnolence?

0 = No.

1 = Yes.

42. Does the patient have symptomatic orthostasis? (record the patient's blood pressure, height, and weight on the scoring form)

0 = No.

1 = Yes.

V. Modified Hoehn and Yahr staging

STAGE 0 = No signs of disease.

STAGE 1 = Unilateral disease.

STAGE 1.5 = Unilateral plus axial involvement.

STAGE 2 = Bilateral disease, without impairment of balance.

STAGE 2.5 = Mild bilateral disease, with recovery on pull test.

STAGE 3 = Mild to moderate bilateral disease; some postural instability; physically independent.

STAGE 4 = Severe disability; still able to walk or stand unassisted.

STAGE 5 = Wheelchair bound or bedridden unless aided.

(continued)

TABLE 1.3 *(continued)*

VI. Schwab and England activities of daily living scale

100% = Completely independent. Able to do all chores without slowness, difficulty, or impairment. Essentially normal. Unaware of any difficulty.

90% = Completely independent. Able to do all chores with some degree of slowness, difficulty, and impairment. Might take twice as long. Beginning to be aware of difficulty.

80% = Completely independent in most chores. Takes twice as long. Conscious of difficulty and slowness.

70% = Not completely independent. More difficulty with some chores. Three to four times as long in some. Must spend a large part of the day with chores.

60% = Some dependency. Can do most chores, but exceedingly slowly and with much effort. Errors; some impossible.

50% = More dependent. Help with half, slower, etc. Difficulty with everything.

40% = Very dependent. Can assist with all chores, but few alone.

30% = With effort, now and then does a few chores alone or begins alone. Much help needed.

20% = Nothing alone. Can be a slight help with some chores. Severe invalid.

10% = Totally dependent, helpless. Complete invalid.

0% = Vegetative functions, such as swallowing, bladder, and bowel functions, are not functioning. Bedridden.

Table 1.3 Unified Parkinson's Disease Rating Scale (UPDRS). From Gancher, S. T. (2002). Quantitative measures and rating scales. In S. A. Factor & W. J. Weiner (Eds.), *Parkinson's disease diagnosis and clinical management* (pp. 115-124). New York: Demos. Reprinted with permission.

TABLE 1.4   Braak Staging of Parkinson's Disease

Braak stage	Pathologic changes/ Lewy body formations	Clinical features
I	Enteric (small intestine) nerve cells	Constipation
II	Medulla (vital functions, special functions); pons (bridge to midbrain)	Sleep-wake dysregulation; REM sleep behavior disorder

(continued)

TABLE 1.4   Braak Staging of Parkinson's Disease (continued)

Braak stage	Pathologic changes/ Lewy body formations	Clinical features
III	Substantia nigra ("home of the dopaminergic cells") and olfactory nuclei	Motor symptoms begin to appear; impaired sense of smell and taste; subtle neurocogntive changes
IV	Prefrontal cortex	Dementia, hallucinations, increasing loss of effect of medications
V	Entire neocortex (most highly evolved brain tissue/functions)	Profound mental and physical impairment; medication intolerance

Adapted from Braak, H., Ghebredmedhin e, Rub, U., Del Tredici, K. (2004). Stages in the development of Parkinson's disease related pathology. *Cell Tissue Research 318*: 123-134.

Subgroups within idiopathic PD began to emerge. Terms like *young-onset, tremor-predominant,* and *postural instability–predominant* disease became common language. Along with these terms, prognostic associations were attached. Young-onset patients tend to have earlier and more severe dystonic and dyskinetic drug reactions (Kostic, Przedborski, Flaster, & Sternic, 1991). Many studies have documented that tremor-predominant PD is more slowly progressive and generally much less disabling than the postural instability–predominant type of PD (Jankovic et al., 1990; Zetusky et al., 1985).

One very helpful point for nursing dealing with patients and families concerned about disease progression is that for the patient with true idiopathic PD (i.e., no atypical features), and for those availing themselves of the best neurologic treatment and state-of-the-art care, patients can live a relatively normal life span and maintain independence for many years, even decades. PD progresses slowly and insidiously. It is important to recognize that PD does not suddenly take a turn for the worse or go into a crisis. When families suspect this, the symptoms can almost always be traced to a medication change or error, concurrent acute illness, or infection. In older adults this sudden change in function can be related to mild dehydration or a urinary tract infection without the classic symptoms or fever that younger patients would experience. Sometimes seemingly minor infections, such as a tooth or skin infection requiring antibiotics, can appear to dramatically worsen PD symptoms. Patients and families must be reassured that this is a temporary response to an acute illness and that the individual with PD is expected to return to baseline once the infection is resolved.

Understanding the progression of PD in the 21st century will undoubtedly be defined by the assistance of neuroimaging studies. To date, limited PET, SPECT, and magnetic resonance imaging (MRI) data are promising in assisting researchers to define loss of dopamine transporter binding, terminal function, and uptake. The ability to monitor these dopaminergic functions will also be a fertile ground for studying disease progression and disease-modifying and neuroprotective strategies to change the course of this progressive neurodegenerative disease.

ATYPICAL PARKINSONISM AND DIFFERENTIAL DIAGNOSES

As with all disorders of health, becoming familiar with the historical context in which they occur, clinical presentations, classic signs and symptoms, and so-called red flags (unusual characteristics) will help differentiate PD from other disorders. Idiopathic PD starts slowly and insidiously, has a prodrome period, and begins asymmetrically. Abrupt onset, symmetrical onset, or history of a trigger, such as a new medication or head trauma, would be a red flag. Onset at an unusually young age or with an atypical feature (Table 1.5) would warrant concern.

Perhaps the most common mistaken diagnosis for PD is essential tremor (ET). ET is the most common of movement disorders, up to 10 times more common than PD. Familial in nature, it is an autosomal dominant trait (Critchley, 1949). Unlike PD, with its myriad of signs and symptoms, ET is characterized by a monosymptom: tremor. The tremor is seen posturally and kinetically (i.e., with action). For example, ask the patient to hold his or her hand in front outstretched and still, and then have the patient use that extremity to lift a coffee cup to his or her mouth. Voice and head tremors may also be seen. Note that this tremor is much different than the resting tremor seen in PD.

Another common entity in the differential diagnosis of PD is the presentation of cognitive decline or dementia. Dementia as a presenting symptom (rather than tremor, bradykinesia, or cogwheel rigidity) should

TABLE 1.5 Atypical Features and Possible Differentials

Atypical feature	possibile differential
Absence of tremor	MSA, vascular PD, PD
Myoclonus	Corticobasal degeneration, Creutzfeldt-Jakob disease
Action/postural tremor	Benign essential tremor
Neuropathy	Multiple system atrophy
Oculomotor dysfunction	Progressive supranuclear palsy
Young onset (before age 40)	Wilson's disease
Early dementia	Diffuse Lewy body disease, Creutzfeldt-Jakob disease

Note. Patients present with some features of PD and one or more unusual features.

be a concern. Older people with dementing illnesses often appear slow, bewildered, and need cueing, which can be mistaken for the signs of PD. Those with PD have bradyphrenia (slowness of thought), and those with dementia have confusion or inability to retrieve thoughts. If a person's cognitive decline is due to a multi-infarct state, he or she may have a gait apraxia, which can be confused with the shuffling gait and postural instability of PD.

Previously thought to be a variant of PD, diffuse Lewy body disease (DLBD) is now considered by many to be a distinct entity (Oertel & Moller, 2004). Characterized by extensive Lewy body formation as well as neuro-pathological findings of plaques and tangles, such as seen in Alzheimer's disease, the patient presents with cognitive decline and parkinsonian features (McKeith et al., 1996). Patients with DLBD have fluctuating attention, hallucinations, sleep and behavioral disorders, neuroleptic sensitivity, and often paradoxical reactions to neuroleptics. Patients with DLBD tend to progress rapidly and are challenges for families to maintain at home due to the severity of their sleep and behavioral disorders.

There are also a host of neurodegenerative disorders that, over the years, have been called the *Parkinson-plus syndromes* or the *atypical parkinsonisms*. These include disorders such as PSP, MSA, corticobasal ganglionic degeneration, olivopontocerebellar atrophy, and SDS. Often, these disorders present early on appearing very much like PD without tremor. Sometimes they even transiently respond to levodopa, only to lose the response and deteriorate with profound and more expansive neurodegenerative symptoms. The Practice Parameter of the American Academy of Neurology considers six findings worthy of consideration as parkinsonian syndromes rather than as true idiopathic PD. These include (a) falls at presentation or early in the course of disease, (b) poor response to levodopa, (c) symmetry at onset, (d) rapid progression (i.e., to Hoehn and Yahr Stage III within 3 years), (e) lack of tremor, and (f) dysautonomia (Suchowersky et al., 2006). Table 1.6 lists some of these disorders and their most notable features.

LOOKING TOWARD THE FUTURE

Basic science and management of PD have grown exponentially in the last 50 years. Future goals, of course, are to find the cause and cure, or a cause and mechanism to prevent the development of PD so that no one has to suffer with this progressive neurodegenerative disorder. Immediate ongoing scientific efforts include attempts to expand the animal model beyond the MPTP paradigm, which is highly specific for the dopaminergic system alone. Genetic research is attempting to find more clues as to what triggers the mutations and aggregations of abnormal proteins. Antioxidants, scavengers for toxic byproducts, are under study in the hope of inhibiting mitochondrial dysfunction. Neurotropic factor infusions will be attempted. Research is prevalent in treating current patients with better methods of continuous receptor stimulation and in attempting to find neuroprotective agents. New receptors are being targeted, such as adenosine and glutamate, to determine their role in managing PD symptoms. Stem cell research will continue to hold new promise for future therapeutics.

SUMMARY

In approximately 10 years (2017) we will be recognizing the 200th anniversary of Dr. James Parkinson's *An Essay on the Shaking Palsy,* the first published description of the disorder that today bears his name. When we reflect back on the scientific advances made in the understanding of PD, the last 50 years have been the most productive in gaining knowledge into the mysteries of the disease and treatment. Several landmark findings have occurred that have pushed research to the next level, and undoubtedly, there

TABLE 1.6 Common "Parkinsonisms": Common Features and Distinguishing Characteristics

Disorder	Common features
Vascular parkinsonism	Acute or stepwise progression, akinesia, documented vascular risk factors, axial/nuccal rigidity, fixed facies, dementia, dysarthria, gait apraxia, seborrhea, "lower body PD"
LUBAY	First, focal dystonia, then generalized within 5 years, followed by parkinsonism
Creutzfeldt-Jakob disease	EEG abnormalities, rapid progression over months, startle myoclonus, dementia, psychiatric disturbances
Diffuse Lewy body disease	Fluctuating attention, sleep and behavioral disorders, neuroleptic sensitivity with paradoxical response to neuroleptics, hallucinations
Corticobasal degeneration	Progressive asymmetric motor dysfunction, myoclonus, apraxia, cortical sensory loss, alien limb, late-onset dementia, frontal release signs, apathy
Multiple system atrophy	Cerebellar, autonomic, and extrapyramidal disorders
(1) Olivopontocerebellar atrophy	(1) truncal and gait apraxia, opthalmoparesis
(2) Shy-Drager	(2) orthostatic hypotension, impotence, urinary incontinence, and anhydrosis
(3) Striatal nigral degeneration	(3) dysarthria, syncope, incontinence, impotence, brisk reflexes

will be more to come. While we continue to look for the causes and cures for this devastating disorder, nurses will continue to take care of patients in all stages of the disease throughout the continuum of care. By understanding where we have been and where we are headed in the understanding of PD, nurses will be ready to meet the challenge of providing excellence of care for patients and their families in a variety of settings to enhance quality of life for all people living with PD.

REFERENCES

Ascherio, A. (2006). Pesticide exposure and risk for Parkinson's disease. *Annals of Neurology, 60,* 197–203.

Ascherio, A., Zhang, S. M., Hernán, M. A., Kawachi, I., Colditz, G. A., Speizer, F. E., et al. (2001). Prospective study of caffeine consumption and risk of Parkinson's disease in men and women. *Annals of Neurology, 50,* 50–63.

Beneditti, M. D., Bower, J. H., Maraganore, D. M., McDonnell, S. K., Peterson, B. J., Ahlskog, J. E., et al. (2000). Smoking, alcohol, coffee consumption preceding Parkinson's disease: A case control study. *Neurology, 55,* 1350–1358.

Braak, H. (2005, March). *Six stages of Parkinson's disease.* Paper presented at the Ninth International Congress of Parkinson's Disease and Movement Disorders, New Orleans, LA.

Braak, H., Ghebredmedhin, E., Rub, U., & Del Tredici, K. (2004). Stages in the development of Parkinson's disease related pathology. *Cell Tissue Research, 318,* 123–134.

Brissaud, E. (1895). *Leçons sur les maladies nerveuses.* Paris: Salpetriere.

Brooks, D. (2004). Neuroimaging of movement disorders. In R. L. Watts & W. C. Koller (Eds.), *Movement disorders: Neurologic principles and practice* (pp. 36–41). New York: McGraw-Hill.

Brotchie, J. M. (2005). Nondopaminergic mechanisms in levodopa-induced dyskinesias. *Movement Disorders, 20,* 919–931.

Christensen, J. H. (2006, Summer). Still waters run deep: Parkinson disease and the thief of expression. *Care Advantage,* 21–23.

Critchley, M. (1949). Observations of essential (heredofamilial) tremor. *Brain, 72,* 113–139.

Dickman, M. S. (2001). Von Economo encephalitis. *Archives of Neurology, 58,* 1696–1698.

Duvoisin, R. C. (1987). History of parkinsonism. *Pharmacology and Therapeutics, 32,* 1–17.

Fahn, S. (2003). Foreword. In S. M. Pulst (Ed.), *Genetics of movement disorders* (p. xix). San Diego, CA: Elsevier Science.

Fahn, S., Elton, R. L., & Members of the UPDRS Development Committee. (1987). United Parkinson Disease Rating Scale. In S. Fahn, C. D. Marsden, D. B. Calne, & M. Goldstein (Eds.), *Recent developments in Parkinson's disease* (Vol. 2, pp. 293–304). Florham Park, NJ: Macmillan.

Firestone, J. A., Smith-Weller, T., Franklin, G., Swanson, P., Longstreth, W. T., & Checkoway, H. (2005). Pesticides and risk of Parkinson disease. *Archives of Neurology, 62,* 91–95.

Gancher, S. T. (2002). Quantitative measures and rating scales. In S. A. Factor & W. J. Weiner (Eds.), *Parkinson's disease diagnosis and clinical management* (pp. 115-124). New York: Demos.

Gowers, Sir W. R. (1903). *A manual of the diseases of the nervous system.* Philadelphia: Blaksiton's.

Hoehn, M. M., & Yahr, M. D. (1967). Parkinsonism: Onset, progression and mortality. *Neurology, 17,* 427.

Hughes, A. J., Ben-Shlomo, Y., Daniel, S. E., & Lees, A. J. (1992). What features improve the accuracy of clinical diagnosis in Parkinson's disease: A clinicopathologic study. *Neurology, 42,* 1142–1146.

Hughes, A. J., Daniel, S. E., Ben-Shlomo, Y., & Lees, A. J. (2002). The accuracy of diagnosis of parkinsonian syndromes in a specialty movement disorder service. *Brain, 125,* 861–870.

Hughes, A. J., Daniel, S. E., Kilford, L., & Lees, A. J. (1992). Accuracy of clinical diagnosis of idiopathic Parkinson's disease: A clinical-pathological study of 100 cases. *Journal of Neurology, Neurosurgery, and Psychiatry, 55,* 181–184.

Jankovic, J., McDermott, M., Carter, J., Gauthier, S., Goetz, C., Golbe, L., et al. (1990). Variable expression of Parkinson's disease: A base-line analysis of the DATATOP cohort. The Parkinson Study Group. *Neurology, 40,* 1529–1534.

Klein, C., & Schlossmacher, M. G. (2006). The genetics of Parkinson disease: Implications for neurological care. *Nature Clinical Practice Neurology, 2,* 136–146.

Kolata, G. (1999). *The story of the great influenza pandemic of 1918 and the search for the virus that caused it.* New York: Farrar, Straus, and Giroux.

Kostic, V., Przedborski, S., Flaster, E., & Sternic, N. (1991). Early development of levodopa-induced dyskinesias and response fluctuations in young-onset Parkinson's disease. *Neurology, 41*(Pt. 1), 202–205.

Kurland, L. (1958). Epidemiology: Incidence, geographic, distribution and genetic considerations. In W. Field (Ed.), *Pathogenesis and treatment of Parkinson disease.* Springfield, IL: Charles C. Thomas.

Lang, A. E. (2005). Selected basic and clinical research developments over the past decade. *Parkinson Report, 16,* 6–11.

Langston, W. (1995). *The case of the frozen addict: Working at the edge of the mysteries of the human brain.* London: Vintage.

Malecki, E. A., Vaughan, C. G., & Anderson, K. E. (2004, April). *What symptoms are most troubling to patients with Parkinson's disease?* Paper presented at the 56th Annual Meeting of the American Academy of Neurology, San Francisco.

Marras, C., & Tanner, C. M. (2004). Epidemiology of Parkinson disease. In R. L. Watts & W. C. Koller (Eds.), *Movement disorders: Neurologic principles and practice* (pp. 177–195). New York: McGraw-Hill.

McKeith, I., Galasko, D., Kosaka, K., Perry, E. K., Dickson, D. W., Hansen, L. A., et al. (1996). Consensus guidelines for the clinical and pathologic diagnosis of dementia with Lewy bodies (DLB): Report of the consortium on DLB international workshop. *Neurology, 47,* 1113–1124, 1196.

National Parkinson Foundation. (2006). *About Parkinson disease.* Retrieved August 5, 2006, from http://www.parkinson.org

Nefzinger, M., Quadfasel, F., & Karl, V. (1968). A retrospective study of smoking and Parkinson's disease. *American Journal of Epidemiology, 88,* 149–158.

Oertel, W. H., & Moller, C. (2004). Rare degenerative syndromes associated with parkinsonism. In R. L. Watts & W. C. Koller (Eds.), *Movement disorders: Neurologic principles and practice* (pp. 403–419). New York: McGraw-Hill.

Parkinson, J. (1817). *Essay on the shaking palsy.* London: Neely and Jones.

Paulson, H. L., & Stern, M. B. (2004). Clinical manifestations of Parkinson's disease. In R. L. Watts & W. C. Koller (Eds.), *Movement disorders: Neurologic principles and practice* (pp. 233–245). New York: McGraw-Hill.

Priyadarshi, A., Khuder, S. A., Schaub, E. A., & Shrivastava, S. (2000). A meta-analysis of Parkinson's disease and exposure to pesticides. *Neurotoxicology, 21,*435–440.

Ross, G. W., Abbott, R. D., Petrovitch, H., Morens, D. M., Grandinetti, A., Tung, K. H., et al. (2000). Association of coffee and caffeine intake with the risk of Parkinson's disease. *Journal of the American Medical Association, 283,* 2674–2679.

Stern, M. B. (1993). Parkinson's disease. In M. B. Stern & W. C. Koller (Eds.), *Parkinsonian syndromes* (pp. 3–29). New York: Marcel Dekker.

Stern, M. B. (1994). Olfactory function in Parkinson's disease subtypes. *Neurology, 44,* 266–268.

Suchowersky, O., Reich, S., Perlmutter, J., Zesiewicz, T., Gronseth, G., & Weiner, W. (2006). *Practice Parameter: Diagnosis and prognosis of new onset Parkinson disease (an evidence based review): Report of the Quality Standards Subcommittee of the American Academy of Neurology.* St. Paul, MN: American Academy of Neurology.

Vila, M., & Przedburski, S. (2004). Genetic clues to the pathogenesis of Parkinson's disease. *Nature Medicine, 10,* S58–S62.

von Economo, K. (1917). Encephalitis lethargica. *Wiener Klinische Wochenschrift, 30,* 581–585.

Ward, C. D., Hess, W. A., & Calne, D. B. (1983). Olfactory impairment in Parkinson's disease. *Neurology, 33,* 943–946.

Zetusky, W. J., Jankovic, J., & Pirozzolo, F. J. (1985). The clinical heterogeneity of Parkinson's disease: Clinical and prognostic implication. *Neurology, 35,* 522–526.

2

Theoretical Approach to the Clinical Care of Parkinson's Disease

Amy M. Sawyer, PhD(C), RN

Health care in the 21st century has been transformed by the increasing prevalence of chronic diseases in our society. According to the World Health Organization, chronic diseases account for 60% of global deaths and almost one-third of the global *burden* of disease. As such, the delivery of health care around the world has necessarily moved from acute-care models to chronic-care models. Acute-care models of health care have traditionally relied on the expertise of the medical providers and the passivity of the patient and family. In contrast, chronic-care models of health care recognize the patient and family as experts of daily care delivery and recognize medical and health professionals as partners in care delivery, offering health information, disease therapeutics, and resources for attaining specialized care. This paradigm shift has gradually emerged as chronic diseases in our society have evoked greater morbidity and disability among those afflicted with chronic disease and have consumed an ever-increasing percentage of resources. In the United States alone, chronic disease serves as the main reason for health care seeking and contributes to 70% of health care spending (Holman & Lorig, 2000). Furthermore, the effectiveness of the traditional acute-care model of health care delivery in promoting positive health and quality of life outcomes in chronic disease management has been increasingly recognized as inadequate (Institute of Medicine, 2003).

Parkinson's disease (PD) is both chronic and progressive, significantly contributing to the overall morbidity rate attributable to chronic disease. In the United States, approximately 1,000,000 individuals and their families are afflicted with PD (Noyes, Liu, Li, Holloway, & Dick, 2006). Furthermore, the cost burden of this disease is substantial for both individuals living with PD and society. According to the Parkinson's Disease Foundation (2005), the combined direct and indirect cost in the United States of this chronic disease is estimated at more than $5,600,000,000 per year. Noyes et al. (2006) estimated the financial burden of care for a PD patient living in the community to be approximately $20,000 per year. Likewise, the annual cost of long-term care for an individual with PD is estimated at $47,000, as compared to long-term care residents without PD, costing $45,000 annually.

Aside from monetary costs, Parkinson's disease contributes to progressive impairment and disability in those afflicted, necessitating patient, caregiver, and health professional management efforts to maintain and achieve positive health outcomes. In order to effect positive outcomes in this chronically diseased population, patients and caregivers must become active participants in the daily management of Parkinson's disease and collaboratively work with expert Parkinson's disease health care professionals, exemplifying the paradigm shift from acute-care disease management to chronic-care disease management. Thereby the critical outcome measures, including physiological, psychosocial, and quality of life outcomes, may be supported and achieved.

SOCIAL COGNITIVE APPROACH TO HEALTH BEHAVIOR

Although individual chronic diseases are treated and managed in varying ways, there are commonalities among this collective of diseases that afford clinicians and researchers an opportunity to better define, measure, and construct interventions that promote patient-centered disease management. The commonality is that chronic disease management takes place outside of the health care institution and without the ever-presence of health care professionals. Simply stated, chronic disease management is carried out as an aspect of daily life among those patients and their caregivers who live with the disease. It is from this perspective that caregiving and chronic disease management necessitate the application of a theoretical approach. By applying a theoretical approach to clinical care delivery in chronic disease, the demands of the patient and the significant other caregiving can be supported and enhanced. Furthermore, by applying a social cognitive approach to chronic disease management, the burden on acute-care health delivery may be lessened and the chronically ill provided with resources and self-management techniques that ultimately enhance their own outcomes.

Social cognitive theory posits that health behavior is determined by a core set of determinants, including knowledge of health risks and benefits of health practices, perceived self-efficacy, outcome expectations, health goals, and facilitators and impediments to health behavior changes (Bandura, 2004). Health behavior, or the ability to change a certain health behavior, is a cumulative response to these core determinants. Recognizing that individuals do not live in isolation, the social cognitive approach to health behavior and health promotion encompasses the individual, support persons, and the environment as influential on the individual's ability to change health behavior or adopt effective health management strategies.

The core determinants in social cognitive theory are opportunities through which individuals can effect new or different health behaviors and also open the door to influence from health care providers and significant others to promote behavior change or the adoption of health management behaviors. The first core determinant, knowledge, "creates the precondition for change" (Bandura, 2004, p. 144). In order that health behaviors and management can be changed, the individual needs to have knowledge of the need for change. Yet, as many empiric studies have demonstrated, knowledge alone does not promote change in health behavior. A second core determinant, and the most important, is perceived self-efficacy. Perceived self-efficacy is the belief that one can effect change by one's own actions. According to Bandura, perceived self-efficacy "is the foundation of human motivation and action . . . . Whatever other factors may serve as guides and motivators, they are rooted in the core belief that one has the power to produce desired changes by one's actions" (2004, p. 144).

Outcome expectations are another core determinant in social cognitive theory. This determinant is the process by which individuals can identify how their actions will eventually afford personal benefit. Although often associated only with physical health changes, Bandura (2004) posited that there are also social outcomes and self-evaluative reactions that contribute to how outcome expectations are viewed by the individual. Goals, then, are another core determinant. Although often envisioned by health professionals as long-term goals, the more immediate gratification of short-term goals contribute to the individual's perceived self-efficacy and motivation for continued behavior change (Bandura, 2004). Finally, the core determinants of facilitators and impediments cannot be overlooked. Impediments are a contributing factor to perceived self-efficacy, for with each impediment to health behavior change or promotion, "self-efficacy beliefs must be measured against gradations of challenges to successful performance" (Bandura, 2004, p. 145). Thereby the lower perceived self-efficacy in light of impediments of health behavior change, the greater the actuality of *not* changing or adopting certain health behaviors.

The interaction of these core determinants in social cognitive theory gives rise to the actuality of health behaviors (Figure 2.1). Through a theoretical approach to clinical care the interacting core determinants can not only be measured, but also intervened on to promote health behaviors. As Bandura eloquently states, "Social cognitive theory offers both predictors and principles on how to inform, enable, guide, and motivate people to adapt habits that promote health and reduce those that impair it" (2004, p. 146).

Figure 2.1 Structural Paths of Influence Where in Perceived Self-efficacy Affects Health Habits Both Directly and Through Its Impact on Goals, Outcome Expectations, and Perception of Sociostructural Facilitators and Impediments to Health-promoting Behavior.

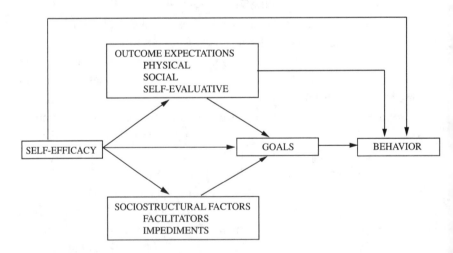

Source: Redrawn From "Bandura, A. (2004). Health Promotion By Social Cognitive Means." Health Education and Behavior, 31(2), 146. Copyright 2004 by Society for Public Health Education. Reproduced With permission Of Sage Publications, Inc.

EMPIRIC EVIDENCE FOR A SOCIAL COGNITIVE APPROACH TO HEALTH BEHAVIOR AND CHRONIC DISEASE MANAGEMENT

Many empiric studies have incorporated Bandura's social cognitive theory in the investigation of health behavior change. Clark and Dodge (1999) conducted a comprehensive review of longitudinal studies focused on chronic disease published in the extant literature specifically addressing the core determinant of self-efficacy and behavior. Although social cognitive theory includes other core determinants, self-efficacy is the most central and influential of the core determinants in the theory. Clark and Dodge (1999) suggested that although many empiric studies have provided evidence of self-efficacy as an associated variable relative to behavior (cross-sectional data), there are a number of longitudinal studies emerging that provide evidence of self-efficacy as a core determinant in health behavior change.

Recognizing that self-efficacy is behavior-specific, empiric studies have examined self-efficacy in relationship to health screening behaviors, exercise, diet, cardiovascular health risk reduction, smoking cessation, medication adherence, HIV risk reduction behaviors, pain behavior and management, and chronic disease management. As Clark and Dodge (1999) summarize, although self-efficacy is not consistently a predictor of all behaviors, the extant literature does support self-efficacy as associated with innumerable health behaviors and as "central" in deconstructing the conditions of health behavior change.

Self-efficacy is behavior-specific and relative to specific goals that are achieved through health-related behaviors. Self-efficacy "specifically implicates the importance of an individual's perception of both his ability and capability to execute as well as to achieve successful and valued behavioral outcomes" (Marks, Allegrante, & Lorig, 2005a, p. 39). Therefore the construct of self-efficacy has most recently been examined as an important interventional opportunity relative to chronic disease management. In chronic disease management the individual and support persons living with the disease must perform daily management behaviors in order to maintain a balance between the disease and their quality of life. Self-efficacy for the behaviors required to manage symptoms, projecting and understanding long-term maintenance requirements of chronic disease management, and identifying goals for a higher quality of life are all important contributing factors to the realized outcomes in chronic disease. As a central tenet, then, self-efficacy is a construct that can be promoted in chronically ill individuals and their support persons to contribute to an overall improved quality of life (Han, Lee, Lee, & Park, 2003). "Baseline self-efficacy for managing health regimens, as well as changes in baseline self-efficacy, are likely to prove fundamental to the individual's ability to set disease management goals" and repeatedly execute behaviors that are health promoting and disease managing (Marks et al., 2005a, p. 40).

Applying self-efficacy-promoting interventions among chronically ill individuals and the management of their disease shows significant promise with regard to improved outcomes and quality of life in chronic disease. Lorig and colleagues (1999) developed and tested a self-management for chronic disease program. The program was constructed based on the principles of social cognitive theory and with particular emphasis on the core determinant of self-efficacy. A randomized control trial, with 952 individuals with heart disease, lung disease, stroke, or arthritis, were randomized to the self-management for chronic disease program or a wait-list control group. The experimental group demonstrated a significant improvement compared with controls at 6 months in the following outcome measures: weekly minutes of exercise ($p < .01$), frequency of cognitive symptom management ($p < .01$), improved communication with their provider ($p < .01$), self-rated health ($p < .02$), disability ($p < .02$), social/role activities limitation ($p < .02$), energy/fatigue ($p < .02$), health distress ($p < .02$), and fewer hospitalizations ($p < .05$; Lorig et al., 1999). There were no significant differences between the treatment and control groups for pain, shortness of breath, or psychological well-being (Lorig et al., 1999). This randomized controlled trial, focusing exclusively on self-efficacy improvement, provides evidence that a chronic disease management program based on self-efficacy promotion improves health behaviors and health status in a heterogeneous group of individuals with chronic disease.

Lorig, Sobel, Ritter, Laurent, and Hobbs (2001) applied their chronic disease self-management program in a longitudinal cohort study that followed 489 subjects over a 1-year period to identify changes in health behaviors, self-efficacy, health status, and health care utilization among participants. Health status, including measures of fatigue, shortness of breath, pain, role function, depression, and health distress; health care utilization, including emergency department visits and self-efficacy; and health behaviors, including exercise, cognitive symptom management, and communication with providers, were measured at 1 year. Statistically significant improvements in health behaviors, self-efficacy, and health status and fewer emergency department visits were identified for participants in the program as compared with nonparticipants (Lorig, et al., 2001).

Although these studies focused on one specific chronic disease management program, there are numerous other studies that have identified self-management programs developed from the theoretical perspective of social cognitive theory and attending to the promotion of self-efficacy in the management of chronic disease that have significant positive findings. To name but a few, the following studies have included chronic disease self-management in a heterogeneous chronic disease group (Farrell, Wicks, & Martin, 2004), a case management approach for coronary risk factor modification after acute myocardial infarction (DeBusk et al., 1994), and an intensive multiple risk factor reduction on coronary artery disease and clinical care events (Haskell et al., 1994). There exist numerous other intervention studies that have measured self-efficacy pre- and postintervention for chronic disease management and risk factor reduction that similarly show positive findings with regard to self-efficacy for the intended behavior and improved outcomes.

From the empiric studies that have been conducted examining self-efficacy as a predictor of particular health behaviors and health promotion activities, there is ample evidence that self-efficacy is indeed a central tenet in health behavior change. Furthermore, the intervention studies that have been rigorously conducted to examine self-efficacy–promoting programs and their effect on behavior modification or change in the management of chronic disease have shown promise with regard to outcomes and perceived health status. "The construct of self-efficacy offers a research-based theoretical construct with which the [health providers] can develop interventions that can positively affect behavioral performance and that will have a significant impact on the human and societal burden created by chronic disease" (Marks et al., 2005a, p. 41).

APPLICATION OF A THEORETICAL APPROACH TO THE CLINICAL CARE OF CHRONIC DISEASE: SELF-MANAGEMENT

Roles, Environments of Interaction, and Self-Management Promotion

Self management, or the "ability of the patient to deal with all that a chronic illness entails, including symptoms, treatment, physical and social consequences, and lifestyle changes" (Coleman & Newton, 2005, pp. 1503–1504), is a process that relies heavily on the patient's self-efficacy for managing his or her own disease and can be influenced and supported by health care providers and educators in the clinical setting. Furthermore, the clinical focus of self-efficacy is a unique viewpoint in a setting that is so often focused on the provider; rather, a self-efficacy focus in care design and delivery of chronic illness care brings attention to the patient's strengths rather than weaknesses and diverts focus from the pathological illness or disease (Keefe, Rumble, Scipio, Giordano, & Perri, 2004), in effect, permitting the individual with chronic disease to become the central figure of care delivery and self-management.

Aside from the central role of the patient in the self-management of chronic disease, Coleman and Newton (2005) coin the provider's role as providing self-management support, expanding the traditional "caregiving" health care provider role to helping patients "build confidence and make choices that lead to improved self management and better outcomes" (pp. 1504–1505). As such, the role of supporting self-management is shared by not only the health provider, but also by support staff, educators, social workers, nurses, physical and occupational therapists, psychologists, and patient family members who interact with the chronically ill patient during outpatient visits, other health-related environments, and within the community or home setting. In this context, there are diversified settings and opportunities to influence the individual's self-efficacy for self-management and promote improved outcomes in health and quality of life.

Beyond the roles that various types of health providers, family members, and the patient play in the self-management of chronic disease, the type of delivered interaction and environment is important to consider. As Bandura (2004) describes, "social cognitive theory extends the conception of human agency to collective agency. People do not operate as isolates. They work together to improve the quality of their lives" (p. 159). This particularly applies to social practices that influence the health of many. Recognizing, though, that individuals living with chronic disease are not isolated and that healthful behaviors from this theoretical perspective are dually promoted through community self-help, the significance of others becomes apparent. Individuals with chronic disease need to be provided with appropriate and needed resources: "guidance to help themselves" (Bandura, 2004, p. 162). Therefore the interactions between the primary health care provider and the patient are complemented by the interactions between patients and other patients experiencing similar disease concerns and resources within the community. Patients helping patients becomes a key strategic environment from which the core self-management skills of problem solving, decision making, and resource identification and utilization are supported.

Various types of interaction opportunities and environments are proposed in the clinical application of self-management of chronic diseases and the promotion of self-efficacy. These include, for example, regularly scheduled office visits with health care providers, patient group visits with providers, systematically delivered phone interactions from health care providers, nurses, or other appropriate health professionals, open telephone call-in time to health providers or other necessary resource persons for self-management, interactive Web-based programs and chat rooms, support groups, and community-based interaction opportunities for patients living with chronic disease. As Holman and Lorig (2000) identify, opportunities to teach and influence health behaviors need to be acceptable to those living with chronic disease. The effectiveness of different types of interaction opportunities and environments for program delivery depends on the content of the program; how the content is taught; the format for delivery; and the patient characteristics of culture, family, and language, to name a few (Holman & Lorig, 2000). By offering choices of interaction opportunities to patients with chronic disease, the patient is exposed to numerous vehicles by which self-efficacy and thereby self-management can be promoted and supported. Furthermore, groups offer the opportunity for peer-to-peer interaction, thereby supporting problem solving and decision making among those living with the disease and forging new roles as a result of the disease.

Practical Applications to Promote Self-Efficacy and the Self-Management of Chronic Disease

What, then, are the necessary steps to take in promoting self-efficacy for self-management of chronic disease in the clinical setting? Moving beyond, but not to the exclusion of the traditional clinical outcome measures of importance specific to each disease (i.e., biomarkers of disease status, such as hemoglobin A1C in diabetes) is first and foremost: refocusing on living each and every day with chronic disease. In this way, what is important to the patient is similarly important to the provider.

From this perspective, self-efficacy-enhancing programs are aimed at the theoretically derived skills necessary for disease self-management: problem solving, decision making, developing effective relationships with health care providers, resource identification and utilization, action planning, goal setting, and self-tailoring. Although certain diseases require a different set of specific skills for the effective management of the disease, there are broad clinical program characteristics that have been empirically identified to enhance self-efficacy.

In their extensive review of self-efficacy-enhancing interventions in chronic disease, Marks et al. (2005b) suggested that the following program characteristics are essential to include in any clinical application of self-efficacy promotion: (a) incorporate a variety of learning strategies while providing mutual aid and support for learning; (b) involve significant others or family members and promote collaborative relationships between patient and health care providers; (c) foster self-management tasks in small increments; (d) supply plenty of encouragement, persuasion, and direct or indirect support for the desired behaviors; (e) encourage self-appraisal of patient responses; (f) encourage self-appraisal of decision making and problem solving; (g) provide and direct to resources for knowledge and skills to deal with disease-related issues across different domains; (h) use trained educators, practice manuals, and multicomponent teaching strategies with content from both other patients and health care providers; and (i) use varied approaches and interaction opportunities (i.e., individual, groups, phone-based, home-based, Web-based) to promote collaborative relationships and active participation.

Coleman and Newton (2005) have further delineated specific clinical practice recommendations that support the chronically ill patient in his self-management regimen. Practice changes and physician (health care provider or others involved in the practice setting) actions include the following:

(1) systematic follow up with patients and family members about established action plans, goals, cognitive symptom management through phone calls, emails, and/or office visits; (2) establish group visits that focus on self-management behaviors/tasks; (3) appointment scheduling should permit time to address self-management tasks; (4) recognize and address health literacy and medical obstacles to self-management; (5) identify problems and concerns from the patient and family perspective; and (6) include goal-setting

(short-term leading to long-term), action planning, and problem-solving strategies to overcome barriers based on the patient's immediate concerns and their perspective. (p. 1505)

These practice changes and action steps are aimed at one particular issue for the chronically ill patient population: helping the individual and his or her family live day-to-day with the disease and obtain the best possible outcomes through self-management.

SUMMARY

Chronic disease is a significant burden for the individual and family living with the disease, health care organizations, and society. Certainly each chronic disease has its own specific health effects; certainly, too, each person afflicted with a chronic disease responds and manages everyday life in a specific manner. Approaching chronic disease from a theoretical perspective, and understanding that effective self-management of the condition is the eventual desired outcome, social cognitive theory provides a conceptual framework and a working model from which to effectively intervene and manage chronic disease. Particularly important is the core determinant of self-efficacy: one's belief in one's own ability to carry out a behavior to achieve a specific goal. Social cognitive theory and the determinant of self-efficacy have been widely applied in both predictor and, more recently, intervention studies.

Although specific disease-oriented interventions may enhance medical outcomes that are desirable to health care providers, the success of psychobehavioral interventions may be more appealing to individuals living with chronic disease. Furthermore, such interventions may improve medical outcomes through the process of enhanced self-management. As such, chronic disease self-management is an important intervention that can be incorporated into clinical practice and provide patients and their families with knowledge, decision-making and problem-solving skills, and collaborative relationship-building skills to afford improved, mutually arrived at medical and daily living goals in chronic disease. It is from this perspective that persons living with chronic disease truly serve as the experts about their own lives and health care providers can truly serve as experts about diseases (Bodenheimer, Lorig, Holman, & Grumbach, 2002). The combined expertise of patients, families, and health care providers can significantly impact on the burden of chronic disease for the individual and family, health care organizations, and society.

REFERENCES

Bandura, A. (2004). Health promotion by social cognitive means. *Health Education & Behavior, 31,* 143–164.

Bodenheimer, T., Lorig, K., Holman, H., & Grumbach, K. (2002). Patient self-management of chronic disease in primary care. *Journal of the American Medical Association, 288,* 2469–2475.

Clark, N. M., & Dodge, J. A. (1999). Exploring self-efficacy as a predictor of disease management. *Health Education & Behavior, 26,* 72–89.

Coleman, M. T., & Newton, K. S. (2005). Supporting self-management in patients with chronic illness. *American Family Physician, 72,* 1503–1510.

DeBusk, R. F., Houston Miller, N., Superko, H. R., Dennis, C. A., Thomas, R. J., Lew, H. T., et al. (1994). A case-management system for coronary risk factor modification after acute myocardial infarction. *Annals of Internal Medicine, 120,* 721–729.

Farrell, K., Wicks, M. N., & Martin, J. C. (2004). Chronic disease self-management improved with enhanced self-efficacy. *Clinical Nursing Research, 13,* 289–308.

Han, K., Lee, P., Lee, S., & Park, E. (2003). Factors influencing quality of life in people with chronic illness in Korea. *Journal of Nursing Scholarship, 35,* 139–144.

Haskell, W. L., Alderman, E. L., Fair, J. M., Maron, D. J., Mackey, S. F., Superko, H. R., et al. (1994). Effects of intensive multiple risk factor reduction on coronary atherosclerosis and clinical cardiac events in men and women with coronary artery disease: The Stanford Coronary Risk Intervention Project (SCRIP). *Circulation, 89,* 975–990.

Holman, H., & Lorig, K. (2000). Patients as partners in managing chronic disease: Partnership is a prerequisite for effective and efficient health care. *British Medical Journal, 320,* 526–527.

Institute of Medicine. (2003). Formulating new rules to redesign and improve care. In *Crossing the quality chasm: A new health system for the 21st century* (pp. 61–68). Washington, DC: National Academy Press.

Keefe, F. J., Rumble, M. E., Scipio, C. D., Giordano, L. A., & Perri, L. M. (2004). Psychological aspects of persistent pain: Current state of the science. *Journal of Pain, 5,* 195–211.

Lorig, K. R., Sobel, D. S., Ritter, P. L., Laurent, D., & Hobbs, M. (2001). Effect of a self-management program on patients with chronic disease. *Effective Clinical Practice, 4,* 256–262.

Lorig, K. R., Sobel, D. S., Stewart, A. L., Brown, B. W., Bandura, A., Ritter, P., et al. (1999). Evidence suggesting that a chronic disease self-management program can improve health status while reducing hospitalization: A randomized trial. *Medical Care, 37,* 5–14.

Marks, R., Allegrante, J. P., & Lorig, K. (2005a). A review and synthesis of research evidence for self-efficacy enhancing interventions for reducing chronic disability: Implications for health education practice (Part I). *Health Promotion Practice, 6,* 37–43.

Marks, R., Allegrante, J. P., & Lorig, K. (2005b). A review and synthesis of research evidence for self-efficacy enhancing interventions for reducing chronic disability: Implications for health education practice (Part II). *Health Promotion Practice, 6,* 148–156.

Noyes, K., Liu, H., Li, Y., Holloway, R., & Dick, A. (2006). Economic burden associated with Parkinson's disease on elderly Medicare beneficiaries. *Movement Disorders, 21,* 362–372.

Parkinson's Disease Foundation. (2005). *Ten frequently-asked questions about Parkinson's disease.* New York: Author.

3

Motor Symptoms and Medication Management

Barbara Fitzsimmons, RN, MS, CNRN
Gwyn M. Vernon, MSN, CRNP
Constance Ward, MSN, RN, BC, CNRN

Parkinson's disease (PD) was first described by James Parkinson nearly 200 years ago. Classic motor features of the disease are resting tremor, rigidity, and bradykinesia. As advances have been made in understanding the pathophysiology of the disease, medications have been developed that target the dopamine deficiency and modify dopamine metabolism. New classes are being developed that may target nondopaminergic brain receptors or offer neuroprotective advantages. Management of the patient's symptoms constantly evolves as the disease progresses and requires an interplay of the beneficial effect and side effect profiles. Often, in early PD, monoamine oxidase (MAO)-B inhibitors, the glutamate antagonist amantadine, anticholinergics, or dopamine agonists are utilized. In moderate PD, symptomatic treatment can be achieved through the administration of carbidopa/levodopa, a precursor of dopamine. Advancing disease can be handled with the addition of dopamine agonists, catecholamine O-methyl transferase (COMT) inhibitors, and newer formulations, such as rapidly dissolving carbidopa/levodopa or a rescue injectable agonist. New methods of delivery, such as transdermal patches and direct gastric infusions, are being investigated. It is essential for nurses caring for patients with PD to have a firm foundation of knowledge in the pharmacological basis of disease management and the complexities of many of the routines prescribed. Nurses play an important role in patient education, compliance issues, and monitoring of effectiveness and for adverse effects.

PD is known as one of the most common neurological disorders of the older adult. Initially described in 1817 by James Parkinson, a London physician, as a "shaking palsy," the observations he made of the disease's symptoms are evident in patients today. Classic signs and symptoms of the disease include resting tremor, muscular rigidity, bradykinesia, and postural instability. Although long recognized for its motor manifestations, PD also has many nonmotor features, such as autonomic manifestations and psychiatric problems (Smith, 2002).

Medications are the mainstay of therapy for PD, yet there are many challenges at every stage of the illness. Over the last 30 years, an increase in the understanding of the pathophysiology of the basal ganglia has resulted in the development of new therapeutic strategies for PD (Tetrud, 2004). Along with this, research has also supported an emphasis on long-term complications and strategies to manage the patient to avoid some of the devastating effects of medication in advanced disease, such as dyskinesias and psychosis. Numerous medications are available for the practitioner to choose from when planning the treatment. The indication, symptom relief properties, and side effect profile need to be carefully considered for each medication or combination prescribed. Furthermore, it is increasingly important to consider potential research implications of neuroprotective agents and alternative receptor targets under clinical study.

Throughout this chapter, treatment approaches for the disease will be explored with discussion of strategies for initial treatment for early disease, management of advancing disease, and therapy in pregnancy and for those with motor fluctuations. Drug classes under investigation will be mentioned. Classes of medications will be explained along with indications for their use. Finally, special considerations about nursing interventions and medication administration in the clinical setting will be addressed. Approaches for promoting adherence to medication schedules will be described.

REVIEW OF MOTOR FEATURES OF PARKINSON'S DISEASE (PD)

An explanation of the motor signs and symptoms of the disease is necessary so that selection of pharmacologic management can be understood. PD is a clinical diagnosis, and the gold standard for diagnosis is the neurological exam. PD at the most basic neuropathological level results from degeneration of dopamine neurons in the substantia nigra, which is located in the midbrain of the brain stem. The loss of nigral cells results in declining levels of striatal dopamine (Miller, 2002). However, as the decades progress, our understanding of the pathological process of this neurodegenerative disease is expanding beyond solely dopaminergic depletion. Nondopaminergic system involvement is now considered mainstream (Brotchie, 2005).

Manifestations of PD become evident once there is a 70% to 80% loss of the nigral neurons. *Resting tremor,* present in 75% of patients, may present as a unilateral symptom and then spread to bilateral involvement. The tremor resolves with purposeful or voluntary motor movement. It is the most visible feature of PD and often the most cosmetically embarrassing to patients (Chapius, 2002).

Muscular rigidity or stiffness of muscles is evident when the patient's extremities are moved through passive range of motion. *Rigidity,* described as a *cogwheel* phenomenon, is the resistance found on passive flexion and extension. In addition to the extremities, rigidity can also be elicited in the patient's neck and trunk (Chapius, 2002).

Bradykinesia, or slowness of movement, is the most disabling feature of PD. Patients may experience difficulty with initiating movements, such as walking, rising from a chair, or turning in bed. All activities slow to a disabling point.

Postural instability is usually a problem with advancing PD and may predispose the patient to falls. The patient's center of gravity changes, and there is forward flexion of the neck and trunk. The gait is short and shuffling, with diminished arm swing. Postural instability can be evaluated by the pull test, wherein the examiner stands behind the patient and pulls on his or her shoulders. The patient should be able to regain balance, but those with impaired balance may fall backward into the examiner's arms (Chapius, 2002).

MEDICATIONS AS MAINSTAY OF MEDICAL THERAPY

Medications are the mainstay of therapy for the patient with PD. The goal of medication therapy is to maximize functioning and optimize the patient's quality of life. Medications usually are not initiated until the patient experiences difficulty with performing activities of daily living (Chapius, 2002). Other issues that will be factored into the decision to start drug therapy are age, employment, and home responsibilities. Medications that are currently available do not halt or alter disease progression, but offer symptomatic relief.

Factors influencing treatment decisions range markedly from one patient to another, one practitioner to another, and one country to another. Some of the variables include age, symptomatic needs, efficacy of agents, safety profile of drug classes, and empirical experience. The patient's personal, cultural, and socioeconomic resources will also need to be considered (Rascol, Payoux, Ferreira, & Brefel-Courbon, 2002). In general, the medications for PD are quite expensive, especially the newer dopamine agonists. Patients may belong to an insurance drug plan that provides a certain level of benefit for one drug over another, which could influence treatment decisions.

In a newly diagnosed patient with PD, the practitioner will face three decisions to be made, ideally with collaboration from the patient and family: (a) At what point have symptoms necessitated intervention? (b) Which class of medication seems appropriate for this individual? and (c) What other services and nonpharmacological approaches might augment treatment of the PD, such as physical therapy?

The decision to initiate therapy and with which agent will be based on a number of considerations. These factors include age, comorbidities, cognitive status, employment status, disease state, household responsibilities, and general side effects that may interfere with the patient's lifestyle (Tetrud, 2004). Ideally, there will be agreement between the practitioner and patient about when medications will be started. For example, if a patient is involved in a profession such as law, education, or pastoral services, where he or she often interacts with the community, the decision to initiate treatment may occur early. In these situations, the patient wants to be symptom free and avoid embarrassment when visible to the public (Tetrud, 2004). In contrast to this situation, in the retired patient, therapy may be delayed because the patient does not carry the stress of work performance. Likewise, an individual's household responsibilities will also contribute to treatment decisions. A woman who is a homemaker with household responsibilities or the mother of young children may need to be treated early to maximize dexterity and functioning in the home (Tetrud, 2004).

Another very important perspective in initiating therapy is based on long-term therapeutic strategies such as those summarized by S. Fahn (personal communication, August 5, 2006). In the early stage of PD, treatment should focus on medication which (a) slow or eliminate the pathological process and subsequent cell death (b) neuroprotection of the surviving dopaminergic neurons, and (c) symptomatic treatment. Currently there is no pharmacologic approach which is proven to slow or delay the pathological process. Approaches to managing PD should therefore focus on protective and symptomatic treatment. Short-term treatment goals are the alleviation of symptoms and reversal of functional disability. The goal of long-term management is to preserve effectiveness of neurons and minimize pharmacologically induced complications. Treatment will be individualized, and the risks and benefits should be considered by the authorized prescriber when initiating treatment for early PD (Miller, 2002). Patients need to be informed that although there is no known cure for the disease, medication may substantially alleviate symptoms and improve quality of life for a period of time (Tetrud, 2004). Additionally, there are challenges, such as motor fluctuations, that present with advancing disease. Management of these challenges will be addressed later in this chapter.

NEUROPROTECTIVE APPROACHES

The arena of neuron protection has long been controversial but may be used as a therapeutic approach that may modify the course of PD. The first medication that was studied for its neuroprotective qualities was selegiline (Deprenyl), known as a MAO-B inhibitor. Studies of this agent were conducted with the Deprenyl and Tocopherol Antioxidatiave Therapy of Parkinsonism trial. The end point of the study was the time to disability and the need for treatment with levodopa. Patients experienced some symptomatic benefit and had a reduced need for levodopa (Ahlskog, 2000c). Tocopherol was found not to be helpful in slowing down the progression of PD. Ongoing studies have shown evidence that early treatment with selegiline is not beneficial in modifying the long-term course of PD. However, it continues to be a medication of interest because it has shown protection in experimental and animal models of PD (Horn & Stern, 2004). Others continue to believe and prescribe it for its symptomatic benefit.

Another agent, coenzyme Q_{10} (CoQ), has been studied in the early stages of PD as another neuroprotective medication. A pilot study conducted with CoQ suggested that it may slow the rate of decline in disability in early untreated PD. CoQ was studied at doses of 300, 600, and 1,200 mg/day and seemingly showed beneficial effect at 1,200 mg/day (Horn & Stern, 2004). However, in longer term studies by the Neuroprotection Exploratory Trials in Parkinson's Disease (NET-PD) group, CoQ was not robust. Further studies and dosages must be studied.

NET-PD is sponsored by the National Institutes of Neurological Disorders and Stroke, a branch of the National Institutes of Health (NIH). The goal of the NET-PD group is to study agents that have the potential to slow, halt, or arrest the progression of PD. A steering committee, the Committee to Identify Neuroprotective Agents in Parkinson's Disease (CINAPS), worked with scientists, neurologists, neuropathologists, and industry representatives to develop criteria on which compounds would be evaluated. To date, futility studies are ongoing. Essentially, compounds are being evaluated to see if they warrant further study. Compounds from a wide variety of mechanisms are being investigated, including antioxidants, mitochondrial stabilizers, trophic factors, glutamate antagonists, adenosine antagonists, anti-inflammatories, and antiapoptotic agents. As the NET-PD group performs their trials, compounds will be gradually eliminated or added as potential neuroprotective agents in PD.

SYMPTOMATIC THERAPY

Treatment Principles

The discovery of dopamine depletion in the striatum of patients with PD in the late 1960s provided the rationale to use levodopa for PD. Today, levodopa remains the gold standard for treating patients with PD. After some years, a question arose about the negative effect of levodopa on the progression of the disease. This was based on the pathophysiological concept that oxidative stress causes neurodegeneration. Owing to this fact, many physicians became reluctant to prescribe levodopa early and deferred use of the drug. This was an attempt to preserve the remaining neurons. The question of levodopa toxicity remains controversial (Rascol et al., 2002).

Of late, another pathophysiological approach has been proposed about how early PD patients should be managed. The concept is known as continuous dopamine stimulation (CDS). Briefly, preclinical data obtained in six OH-treated rats and MPTP-intoxicated monkeys showed that a parkinsonian brain cannot adequately buffer the peak dopamine concentrations elicited by the intermittent administration of short-acting drugs like oral levodopa. This non-physiological pulsatile dopamine stimulation may induce a cascade of abnormal responses in the basal ganglia: dysregulation of striatal dopamine and nondopamine receptors; abnormal intracellular signaling of striatal neurons; abnormal output of the basal ganglia motor loop; and finally, abnormal motor behaviors like the on–off phenomenon and dyskinesias (Rascol et al., 2002).

In consideration of this concept, when patients warrant dopaminergic therapy, practitioners are encouraged to prescribe the most CDS to promote smooth, nonpulsatile delivery. Avoiding the pulsatile, high peak levels of short-acting levodopa will decrease the risk and severity of the long-term motor complications of dyskinesias as the PD progresses. Drugs that may be prescribed to achieve CDS are levodopa/carbidopa-controlled release formulation, COMT inhibitors, and dopamine agonists (Rascol et al., 2002).

Initiation of Therapy

Initial medications for patients include MAO-B inhibitors, amantadine, and anticholinergics. Another option is a dopamine agonist. A combination of the above may be tried. If the desired response is not observed, sustained release carbidopa/levodopa, or carbidopa/levodopa with a COMT inhibitor, should be added. Additionally, adjuvant therapy with amantadine or anticholinergics may be started (Miller, 2002). If, however, the patient is an elderly person with multiple comorbidities and a shortened life span, often, these initial medications are not the optimal choices, and these patients are candidates to go directly to carbidopa/levodopa therapy. As the disease advances, patients will undoubtedly need carbidopa/levodopa coupled with an agonist and often the subtle benefit offered by the addition or continued use of anticholinergics, amantadine, or MAO-B inhibitors. From this overview of medication therapy, each class of medication will now be explored.

DISCUSSION OF SPECIFIC AGENTS IN SYMPTOMATIC THERAPY

Monoamine Oxidase–B Inhibitors

In the brain, liver, and other regions of the body, the enzyme MAO metabolizes chemicals known as amines. Important amines in psychopharmacology include the indolamine neurotransmitter serotonin (5-HT), the catecholamine neurotransmitter norepinephrine (NE), and dopamine (DA). MAO occurs in the body as two subtypes, referred to as MAO-A and MAO-B. MAO-A is primarily located in the gut, liver, and brain. MAO-B is predominately found in the brain. MAO-A is responsible for the metabolism of 5-HT, NE, and epinephrine. DA is metabolized by both MAO-A and MAO-B (Howland, 2006).

MAO-B works in the brain to degrade dopamine. Therefore inhibiting MAO-B is a therapeutic approach for patients with PD. Selegiline (Deprenyl) was the first U.S. Food and Drug Administration (FDA)-approved MAO-B inhibitor. Rasalagiline (Azilect) and selegiline orally disintegrating (Zelepar) came onto the market in 2006. The action of MAO-B inhibitors is to block one of the dopamine degradative pathways, thus inhibiting the B form of monoamine oxidase. This medication does not require special dietary restrictions on red wine and aged cheese like other MAO-A inhibitors if the maximal dose is not exceeded. Above recommended dosages, MAO-B inhibitors may lose their specificity for B inhibition. It should be stressed that patients receiving selegiline should not be given meperidine because of the potential for severe interactions resulting in symptoms of fever, agitation, and fluctuating blood pressure (Ahlskog, 2000b). MAO-B inhibition of platelets takes 5–7 days to reverse. It is not clear how long reversal takes in the brain. To avoid any interactions, it is suggested that selegiline be stopped 10–14 days prior to surgery to avoid this possible interaction. This may also be true of the newer MAO-B inhibitors.

Anticholinergics

Anticholinergic agents such as trihexyphendyl (Artane) and benztropine (Cogentin) reduce tremor, rigidity, and dystonia but are particularly helpful with tremor in early disease. In early tremor-predominant disease, anticholinergics can offer symptomatic relief, especially on a pro re nata basis for the busy professional or socialite. These medications have side effects such as dry mouth, impaired memory, blurred vision, urinary retention, and constipation, especially at high doses (Ahlskog, 2000b). Anticholinergics reestablish motor function by blocking muscarinic cholinergic receptors within the striatum. They are helpful in patients who have tremor as a predominant symptom but do not help considerably with the management of other motor features of PD, such as bradykinesia and shuffling gait. They should be used with caution in the elderly due to their ability to cause cognitive impairment. Adverse effects of these drugs may limit their usefulness, especially in the elderly (Miller, 2002).

Amantadine

Amantadine (Symmetrel) is a medication that has been traditionally classified as a dopaminergic but more correctly is a glutamate antagonist. Patients with early PD obtain symptomatic benefit from this drug and may be maintained for months or a few years with this monotherapy. In advanced, fluctuating disease, amantadine helps smooth out the carbidopa/levodopa response and appears to decrease dyskinesias (Adler, Stern, Vernon, & Hurtig, 1997). Evidence suggests that this drug blocks the N-methyl-D-aspartate subtype of glutamate receptor in the brain. Side effects include swelling of the legs and livedo reticularis, which is a reddish purple fishnet mottling of the skin on the legs (Ahlskog, 2000a). Women may find the appearance of livedo reticularis on their lower extremities cosmetically embarrassing.

Dopamine Agonists

Initially, these medications were prescribed as an adjuvant therapy for patients with advancing PD. In the past 10 years they have been found to be helpful early in the disease and are often used as monotherapy in initial treatment. In fact, for many patients, the dopamine agonist would be considered standard of care choice of medication to introduce in early disease when symptoms warrant treatment. Dopamine agonists are medications that replicate the action of dopamine in the brain. They directly stimulate postsynaptic dopamine receptor sites. Patients may benefit from the use of dopamine agonists for a number of years. Use of dopamine agonists rarely results in the development of dyskinesia, which is an abnormal writhing movement that a patient may experience when taking levodopa (Samii, Nutt, & Ransom, 2004).

Patients may be on a dopamine agonist as monotherapy for as long as the motor symptoms can be controlled. The agonist is introduced at a very low dose and is slowly increased to minimize side effects. As a monotherapy, dopamine agonists will be titrated to the higher end of the dosage range. Medications in this class include bromocriptine (Parlodel; seldom used any longer), pergolide (Permax), pramipexole (Mirapex), and ropinirole (Requip), (Ahlskog, 2000b). Bromocriptine and pergolide, older dopamine agonists, are ergot derivatives. Recent studies have demonstrated an increase risk of valvular heart disease in patients being treated with ergot-derived dopamine receptor agonists. Researchers conclude that

"The frequency of clinically important valve regurgitation was significantly increased in patients taking pergolide or cabergoline, but not in patients taking non-ergot-derived dopamine agonists, as compared with controls" (Zanettini, Antonini, Gatto, Gentile, Tesei, Pezzoli, 2007, p.39). On March 29, 2007 the US Food and Drug Administration announced that pergolide (Permax) was voluntarily withdrawn from the US market related to the risk of developing heart valve damage and regurgitation. Pergolide will be slowly taken off the US market to provide health care providers an opportunity to switch patients from pergolide to nonergot dopamine agonist, such as pramipexole or ropinirole. Parkinson's disease patients should not abruptly stop taking pergolide, but should gradually decrease their pergolide dose, under the direction of a health care provider (US Food and Drug Administration, 2007a,b).

Patients should be cautioned about the side effects that are seen with the use of dopamine agonists. These include nausea, hypotension, leg edema, vivid dreams, hallucinations, somnolence, and sleep attacks (Samii et al., 2004). Recent attention has focused on agonists and compulsive behaviors like gambling. The medication pramipexole was recently associated with potentially reversible pathological gambling (Dodd et al., 2005).

Levodopa

Levodopa remains the mainstay of medication management for patients with PD. Although neuroscientists are beginning to appreciate PD as a complex neurophysiological disorder, for many decades a deficiency of dopamine had been considered the sole underlying problem contributing to the motor features. Treatment with levodopa targets the reversal of this dopamine deficiency. Levodopa is generally prescribed as an initial treatment for the patient over 70 years of age and is used in others when there is significant impairment of the ability to perform activities of occupational or daily living (Ahlskog, 2000b).

Levodopa is available in a variety of formulations as a combination tablet of carbidopa/levodopa (Sinemet). Initially, when levodopa therapy was introduced in the 1960s, patients often experienced nausea and vomiting, which limited therapy. When levodopa is administered, it is converted to dopamine in the periphery, and only small amounts are available for transport into the central nervous system. This necessitates large doses in order to achieve a therapeutic response. Because the peripheral dopamine is responsible for the majority of adverse effects, namely nausea, vomiting, and orthostatic hypotension, these increased doses make side effects worse. Carbidopa, a peripheral inhibitor of dopa decarboxylase, prevents breakdown of levodopa in the periphery, therefore increasing the amount of unmetabolized drug that is available to cross the blood–brain barrier (Ahlskog, 2000b). In this process the peripheral side effects of nausea and vomiting are minimized or eliminated for most patients.

Formulations of carbidopa and levodopa include an immediate release tablet of 10/100, 25/100, 25/250. The numerator reflects the milligrams of carbidopa in the tablet, while the denominator indicates the milligrams of levodopa. Patients will require between 75 and 150 mg/day of carbidopa to block the peripheral breakdown of the levodopa. Patients may require up to 1,000 mg/day of levodopa in divided dosages. There are some patients with PD who require doses in excess of 1,000 mg/day; however, in general, for those who do not respond to high doses of levodopa (greater than 1,000 mg), careful assessment for an atypical parkinsonism should be considered (Olanow, Watts, & Koller, 2001).

Carbidopa/levodopa is also manufactured as a controlled release (CR) formulation of 25/100 and 50/200 tablets. For many, this formulation provides a more even response of continuous dopamine stimulation. These tablets may not be crushed for administration as it breaks the matrix that allows the slow release of the drug. When the immediate release formula is utilized, patients often feel that the medication is working within 30 min of administration. The immediate release carbidopa/levodopa peaks not only faster, but at a higher level. However, it also does not last as long. With the CR formulation, there is often a delayed onset of action and a lower peak. Patients often note this most profoundly in the morning response. With a lower peak effect, patients may complain of a lack of the same dramatic improvement of motor symptoms compared to the immediate release. The provider may prescribe a daily combination of immediate and CR tablets (Ahlskog, 2000a). CR carbidopa/levodopa is useful when administered at the hour of sleep because it has a longer duration of action.

Side effects of carbidopa/levodopa include nausea, dyskinesia, orthostatic hypotension, and hallucinations. Most patients started on carbidopa/levodopa do not experience nausea. If it does occur, it usually resolves as the medication continues. Pharmacists may instruct patients to take the medication with food to avoid nausea. Patients taking the immediate release formulation usually achieve the best response when taking it on an empty stomach as food may decrease the peak serum concentrations, but not total absorption. In addition, the amino acids of dietary protein can compete for the uptake of the levodopa. A meal high in protein can reduce levodopa absorption and limit its crossing the blood–brain barrier (Samii et al., 2004). For these reasons it is important to take caribdopa/levodopa consistently with regard to meals.

Dyskinesia, an abnormal involuntary movement, can appear in advanced disease after administration of carbidopa/levodopa. It reflects an effect of excessive levodopa and hypersensitized neurons. There are many dosing strategies that can be employed, such as lower doses taken more frequently, to ameliorate this effect (Ahlskog, 2000a). The next section of this chapter will deal with challenges of treating advancing disease.

CHALLENGES OF TREATING MOTOR FLUCTUATIONS WITH ADVANCING DISEASE

As PD advances, challenges develop in the management of the disease. Patients may not have an optimal response to tablets of carbidopa/levodopa. Therapeutic challenges arise in establishing a smooth response to the medication, maximizing mobility, and minimizing side effects. Motor fluctuations often occur after 5 years of therapy with carbidopa/levodopa. They include (a) freezing, (b) the on–off phenomenon, and (c) peak-dose dyskinesia with end-of-dose failure (Samii et al., 2004).

Freezing episodes are characterized by periods of unpredictable immobility, where the patient's feet are actually stuck to the floor. These are brief, transient, and often situational. For example, freezing often occurs in tight spaces, such as bathrooms, or when crossing thresholds, such as coming out of elevators. With the on–off phenomenon, patients experience sudden switches between periods of mobility to sudden immobility. Most on–off phenomena can be tracked to a wearing off or end-of-dose pattern. However, random on–off phenomena can occur. Patients with peak-dose dyskinesia may experience mild movements to wild flailing movements of the extremities, followed by a wearing off of levodopa (Ahlskog, 2000a).

There are several medication management strategies that may be employed for the patient with advancing PD. One of the first adjustments can be to increase the overall daily dosage of carbidopa/levodopa. If this results in the development or worsening of dyskinesia, a second approach is to decrease the amount of time between each dose of the carbidopa/

levodopa tablet. Additional daily dosages can help to provide coverage of the symptoms. This may be an appropriate time to initiate use of the CR carbidopa/levodopa if it has not been previously used.

Another approach is to add one of the dopamine agonists to the medication schedule. Selection of a medication such as pramipexole or ropinirole will help to smooth out the motor fluctuations in the patient who is only responding to carbidopa/levodopa for a short period of time. Initially, the dopamine agonist will be administered in low doses and slowly titrated to effect over several weeks. As the daily dosage of the dopamine agonist is increased, it may be necessary to reduce the total daily dose of carbidopa/levodopa to avoid adverse effects and dyskinesias (Ahlskog, 2000a).

In recent years, another class of medications called COMT inhibitors has come to market. The agents currently available are tolcapone (Tasmar) and entacapone (Comtan). COMT is a dopamine degradative enzyme. The inhibition of this enzyme will increase the potency of levodopa. Therefore any side effects of levodopa the patient may experience, including an increase in dyskinesias, can occur, and the overall drug dosage may need to be adjusted. The patient on tolcapone will also need to have liver functions monitored on a regular basis due to the potential for fatal fulminant liver failure. The other COMT inhibitor, entacapone, has not been shown to cause liver failure, but diarrhea and urine discoloration are common adverse effects (Ahlskog, 2000a).

In addition to being used early in the treatment of PD, amantadine decreases levodopa-induced dyskinesias in advanced PD. Amantadine is a glutamate antagonist, and recent studies show that enhanced stimulation of striatal glutamate receptors contributes to the development of levodopa-induced dyskinesias (Brotchie, 2005). When given in advanced disease at 100–200 mg/day, amantadine adds a subtle antiparkinson effect and diminishes disabling dyskinesias (Adler et al., 1997).

New Medication Formulations

Presently, a new formulation of carbidopa/levodopa has been introduced with entacapone. This medication is known as Stalevo and is associated with a lower risk of motor complications in PD (Schapira, 2005). This allows one dose of medication to be given in place of two separate medications. The levodopa will manage the symptoms of PD, while entacapone will extend the time that levodopa is active in the brain and help avoid the pulsatile dopamine stimulation of carbidopa/levodopa when given alone. In essence, this is an attempt to accomplish CDS.

Another formulation that is now available is a rapidly disintegrating tablet of carbidopa/levodopa known as Parcopa. This medication can be taken without water and rapidly disintegrates in the patient's mouth. It is convenient because it can be kept on the bedside table for the patient to take on awakening in the morning. It will assist the patient with getting started for the day. Another advantage is that the patient may feel less self-conscious about taking medications when out in public. It may also be ordered when a patient's status is nothing by mouth (NPO) prior to a test or procedures and in advanced disease patients who have dysphagia. In general, this formulation is helpful in some patients because it is convenient, easy to use, and provides rapid access to medication (Nausieda et al., 2005).

Apomorphine (APOKYN) is an injectable dopamine agonist that was approved in 2004 by the FDA as a rescue medication for PD patients who experience unpredictable off episodes or hypomobility. Apomorphine is used as an adjunct to prescribed oral PD medications, not as a replacement. Initiation of treatment with apomorphine requires close nursing assessment and antiemetic prophylaxis.

Apomorphine is given by subcutaneous injection into the abdomen, arms, or thighs with an autoinjector pen device that holds several doses of apomorphine, making as-needed injections readily available. The pen device uses a 29-gauge, one-half-inch needle, much like the insulin delivery systems. Thoughtful nursing education is required to provide the patient and caregiver with information on action of medication, indication for use, aseptic technique, subcutaneous injection technique, and side effects. Common side effects include nausea, vomiting, sedation, dyskinesias, dizziness, hallucinations, and depression (Mylan Bertek Pharmaceuticals, Inc., 2005). Patients should be informed about drowsiness and should be discouraged from driving or engaging in other potentially hazardous activities until the patient knows how he or she tolerates the apomorphine dose. Yawning is commonly seen before the onset of the apomorphine effect and should not be misinterpreted as the onset of drowsiness (Chen & Obering, 2005). Yawning is an indication that the PD patient is moving from the off to the on state.

At the time of the initial dosing and educational session the patient or caregiver will administer the apomorphine injection as a return demonstration, and the nurse will monitor orthostatic blood pressure for signs of hypotension. Three days prior to the initial administration of apomorphine, the patient should be prescribed trimethobenzamide (Tigan) to prevent nausea and vomiting. Trimethobenzamide is usually continued for 2 months after the first dose of apomorphine and then discontinued. Apomorphine peak plasma levels are reached within 5–15 min and cerebrospinal peak concentrations within 15–25 min. The benefit of increased mobility from apomorphine injection ranges from 30 to 90 min (Chen & Obering, 2005).

PD Medications and Pregnancy

Although many individuals diagnosed with PD are over the age of 60, there is a subset of younger people with PD. Life issues for the younger age group differ from those near retirement age. One of the concerns for the younger patient is reproduction. Pregnancy in patients with PD is rare, and reports from retrospective analysis suggest that pregnancy may have a deleterious effect on PD (Shulman, Minagar, & Weiner, 2000). Currently, there is limited research data available on the topic of pregnancy in PD, with most of the literature describing individual case reports.

One article cites that the use of amantadine during the first trimester of pregnancy was associated with obstetrical complications, including miscarriage (Golbe, 1987). Shulman et al. (2000) provided a report about a 33-year-old woman during the prepartum, intrapartum, and postpartum periods. She was followed by a neurologist for her PD prior to becoming pregnant. She received carbidopa/levodopa during her pregnancy. She delivered a normal, full-term infant. The patient experienced a worsening of motor symptoms during pregnancy, during which time her dose of levodopa was increased. This patient's motor symptoms did not return to her prepregnancy state within 15 months after giving birth. From this experience the authors concluded that pregnancy may exacerbate the illness and have a long-term negative impact on PD.

In an article by Chen and Obering (2005) it is cited that apomorphine has not been evaluated during pregnancy or lactation. It further states that the drug should not be used in pregnant or nursing women unless there is a clear need.

At this time, there is limited research on the safety of anti-PD medications for the pregnant woman or fetus. All common classes of anti-PD medications are FDA classified as category C. This means that the drugs should only be given if the potential benefit justifies the potential risk to the fetus or that no controlled trials in women have been done.

NURSING CONSIDERATIONS WHEN ADMINISTERING MEDICATIONS

Patients with PD will be encountered in a variety of health care settings, such as acute care, long-term care, rehabilitation, and home care. On entry into the health care system, an accurate history of all PD medications should be obtained, along with any alternative or complementary medications the patient is taking. The medication regimen that patients follow should be adhered to as closely as possible when they are admitted to an inpatient setting. Many of the medications are titrated to maximize the patient's functional effect, and deviations can result in periods of extreme immobility. Often, patients are meticulous about their medication schedules and will enlist assistance of the nurse to receive the medication in a timely manner. When medication doses are missed or late, the patient may experience painful dystonia, shortness of breath, panic, or anxiety. Additionally, discontinuation of the medications will result in immobility, which increases the risk of aspiration and deep vein thrombosis. Neuroleptic malignant syndrome, frequently fatal, has been reported due to sudden cessation of anti-PD medications and is described in detail below.

A medication reference table has been compiled that names the class of medication, typical dosage, indications for use, and common side effects (Table 3.1). It is important for the nurse to be knowledgeable about these medications and alert to side effects since many patients receive polypharmacy.

Currently, new electronic order entry and medication administration systems are being used in most health care facilities. These systems may be a detriment for the person with PD. For example, if a medication is ordered 4 times a day, there will be a default to the standard administration times, which could be 10 a.m., 2 p.m., 6 p.m., and 10 p.m. This schedule could dramatically impact a PD patient's performance of activities of daily living in the morning. Nurses need to be advocates and collaborate with the patient, ordering physicians and pharmacists to assure that there are mechanisms to allow for deviation on set computer default administration times.

TABLE 3.1 Medications for Parkinson's Disease

Drug Classification	Typical Daily Dose*	Indications for Use	Side Effects
Anticholinergics			
Trihexyphenidyl (Artane®)	1 mg two times a day to 2 mg three times a day	Tremor Rigidity Drooling	Impaired memory, dry mouth, constipation, blurred vision, urinary retention, mental confusion
Benztropine (Cogentin®)	1 – 2 mg two times a day		
Glutamate antagonist			
Amantadine (Symmetrel®) (Note: Formerly classified as a dopaminergic; may be reclassified as a glutamate antagonist)	100 mg two times a day	Tremor Rigidity Bradykinesia Dyskinesias in advanced disease	Leg edema, dizziness, insomnia, nervousness, livedo reticularis, hallucinations, mental confusion
Dopaminergics			
Carbidopa/levodopa (Sinemet®) Immediate release 10/100, 25/100, or 25/250 tablets	One 25/100 tablet three to four times a day	Tremor Rigidity Bradykinesia (Also is helpful in treating nonmotor symptoms, such as, drooling and pain)	Initial therapy: Anorexia, nausea, vomiting, hypotension. Long term therapy: Motor fluctuations, dyskinesias, mental confusion, hallucinations
Carbidopa/levodopa (Sinemet®) Controlled release 25/100 or 50/200 tablets	One 50/200 tablet three times a day *Note: Sinemet CR should not be chewed or crushed but can be broken in half*		

TABLE 3.1 Medications for Parkinson's Disease *(continued)*

Drug Classification	Typical Daily Dose*	Indications for Use	Side Effects
Carbidopa/levodopa (Parcopa®) 10/100, 25/100, or 25/250 tablets [Orally disintegrating]	One 25/100 tablet three times a day	Tremor Rigidity Bradykinesia	Hypotension, nausea, mental confusion, dry mouth, dyskinesia, and dizziness
Carbidopa/levodopa/ entacapone			
Stalevo® 50 (12.5/50/200 mg) Stalevo® 100 (25/100/200 mg) Stalevo® 150 (37.5/150/200 mg)	One 25/100/200 tablet three times a day	Motor symptoms of PD, and attempts to provide continuous dopamine stimulation	Abdominal pain, diarrhea, nausea, mental confusion, brownish-orange urine
Note: Tablets contain # mg carbidopa /# mg levodopa/ 200 mg entacapone each			
First Generation Dopamine Agonists			
Bromocriptine (Parlodel®) Note: bromocriptine is not currently recommended for treatment of PD	5 mg three times a day to 10 mg three times a day	Motor fluctuations in Parkinson's disease (wearing off, dyskinesias, dystonia)	Hallucinations, mental confusion, orthostatic hypotension, nausea, cardiac valvular dysfunction
Pergolide (Permax®) Note: FDA voluntarily withdraws from U.S. markets March 29, 2007	1 mg three times a day	Motor symptoms of PD. Can be used as initial therapy or in combination with levodopa	Orthostatic hypotension, mental confusion, nausea, dyskinesia, cardiac valvular dysfunction

Second Generation Dopamine Agonists

	Dose	Use	Side Effects
Pramipexole (Mirapex®)	0.5 - 1.5 mg three times a day	Monotherapy in early Parkinson's disease; added to L-dopa in patients who are not well controlled and/or have motor fluctuations	Nausea, vomiting, hypotension, ankle edema, daytime sleepiness, compulsive behavior, mental confusion, hallucinations
Ropinerole (Requip®)	3 – 8 mg three times a day	Monotherapy in early Parkinson's disease; added to L-dopa in patients who are not well controlled and/or have motor fluctuations	Nausea, vomiting, hypotension, ankle edema, daytime sleepiness, compulsive behavior, mental confusion, hallucinations
Apomorphine (Apokyn®) Note: Apokin dose: 1 mg = 0.1 ml	5.4 mg subcutaneous injection two to three times a day	Rescue drug for episodes of hypomobility and sudden *off* symptoms	Reaction at injection site, nausea, vomiting, orthostatic hypotension, yawning, drowsiness
COMT Inhibitors (Note: Must be given with carbidopa/levodopa, no independent action)			**See full prescribing information for tasmar.**
Tocapone (Tasmar®) [Hepatotoxicity has limited prescriptive use]	100–200 mg three times a day	Decrease motor fluctuations. Supplement to L-dopa in the treatment of PD.	Dyskinesia, nauseas, vomiting, sleep disorder, excessive dreaming, anorexia, orthostatic hypotension, mental confusion, diarrhea, urine discoloration, **fatal hepatic failure** (requires liver monitoring)

(continued)

TABLE 3.1 Medications for Parkinson's Disease *(Continued)*

Drug Classification	Typical Daily Dose*	Indications for Use	Side Effects
Entacapone (Comtan®)	200 mg with each dose of carbidopa/levodopa, not to exceed 6 doses per day	Decrease motor fluctuations. Supplement to L-dopa in the treatment of PD.	Nausea, vomiting, ortho-static hypotension, excessive dreaming, anorexia, mental confusion, diarrhea, brownish-orange urine discoloration
MAO Inhibitor (Type B)			
Selegeline hydrochloride (Eldepryl®)	5 mg one or two times a day	Newly diagnosed PD, motor fluctuations in PD and ad-junct to carbidopa/levodopa	Abdominal pain, dry mouth, nausea, dizziness, mental confusion, visual hallucinations worsening dyskinesias
Selegeline hydrochloride (Zelapar®) [Orally disintegrat-ing tablet]	1.25 mg sublingual tablet two times a day		
Rasagiline (Azilect®)	0.5 mg two times a day	Monotherapy for early Parkin-son's disease and as adjunc-tive therapy later in disease	Orthostatic hypotension, rash, weight loss, constipation, ataxia, depression, bundle branch block, GI hemorrhage

* **Typical Daily Dose** reflects the average prescription dose for the treatment of PD symptoms. However, doses may be higher or lower depending on patient response to medications, severity of disease, and types of symptoms targeted for treatment.

* Adapted from: Micromedex HealthCare Series: DRUGDEX Drug Point Summary (online reference)

* http://www.thomsonhc.com/hcs/librarian

Nutt, J. & Wooten, F. (2005). Diagnosis and initial management of Parkinson's disease. *The New England Journal of Medicine, 353* (10), 1021-1027.

Dewey, R., Hutton, J., LeWitt, P., & Factor, S. (2001). A randomized, double-blind, placebo-controlled trial of subcutaneously injected apomorphine for parkinsonian off-state events. *Archives of Neurology, 58*(9), 1385-1392.

Admission to the hospital can also present special challenges to obtaining necessary medications. All medications may not be stocked through the hospital pharmacy system, called the *hospital formulary*. Patients should be encouraged to take medications with them to the hospital in the event they need to be given medications from their personal supply. Patients are carefully titrated on their medications, and this balance should not be interrupted during a hospitalization.

The patient with PD who is undergoing a diagnostic test or surgery also presents special challenges. It is helpful to confer with the physician ordering the test and with the anesthesiologist to see if the patient may take his or her antiparkinson medications with a small sip of water. Parcopa is an option for the patient on carbidopa/levodopa because it can be taken without water. With postoperative orders, medications such as metoclopramide (Reglan) and prochlorperazine (Compazine) should be avoided because they are dopamine-blocking agents and therefore will worsen PD. Other antiemetics, such as ondansetron (Zofran), could be utilized (Doyle & Kremer, 2003). Additionally, haloperidol (Haldol), often prescribed for agitation, should be avoided due to its dopamine-blocking qualities. Following surgery, as the patient moves from intensive care to the inpatient unit and then rehabilitation, medication reconciliation needs to be accomplished at each level of care so that no medication is overlooked.

Neuroleptic malignant syndrome (NMS) is a potentially life-threatening condition that can develop in the patient with PD if long-term dopaminergic medications are suddenly discontinued or moderately reduced. Clinical signs of NMS include autonomic dysfunction, namely hyperthermia, tachycardia, tachypnea, and diaphoresis; a change in level of consciousness; and hypertension or hypotension. Rigidity, leukocytosis, tremors, and elevation of serum creatinine kinase are also noted. Rhabdomyolysis, an acute fulminating and potentially lethal disease of skeletal muscles that damages muscle tissue, is a serious complication of NMS. One account in the literature described a patient with PD who developed NMS one month after receiving a deep brain stimulator implant. He presented to the hospital with fever, diminished mental status, rigidity, and stiffness. A review of his record indicated that in his postoperative course, after the implant was turned on, the patient's carbidopa/levodopa was reduced, and selegiline was stopped (Ward, 2005). Another case of severe NMS involved a patient with PD who fell and could not reach her medications for 48 hours. This resulted in a head injury, NMS, and prolonged coma. The outcome at this point is uncertain (G. M. Vernon, personal communication, September 30, 2006).

The nurse is in the unique position to recognize that NMS is a potential complication that can develop with the withdrawal of dopaminergic agents. The condition poses a considerable risk of mortality to the patient. Nurses need to be knowledgeable about the cause and symptoms because even a moderate withdrawal of dopaminergic medication in a patient with PD may result in NMS (Ward, 2005).

Medication Administration Challenges in Advancing Disease

As the disease advances, patients with PD may require a nasogastric tube or a permanent tube, such as a percutaneous esophageal gastrostomy or a percutaneous esophageal gastrostomy (PEG)/jeujunostomy tube. If the medication is not available in a liquid form (like amantadine), a tablet may be crushed only after consulting a pharmacist or clinical reference to see if the medication may be crushed. For example, the CR formulation of carbidopa/levodopa may not be crushed.

Management challenges will also arise as the patient crosses care settings in the hospital. Carbidopa/levodopa formulations and dopamine agonists are not available as an IV, IM, or rectal suppository formulation. Diphenhydramine (Benedryl) and benztropine (Cogentin) are available for IV or IM injection. Rotigotine, a dopamine agonist, is being explored currently for delivery in a transdermal patch delivery system. Zelapar and Parcopa are available as sublingual tablets, offering an advantage to the patient who is NPO or has dysphagia. Table 3.1 lists currently available medications, and Table 3.2 lists drugs close to market.

Considerations of Medication Administration in the Elderly

The patient who is over 60 years of age may be receiving medications for other complex comorbidities. Owing to this fact, there needs to be a careful balance of monitoring the patient for side effects and drug interactions. In many instances with polypharmacy, it may be difficult to detect which

TABLE 3.2 Medications for Parkinson's Disease Under Development (Near Market)

L-dopa

  Duodopa (Solvay Pharmaceuticals)

    Available in Sweden since 2004

    Infused via PEG for advanced, fluctuating PD

    Side effect profile that of carbidopa/levodopa

    Attempts to provide continous dopamine stimulation (CDS)

Dopamine agonist

  Rotigotine (Neupro) (Swartz Pharma)

    Transdermal patch delivery system

    8–12 mg/day

    Used in early disease as monotherapy and advanced
      fluctutating disease

    Side effect profile similar to other agonist, plus patch site reactions,
      nausea, somnolence, and dizziness

Adenosine A (2a) antagonist

  Istradefylline

    Appears to increase on time in advanced fluctuating PD patients

    Has been studied in early PD

    Dosage range 20–60 mg/daily

On the horizon: Glutamate antagonists

medication is causing the adverse effect. The elderly are more sensitive to side effects of orthostasis, psychosis, and constipation. Renal compromise in the older adult may also impact clearance of the medication. Finally, financial constraints can pose challenges when patients are taking multiple medications, which may be costly. The cost of some medications may be prohibitive for a patient on a fixed retirement income. Prescribing generic medications and referring patients to resources such as mail-order pharmacies, state pharmacy assistance plans, or the Veterans Administration (if appropriate) may help with cost containment. Nurses are in the position to act as a patient advocate when new medications are tried. After a sufficient interval, if the patient is not demonstrating benefit from the drug, the nurse should collaborate with the prescriber and recommend that unnecessary drugs be discontinued.

PATIENT EDUCATION AND ADHERENCE STRATEGIES

Strategies need to be employed to promote adherence to medication. Adherence is a concept that recognizes the autonomy of the patient and requires his or her agreement to follow instructions given by the prescriber. In populations where there are multiple morbidities, like the elderly, nonadherence can result in poor disease control and impaired quality of life. Medication adherence problems account for up to 69% of medication-related hospitalizations per year at a cost of $100,000,000 (McDonnell & Jacobs, 2002). The practice of taking medications is one of the most intriguing and complex behaviors demonstrated by patients. Administration schedules should be simplified so that several medications may be taken at one time. Unnecessary medications should be eliminated. Assistive devices, such as pillboxes, alarm watches, or personal assistive devices, all play a role in medication adherence (Hughes, 2004). Patients should be encouraged to carry doses of medication with them when they leave home, along with a water bottle.

Patients and caregivers require education about the disease process and the actions of the medications. Sessions should be planned so that patients and caregivers are instructed on (a) names of medications, (b) times and doses, (c) side effects, (d) basic understanding of how medications should be administered, and (e) possible interactions between PD medications and commonly taken supplements or over-the-counter medications (O'Maley, O'Sullivan, Wollin, Barras, & Brammer, 2005).

Multiple teaching sessions may need to be arranged. Verbal instructions can be reinforced with written materials (O'Maley et al., 2005). Patients need to be able to differentiate between side effects of the medications, such as dyskinesias, and effects of the disease, such as tremor. Patients should be encouraged to communicate openly with their health care providers so that medications can be titrated to maximize mobility. They should be discouraged from making changes independently. It may be suggested that the patient keep a diary of daily on times to reflect total hours per day of good-quality mobility. This may range from a simple paper and pencil record to a more elaborate spreadsheet reflecting hourly fluctuations in functional mobility. With a provider's guidance a simple diary can be devised to chart fluctuations and response to medications. Guidance should be given about missed doses of medications.

A multidisciplinary approach to disease management at specialty centers can assist the nurse in patient education. Pharmacists, social workers, case workers, and physical and occupational therapists all contribute to the goal of optimal patient functioning. Additionally, patients and families can be referred to national organizations such as the American Parkinson Disease Association (APDA) or the National Parkinson Foundation (NPF) for online and written materials. These national organizations also sponsor regional and national patient education meetings. Finally, referral to local support groups so that patients and families can learn from each other in managing the disease can be invaluable. Strategies for disease management and coping can be shared by individuals who are newly diagnosed as well as individuals who are further along in the course of the disease.

Important to note is that nurses play a vital role in educating patients that the goal of treatment is to promote independent function and mobility, not to eliminate all signs and symptoms of the disease (Miller, 2002). PD is a chronic condition requiring ongoing attention. Motor symptoms change, and medications must be changed. Patients should be instructed to always carry an accurate, up-to-date list of their medications at all times, which should include any complementary or alternative medications that they are taking. This list should contain current doses and times medications are taken as PD drugs are frequently adjusted for optimal effect. A complete medication list is helpful as the patient sees other health care consultants or has to be suddenly hospitalized.

SUMMARY

As a mainstay of therapy for PD, medications play a vital role in ameliorating the signs and symptoms of the disease and thereby maximizing the patient's daily functional independence. New symptomatic treatments for PD have improved the range of drug therapies available to manage the patient. Strides are being gained in new delivery systems. Research in neuroprotection and new receptor targets are ongoing as we write this book. Nurses in all settings along the care continuum are integral members of the multidisciplinary team and those often working closest with patients and their medications. When caring for patients with PD, nurses require a strong foundation in understanding the pharmacology used in disease management and the complex multidrug regimens and meticulous schedules needed for optimal management. Working together with patients and their health care team, therapy can be properly monitored, and response to therapy can be optimized.

REFERENCES

Adler, C. A., Stern, M. B., Vernon, G. M., & Hurtig, H. I. (1997). Amantadine in advanced Parkinson's disease: Good use of an old drug. *Journal of Neurology, 244,* 336–337.

Ahlskog, J. E. (2000a). Advancing Parkinson's disease and treatment of motor complications. In C. H. Adler & J. E. Ahlskog (Eds.), *Parkinson's disease and movement disorders* (pp. 129–149). Totowa, NJ: Humana Press.

Ahlskog, J. E. (2000b). Initial symptomatic treatment of Parkinson's disease. In C. H. Adler & J. E. Ahlskog (Eds.), *Parkinson's disease and movement disorders* (pp. 115–128). Totowa, NJ: Humana Press.

Ahlskog, J. E. (2000c). Medication strategies for slowing the progression of Parkinson's disease. In C. H. Adler & J. E. Ahlskog (Eds.), *Parkinson's disease and movement disorders* (pp. 101–114). Totowa, NJ: Humana Press.

Brotchie, J. M. (2005). Nondopaminergic mechanisms in levodopa-induced dyskinesia. *Movement Disorders, 20,* 919–931.

Chapius, T. (2002). Parkinson's disease manifestations and management. *Clinician Reviews, 12,* 62–69.

Chen, J. J., & Obering, C. (2005). A review of intermittent subcutaneous apomorphine injections for the rescue management of motor fluctuations associated with advanced Parkinson's disease. *Clinical Therapeutics, 27,* 1710–1724.

Dodd, M., Klos, K., Bower, J., Geda, Y., Josephs, K., & Ahlskog, J. E. (2005). Pathological gambling caused by drugs used to treat Parkinson disease. *Archives of Neurology, 62,* 1–5.

Doyle, S. R., & Kremer, M. J. (2003). Update for nurse anesthetists: Parkinson disease. *AANA Journal, 71,* 229–234.

Golbe, L. I. (1987). Parkinson's disease and pregnancy. *Neurology, 37,* 1245–1249.

Horn, S., & Stern, M. B. (2004). The comparative effects of medical therapies for Parkinson's disease. *Neurology, 63*(Supplement. 2), 7–12.

Howland, R. H. (2006). MAOI antidepressant drugs. *Journal of Psychosocial Nursing, 44,* 9–12.

Hughes, C. M. (2004). Medication non-adherence in the elderly: How big is the problem? *Drugs and Aging, 21,* 793–811.

McDonnell, P. J., & Jacobs, M. R. (2002). Hospital admissions resulting from preventable adverse reactions. *Annals of Pharmacotherapy, 36,* 1331–1336.

Miller, J. L. (2002). Parkinson's disease primer. *Geriatric Nursing, 23,* 69–75.

Mylan Bertek Pharmaceuticals, Inc. (2005). *All about APOKYN: Why to use it and what to expect* [Brochure]. Research Triangle Park, NC: Author.

Nausieda, P., Pfeiffer, R., Tagliati, M., Kastenholz, K., DeRoche, M., & Slevin, J. (2005). A multicenter, open-label, sequential study comparing preferences for carbidopa-levodopa orally disintegrating tablets and conventional tablets in subjects with Parkinson's disease. *Clinical Therapeutics, 27,* 58–63.

Olanow, C. W., Watts, R. L., & Koller, W. C. (2001). An algorithm (decision tree) for the management of Parkinson's disease: Treatment guidelines. *Neurology, 56*(Suppl. 1), 88.

O'Maley, K., O'Sullivan, J., Wollin, J., Barras, M., & Brammer, J. (2005). Teaching people with Parkinson's disease about their medication. *Nursing Older People, 17,* 14–20.

Samii, A., Nutt, J. G., & Ransom, B. R. (2004). Parkinson's disease. *Lancet, 363,* 1783–1793.

Schapira, A. (2005). Present and future drug treatment for Parkinson's disease. *Journal of Neurology, Neurosurgery, and Psychiatry, 76,* 1472–1478.

Shulman, L. M., Minagar, A., & Weiner, W. J. (2000). The effect of pregnancy in Parkinson's disease. *Movement Disorders, 15,* 132–135.

Smith, L. P. (2002). Steady the course of Parkinson's disease. *Nursing, 32,* 43–45.

Tetrud, J. (2004). Treatment challenges in early stage Parkinson's disease. *Neurologic Clinics, 22,* S19–S33.

US Food and Drug Administration. (2007a, March). FDA Announces Voluntary Withdrawal of Pergolide Products. Retrieved April 2, 2007, from US Food and Drug Administration Announcements Online via access: http://www.fda.gov/bbs/topics/NEWS/2007/NEW01596.html

US Food and Drug Administration. (2007b, March). FDA Public Health Advisory: Pergolide (marketed as Permax). Retrieved April 2, 2007, from US Food and Drug Administration Announcements Online via access: http://www.fda.gov/cder/drug/advisory/pergolide.htm

Ward, C. (2005). Neuroleptic malignant syndrome in a patient with Parkinson's disease: A case study. *Journal of Neuroscience Nursing, 37,* 160–162.

Zanettini, R., Antonini, A., Gatto, G., Gentile, R., Tesei, S., & Pezzoli, G. (2007). Valvular heart disease and the use of dopamine agonists for Parkinson's disease. New England Journal of Medicine. 356(1), 39-46.

4

The Psychiatric Realm of Parkinson's Disease

Rebecca Martine, APRN, CS, BC

Parkinson's disease (PD) is a complex neurodegenerative disorder that exposes the intricate wiring of the human brain. The interplay of the motor, cognitive, and behavioral systems is objectified by the wide spectrum of neurological and psychiatric manifestations of PD. Once defined as a neurological illness, PD is now conceptualized as a neuropsychiatric disorder that commands multifaceted psychiatric and neurological care.

In his first description of the "shaking palsy," Dr. James Parkinson provided a brief glimpse into the psychiatric realm of PD. He acknowledged the presence of depression by noting, "A more melancholy object I never beheld" (Parkinson, 1817, p. 40). However, Dr. Parkinson concurrently dismissed the role of psychological dysfunction with the statement "by the absence of any injury to the senses and to the intellect, we are taught that the morbid state does not extend to the encephalon" (Parkinson, 1817, p. 34). It has taken the scientific community almost two centuries to uncover the extent of psychiatric dysfunction induced by PD. These symptoms have been unappreciated, leaving the Parkinson community to suffer from depression, anxiety, psychosis, dementia, and a host of other psychiatric disorders. Notable strides have been made over the past decade to properly acknowledge and address the psychiatric complications of parkinsonism. Research is increasingly focused on the nonmotor symptoms of the disease, with a strong focus on psychiatric comorbidity. Despite this trend, the basis for psychiatric dysfunction in PD remains obscure.

The psychiatric complications of PD are associated with excess disability, worse quality of life, poorer outcomes, and caregiver distress (Weintraub & Stern, 2005). These symptoms represent a distinct subset of illness that requires tactful evaluation and treatment in addition to strong professional and community support. As frontline providers, nurses are in the optimal position to unlock this area of distress through the delivery of comprehensive assessment and care. In this chapter we will further examine the neuropsychiatric aspects of PD, concentrating on symptom presentation, assessment, diagnostic considerations, and treatment options. Most importantly, we will explore the role of the nurse and highlight the importance of mental health awareness and advocacy for the Parkinson community.

THE PARKINSONIAN PERSONALITY

To begin this discussion, let us first reflect on the idea of the parkinsonian personality. Researchers and clinicians have detected a set of inherent personality traits that are frequently observed in individuals affected by PD. Studies as early as 1913 have suggested a personality type associated with PD (Ishihara & Brayne, 2006). Characteristics of this personality include being rigid, depressed, inflexible, and introverted (Poewe, Karamat, Kemmler, & Gerstenbrand, 1990). A retrospective study was performed at the Mayo Clinic examining the risk of PD in healthy individuals based on personality profile. The results supported the hypothesis that anxiety-prone individuals are at higher risk of developing PD up to several decades later (Bower et al., 2005). The perception of a parkinsonian personality implies an intrinsic association between premorbid mental health and PD. This theory remains controversial and requires greater research.

DEPRESSION

Background

Depression is the most well-studied neuropsychiatric, and perhaps nonmotor, complication associated with PD. Prevalence estimates vary widely, with rates between 20% and 40%, ranging from milder depression (e.g., dysthymia and minor depression) to major depressive disorder (Marsh et al., 2004; Weintraub, Moberg, Duda, Katz, & Stern, 2004). Epidemiological studies have proposed risk factors, including female sex, predominantly right-sided motor features, personal history of depression, early-onset PD, and atypical parkinsonism (rigid or bradykinetic-predominant disease; Weintraub & Stern, 2005). Depression in PD (dPD) commonly overlaps with other neuropsychiatric symptoms, such as cognitive impairment, psychosis, fatigue, insomnia, impaired executive functioning, and particularly anxiety (Rabinstein & Shulman, 2000). Ultimately, it remains unclear why some PD patients develop depression, while others go unaffected throughout the course of illness (Thanvi, Munshi, Vijaykumar, & Lo, 2003). It is not unusual for depressive symptomatology to occur in the years prior to the onset of motor symptoms, leaving some to speculate that depression is either a risk factor or a prodromal symptom for some PD patients.

Adjustment to the diagnosis of a chronic illness undoubtedly contributes to the development of mood disturbances in PD. A recent study suggested that maladaptive metacognitive style, or a negative belief system with a strong tendency to worry, directly impacts the risk of depression in this population (Allott, Wells, Morrison, & Walker, 2005). However, dPD most likely stems from a fusion of psychological factors and neurobiological dysregulation. It is thought that several areas of the brain are implicated in the neuropathology of dPD, including (a) subcortical nuclei and the frontal lobes, (b) striatal-thalamic-frontal neural circuitry, and (c) brain stem monoamine and indolamine systems. Functional brain imaging studies suggest interference in the pathways connecting these regions. This may lead to a complex disruption of serotonin as well as dopamine, norepinephrine, and acetylcholine (Weintraub & Stern, 2005).

Symptom Presentation

Depression in PD is easily overlooked due to shared symptomatology with classic parkinsonism. Psychomotor retardation, appetite and sleep alterations, cognitive impairment, poor concentration, lethargy, and restlessness are anticipated symptoms of PD that mutually characterize depression. Such symptoms of depression can manifest before or after the onset of motor dysfunction with progression and periods of exacerbation throughout the disease process. In addition to the above symptoms, depressed PD patients can experience or exhibit signs of anhedonia, pessimism, and hopelessness. In some respects, dPD is atypical, with greater anxiety but less self-punitive behavior, guilt, and suicidal ideation as compared with general depression (Thanvi et al., 2003).

Affective changes have been linked to motor fluctuations, with reports of dysphoria and anxiety when medications begin to lose effect. Patients will sometimes report a shift in mood with feelings of doom when approaching an off period. True nonmotor fluctuations that are related to medication response will rebound during on time. There is uncertainty whether this phenomenon is biologically or psychologically driven. Interestingly, optimal treatment of motor symptoms is not associated with improved mood, but successful treatment of depression is associated with improved motor function (Marsh, 2000b).

Assessment and Diagnostic Considerations

Lack of symptom differentiation for PD and depression can lead to misdiagnosis of the nondepressed PD patient but, more commonly, delayed diagnosis and treatment of the depressed PD patient. Shulman, Taback, Rabinstein & Weiner (2002) conducted a study examining the diagnostic accuracy of nonmotor symptoms by movement disorder specialists. While 41% of subjects met diagnostic criteria for depression, only 21% were properly recognized and diagnosed by the specialist. Alternatively, individuals who appear objectively depressed or meet strict diagnostic criteria do not always endorse feelings of depression. Weintraub et al. (2004) found that 46% of PD subjects who met diagnostic criteria for a depressive disorder did not consider themselves depressed. This endorses the need for tactful clinical evaluation as PD patients may not experience depression in a typical manner. Additionally, it underscores the value of caregiver input to increase sensitivity in detecting subtle changes in mood and personality.

Assessment and diagnosis of dPD can be further complicated by ambiguous psychiatric comorbidity. This is commonly seen with dementia, which can both mask and mimic symptoms of depression. As PD progresses, it becomes increasingly difficult to discern blended psychiatric illness. Individualized, creative questioning can be useful when distinguishing specific symptoms of depression, anxiety, and cognitive impairment.

Evaluation of possible depression should take place during routine visits via screening and direct questioning. A specific dPD assessment tool has not yet been developed. The American Academy of Neurology (AAN) recently validated use of the Beck Depression Inventory and the Hamilton Depression Rating Scale for dPD (Miyasaki et al., 2006). The Montgomery–Asberg Depression Rating Scale and the 15-item Geriatric Depression Scale have also been endorsed by several studies (Weintraub,

Oehlberg, Katz, & Stern, 2006a). Diagnosis of dPD is based on standard criteria for depression, as cited by the *DSM–IV* (American Psychiatric Association, 1994b).

It is strongly advised that the clinician assess for suicidal and homicidal ideation during routine assessment. Literature suggests that the risk of suicide resulting from dPD is minimal compared to that in idiopathic depression (Merschdorf et al., 2003). However, a special point of consideration lies with the increased risk of suicide in the older, white, male population (Turvey et al., 2002).

Management and Treatment

Treatment of dPD encompasses the same basic principles and management options as idiopathic depression. Pharmacological management is commonly required due to underlying biologic dysfunction that can be resistant to nonpharmacological intervention. It is estimated that 20% to 25% of PD patients in specialty care are treated with antidepressants, most commonly selective serotonin reuptake inhibitors (SSRIs). This class of drugs includes fluoxetine (Prozac), escitalopram (Lexapro), sertraline (Zoloft), paroxetine (Paxil), and citalopram (Celexa). These medications are often well tolerated with good benefit and are consequently used as first-line therapy (Weintraub, Moberg, Duda, Katz, & Stern, 2003). SSRIs are particularly valuable when treating coexisting anxiety, lessening the burden of polypharmacy. Other antidepressants can be considered for persistent depression or as adjunctive treatment, including venlafaxine (Effexor), mirtazapine (Remeron), bupropion (Wellbutrin), and tricyclic agents like nortriptyline (Pamelor; Rabinstein & Shulman, 2000). The latter must be used with caution in the geriatric and PD population due to possible aggravation of orthostasis, constipation, and cognitive impairment. There has been clinical speculation that dopamine agonists may also improve dPD; however, it is not possible to recommend this treatment strategy until additional research confirms the antidepressant properties of this class of medications (Rektorova et al., 2003). Generally speaking, medications are safe options for this population, but caution must be used when determining dosage and potential adverse effects. It is crucial that the patient and family be well educated on the purpose of the drug, directions for proper administration, and the risk of side effects.

Electroconvulsive therapy (ECT) has been cited as a viable treatment option for dPD. Furthermore, it has been shown to temporarily improve motor symptoms of PD in addition to treating depression (Moellentine et al., 1998). Though ECT offers a proven treatment alternative, it is mostly reserved for severe, refractory depression and is rarely elected by PD patients and providers.

Nonpharmacological management can play a vital role in the treatment of dPD, whether alone or in combination with medications. The role of psychotherapy in dPD remains unclear from a scientific standpoint but is commonly endorsed by patients and caregivers. Recent attention has been paid to cognitive behavioral therapy (CBT) for dPD, which is an interactive and educational approach to addressing negative thoughts. Cole and Vaughn (2005) supported the relevance of CBT for dPD subjects by showing clinically reliable reduction of depressive symptoms, specifically on the cognitive dimensions of guilt, pessimism, and failure. Support groups can also be encouraged for peer support, discussion, and experienced advice. Furthermore, the role of exercise cannot be underestimated for the treatment of all areas of PD, including mood, sleep, and motor management. Yoga, tai chi, or even daily walks can serve as simple approaches to boost mood and energy and promote restful sleep. See Table 4.1 for a quick reference guide to depression in PD.

ANXIETY

Background

Anxiety is a natural response to a stressful situation and is expected when examining the effects of chronic illness. It is assumed that anxiety in PD is partly related to normal psychosocial adaptation. However, prevalence rates in PD, noted at 30% to 40%, exceed those of other medical illnesses with comparable levels of disability (Marsh, 2000a). This substantiates the theory that anxiety is related to the underlying pathology of PD. Changes to the noradrenergic system (e.g., norepinephrine), including cell loss in the locus coeruleus, are likely involved, as are chemical imbalances of dopamine, serotonin, gamma-aminobutyric acid, glutamate, and various neuropeptides (Anderson & Weiner, 2002; Jetty, Charney, & Goddard, 2001). Ultimately, the etiology of anxiety in PD remains unclear and has not been systematically studied to date.

TABLE 4.1 Quick Reference Guide: Depression in Parkinson's Disease

Key assessment questions[a]	• Do you ever feel sad for extended periods of time?
	• Do you ever become tearful?
	• How is your sleep?
	• How is your appetite?
	• How is your motivation?
	• When did these symptoms start or worsen?
Applicable assessment tools	• Beck Depression Inventory (BDI)
	• Hamilton Depression Rating Scale (HDRS)
	• 15-Item Geriatric Depression Scale (GDS–15)
	• Montgomery–Asberg Depression Rating Scale (MADRS)
Differential diagnoses	• Apathy
	• Adjustment disorder
	• Anxiety
	• Cognitive impairment/dementia
	• Sleep disorder
Nonpharmacological approaches	• Psychotherapy (individual, couple, or group)
	• Patient and family education and supportive therapy
	• Exercise
	• Support group participation
Pharmacological approaches	• "Start low and go slow"
	• Consider selective serotonin reuptake inhibitors (SSRIs) as first line agents (e.g., fluoxetine [Prozac], sertraline [Zoloft], paroxetine [Paxil], citalopram [Celexa])
	• Consider tricyclic antidepressants (e.g., nortriptyline [Pamelor])
	• Consider venlafaxine (Effexor)

(continued)

TABLE 4.1 Quick Reference Guide: Depression in Parkinson's Disease *(continued)*

	• Consider mirtazapine (Remeron)
	• Consider bupropion (Wellbutrin)
Medical approaches	• Electroconvulsive therapy (ECT)
Other considerations	• Initiate education of depression shortly after PD diagnosis
	• Screen for depression at every visit
	• Differentiate signs and symptoms of depression from primary signs and symptoms of Parkinson's disease
	• Acknowledge patient and family stigmas and misconceptions
	• Perform suicide/homicide risk assessment
	• Consider psychiatric and social work consultations

ªQuestions can also be directed to the caregiver with the patient's consent.

The onset of anxiety most commonly follows the diagnosis of PD. However, like depression, there is interest in examining patients with a personal history of anxiety preceding PD diagnosis. Some studies have suggested that anxiety can actually precede the development of PD by up to 20 years, tying to the idea of a premorbid parkinsonian personality type (Lauterbach & Duvoisin, 1991). There appears to be significant overlap between dPD and anxiety. Menza, Robertson-Hoffman, and Bonapace (1993) found that 92% of PD patients with anxiety experienced comorbid depression. Likewise, up to 67% of PD patients with depression suffered from comorbid anxiety.

Symptom Presentation

The term *anxiety* does not describe one disorder but rather a constellation of syndromes with different manifestations of anxiety symptoms. According to the *DSM–IV,* specific anxiety disorders include panic disorder, agoraphobia, social phobia, specific phobia, obsessive–compulsive disorder, and generalized anxiety disorder, all of which have been reported in PD. Each disorder represents a unique array of symptoms and clinical considerations. In most cases these disorders are phenomenologically indistinct from idiopathic anxiety disorders. Patients do not typically label their symptoms as anxiety but rather as feelings of nervousness, apprehension, tension, social avoidance, or agitation that is persistent, episodic, or recurrent (Marsh, 2000a). Furthermore, patients may experience symptoms of varied domains, including cognitive, physical, and emotional complaints. Like depression, it is often difficult to differentiate these ambiguous symptoms as they blend together, forming an aggregation of neuropsychiatric illness.

The experience of anxiety in PD has been associated with levodopa levels and related motor control in some patients. Several studies have described anxiety disorders more often in individuals who experience motor fluctuations, specifically in the off state (Henderson, Kurlan, Kersun, & Como, 1992; Stein, Heuser, Juncos, & Uhde, 1990; Vazquez, Jimenez-Jimenez, Garcia-Ruiz, & Garcia-Urra, 1993). There appears to be a reciprocal association between anxiety and off motor symptomatology. Anxiety can trigger and exacerbate off symptoms, most commonly tremor, whereas off symptoms can trigger and exacerbate anxiety. The exact relationship between these events has not been established (Anderson & Weiner, 2002). Regardless of the catalyst, overlapping anxiety and off symptomatology can result in intensified levels of disability and caregiver burden. Charting and diaries are sometimes helpful in uncovering the association and pattern of anxiety and motor fluctuations.

Assessment and Diagnostic Considerations

Anxiety, like depression, tends to go underrecognized and undertreated in the PD population. In addition to poor diagnostic accuracy of depression, Shulman et al. (2002) found that even movement disorder specialists overlooked anxiety in almost half of cases. The cause of clinical neglect implicates not only clinicians, but patients and caregivers alike. Reluctance to discuss mental health problems inhibits proper discussion, diagnosis, and treatment. Nevertheless, it is the responsibility of the clinician to introduce questions regarding anxiety and other mood disturbances to ensure proper acknowledgment of these prominent issues. Such questions should be incorporated in each clinical evaluation.

When anxiety is reported or detected, screening tools can be useful in determining the presence and magnitude of symptoms. A questionnaire has not yet been developed for anxiety in PD. However, universally validated tools, such as the Beck Anxiety Index, are generally appropriate and applied in clinical practice. The clinician can also utilize diaries, to be completed by the patient or caregiver at home, to assess a possible relationship between anxiety and motor fluctuations. Differentiating the type of anxiety disorder will also assist in determination and application of treatment strategies. Diagnosis of anxiety disorders in PD is based on *DSM–IV* diagnostic criteria.

Management and Treatment

The treatment of anxiety in PD is guided by anecdotal experience as research has yet to produce evidence-based recommendations. Before treatment is initiated, the clinician should consider the nature and severity of the presenting symptoms. Nonpharmacological approaches, as discussed later, may be especially helpful for patients with mild symptoms or for those with polypharmacy concerns. Additionally, a clinician may consider adjusting a patient's dopaminergic regimen if the anxiety routinely presents with motor fluctuations. Given the dramatic impact on quality of life, clinicians are often required to introduce antianxiety agents.

SSRIs are the preferred drug class for the treatment for both affective and anxiety disorders in PD. Owing to the serotonergic mechanisms of both depression and anxiety and the high incidence of their co-occurrence in PD, SSRIs serve as versatile and convenient first-line agents (Rabinstein & Shulman, 2000). Selection of the appropriate drug should be individualized and based on the patient's medical history, medication sensitivity, and symptom presentation.

Additional medication classes can be considered in the treatment of anxiety disorders associated with PD. Venlafaxine (Effexor), mirtazapine (Remeron), and bupropion (Wellbutrin) are commonly used in clinical practice. Tricyclic antidepressants can also be appropriate but must be used with caution based on their side effect profile for the geriatric population. Additionally, benzodiazepines remain practical management options, especially for short-term treatment. Medications such as lorazepam (Ativan), alprazolam (Xanax), and clonazepam (Klonopin) can provide timely relief of acute anxiety and panic attacks. Short-acting benzodiazepines can be particularly useful due to rapid absorption for anxiety associated with motor fluctuations and sudden, unpredictable off time. Long-term use of these agents, however, should be avoided in the geriatric population due to the increased risk of falls, sedation, sleep disturbances, cognitive impairment or delirium, and other adverse effects (Marsh, 2000a; Rabinstein & Shulman, 2000).

Nonpharmacological approaches can provide substantial benefit of anxiety, whether alone or in combination with drug therapy. The focal point of nonpharmacological management is patient and family education. While some patients may be resistant to alternative health modalities, others appreciate these less invasive and holistic approaches to care. Physical activity and exercise (yoga, tai chi, walking, etc.) as well as relaxation techniques (progressive relaxation, imagery, massages) can be suggested as safe and effective treatment options for anxiety. Psychotherapy can also be beneficial in identifying the source of the anxiety, while incorporating individualized treatment strategies. See Table 4.2 for a quick reference guide to anxiety in PD.

APATHY

Background

Apathy is a Greek word meaning "without passion." This affective disturbance represents a triad of behavioral, emotional, and motivational features. Prevalence rates vary between 17% and 51% in the PD population (Kirsch-Darrow, Fernandez, Marsiske, Okun, & Bowers, 2006). Apathy is becoming increasingly recognized in both neurological and psychiatric disorders, particularly in those associated with frontal-subcortical dysfunction. The exact etiology remains unclear; however, disruptions to the limbic pathway as well as dopamine and nonadrenergic functions are likely related (Pluck & Brown, 2002). While it is generally assumed that apathy is a result of underlying pathological changes, psychological reactions and adaptations to chronic disease are also implicated. Apathy contributes significantly to caregiver burden and has a negative impact on long-term outcome (Krupp, 1997).

Symptom Presentation

Symptoms of apathy consist of reduced interest, lack of motivation and initiation, lack of concern or indifference, flat affect, and changes in mood and thinking (Isella et al., 2002). Patients typically present as disinterested, with little or no goal-directed behavior. Apathy overlaps both conceptually

TABLE 4.2 Quick Reference Guide: Anxiety in Parkinson's Disease

Key assessment questions[a]	• Do you worry excessively?
	• Do you ever experience panic attacks?
	• Do you lose sleep over your worries/fears?
	• Do you avoid social situations because of your worries/fears?
	• Do you repeat certain actions or behaviors that are out of your control?
	• Do these symptoms correspond to changes in your motor state?
Applicable assessment tools	• Beck Anxiety Inventory (BAI)
	• Patient diaries
Differential diagnoses	• Depression
	• Apathy
	• Adjustment disorder
	• Cognitive impairment/dementia
	• Sleep disorder
Nonpharmacological approaches	• Psychotherapy (individual, couple, or group)
	• Patient and family education and supportive therapy
	• Physical activity and exercise
	• Relaxation techniques, imagery
	• Support group participation
Pharmacological approaches	• "Start low and go slow"
	• Consider selective serotonin reuptake inhibitors (SSRIs) for long-term benefit (e.g., fluoxetine [Prozac], fluvoxamine [Luvox], sertraline [Zoloft], paroxetine [Paxil], citalopram [Celexa])
	• Consider benzodiazepines for short-term benefit (e.g., lorazepam [Ativan], clonazepam [Klonopin], alprazolam [Xanax])

(continued)

TABLE 4.2   *(continued)*

	• Consider other antidepressant classes (e.g., venlafaxine [Effexor], mirtazapine [Remeron], bupropion [Wellbutrin], tricyclics)
Other considerations	• Initiate education of anxiety shortly after PD diagnosis
	• Screen for anxiety at every visit
	• Differentiate signs and symptoms of anxiety from primary signs and symptoms of Parkinson's disease
	• Assess relationship to motor fluctuations
	• Consider psychiatric and social work consultations

aQuestions can also be directed to the caregiver with the patient's consent.

and clinically with a wide variety of psychiatric comorbidities, confounding diagnosis and treatment. Greatest consideration must be paid to the deep entanglement of depression and apathy. While symptoms are analogous and often converge, it is thought that apathy and depression are two distinct syndromes that do not always coexist. A recent study suggested that apathy can occur in PD without depression in up to 28% of cases (Kirsch-Darrow et al., 2006). Similar to depression, apathy is associated with impaired functioning due to the extent of executive deficits, verbal memory impairment, and *bradyphrenia* (slowed thinking) (Isella et al., 2002; Starkstein et al., 1992).

Assessment and Diagnostic Considerations

The assessment and diagnosis of apathy is often complicated by superficial overlap with other psychiatric syndromes. Poignant questions will assist the clinician in differentiating manifestations of depression, dementia, delirium, and apathy. Patients with pure apathy do not typically endorse classic symptoms of depression, such as sadness, hopelessness, and guilt. Apathy will instead be perceived as a neutral mood with poor initiation and interest (Richard, 2006). Affected patients often experience diminished self-awareness and will deny health concerns. Consequently, caregivers commonly serve as primary informants. Phrases like *lazy, bored,* or *difficult to motivate* are frequently used when describing an apathetic patient. Clinicians may find it helpful to explore the patient's personality profile. For example, has he or she always been introverted, quiet, or indolent? There is speculation that the presentation of apathy may be related to the parkinsonian personality (Pluck & Brown, 2002). In addition to clinical interview, the Apathy Evaluation Scale and the Apathy Scale are validated tools for use in PD (Marin, Biedrzycki, & Firinciogullari, 1991; Starkstein et al., 1992).

Moreover, it is important to consider the shared features of apathy and classic parkinsonism. Bradykinesia, masked face, and low voice can mimic as well as mask symptoms of apathy. It is again for these reasons that a comprehensive subjective report is critical for proper assessment and diagnosis.

Management and Treatment

The treatment of apathy continues to take form as this disorder becomes better understood. There has been no specific treatment study for apathy in PD to date. However, clinical experience has provided anecdotal recommendations, which will be discussed in this section. Comorbid psychiatric illnesses, such as depression, should be treated initially. On the basis of the proposed neuropathophysiology of apathy, antidepressants and other medications that increase dopamine or norepinephrine activity may be beneficial (Marin, Fogel, Hawkins, Duffy, & Krupp, 1995). Movement disorder specialists are trying stimulants (e.g., methylphenidate [Ritalin]), stimulant-related compounds (e.g., modafinil [Provigil]), and atomoxetine (Strattera) in the treatment of apathy in PD. There are also early indications that dopamine agonists and cholinesterase inhibitors may be efficacious (Pluck & Brown, 2002).

Nonpharmacological treatment relies most heavily on education, with special attention to caregivers. Apathy is often misunderstood by caregivers, who may experience frustration and aggravation surrounding these changes in behavior and personality. This is especially true when the patient denies feelings of depression but restricts communication and activity. Common assumptions suggest that the patient is defiant, lazy, or dissatisfied in his or her relationship with the caregiver. It is important to address these ideas and assist the caregiver in appreciating the biological basis of this syndrome. Behavioral strategies for patients may not be successful due to the fundamental nature of apathy, including diminished goal-directed behavior and motivation. See Table 4.3 for a quick reference guide to apathy in PD.

TABLE 4.3. Quick Reference Guide: Apathy in Parkinson's Disease

Key assessment questions[a]	• How do you spend your day? Can you give me an example of your daily activities?
	• Do you take pleasure in hobbies or activities?
	• How is your mood? Do you feel sad, hopeless, or guilty?
	• How is your memory?
	• How is your motivation?
	• Has your personality changed following diagnosis of PD? If so, how?
Applicable assessment tools	• Apathy Evaluation Scale
	• Apathy Scale
Differential diagnoses	• Depression
	• Adjustment disorder
	• Cognitive impairment/dementia
	• Sleep disorder (e.g., excessive daytime sleepiness)
	• Delirium
Nonpharmacological approaches	• Patient and family education and supportive therapy
	• Physical activity and exercise
	• Support group participation
Pharmacological approaches	• Treat coexisting psychiatric illnesses first (e.g., antidepressants)
	• Consider psychostimulants (e.g., methylphenidate [Ritalin])

(continued)

TABLE 4.3   Quick Reference Guide: Apathy in Parkinson's Disease *(continued)*

	• Consider stimulant-related compounds (e.g., modafinil [Provigil])
Other considerations	• Initiate education of apathy shortly after PD diagnosis
	• Screen for apathy at every visit
	• Differentiate signs and symptoms of apathy from signs and symptoms of other psychiatric disorders (e.g., depression)
	• Differentiate signs and symptoms of apathy from primary signs and symptoms of Parkinson's disease
	• Address caregiver frustration and misconceptions
	• Provide family support and guidance
	• Consider psychiatric consultation

aQuestions can also be directed to the caregiver with the patient's consent.

COGNITIVE DYSFUNCTION

Background

Cognitive dysfunction is an anticipated component of PD, with symptoms ranging from subtle deficits in select cognitive domains to advanced dementia. It is common for patients to report general cognitive changes, such as poor complex task planning and completion, word finding difficulties, and bradyphrenia, even in early disease. While these symptoms can remain mild with limited functional impact, up to 80% of PD patients will ultimately develop overt dementia according to a recent longitudinal study (Aarsland, Andersen, Larsen, Lolk, & Kragh-Sorensen, 2003). The Parkinson population has an almost sixfold increased risk of developing dementia compared to healthy controls (Aarsland et al., 2001). Dementia is directly associated with increased morbidity and mortality in the PD population. Identified risk factors for Parkinson's disease with dementia (PDD) include increasing age, increasing severity of disease, akinetic-rigid-predominant symptoms, gait-predominant symptoms, atypical parkinsonism, psychosis, depression, early occurrence of drug-related hallucinations, impaired verbal fluency at baseline, symmetrical disease presentation, and poor to moderate response to levodopa (Emre, 2003).

PDD is traditionally defined as a subcortical dementia, suggesting that significant pathological changes occur below the cerebral cortex. However, PDD is associated with diffuse subcortical as well as cortical Lewy body disease pathology. Degeneration of the neural circuits connecting the basal ganglia and cortical regions, including the prefrontal cortex, are thought to contribute to overall cognitive impairment in PD. Additionally, there is a strong chemical component with a combined effect from several neurotransmitter deficiencies. It has been hypothesized that cholinergic deficits result primarily in memory impairment, dopaminergic deficits affect executive dysfunction, noradrenergic deficits contribute to impaired attention, and serotoninergic deficits lead to depressed mood (Emre, 2003).

It is important to appreciate the shared and diverse characteristics of PDD and other forms of dementia, such as Alzheimer's disease (AD) and dementia with Lewy bodies (DLB). Diagnostic criteria separate these disorders, but there is known overlap in symptom presentation and pathology. AD is generally defined as a cortical dementia, representing a stronger presence of memory and language abnormalities, with less executive dysfunction, compared with PDD (Cahn-Weiner, Grace, Ott, Fernandez, & Friedman, 2002). Surprisingly, up to 40% of PD patients have AD-related neuropathological changes on autopsy, with a positive correlation to the severity of PDD symptomatology (Weintraub & Stern, 2005). DLB presents more closely to PDD than AD, with pronounced parkinsonian features accompanied by dementia with prominent subcortical features. Both these disorders involve the accumulation of Lewy bodies, or abnormal aggregates of protein that develop inside nerve cells, with a more widespread pathological process linked to DLB (Noe et al., 2004). The relationship between PDD and DLB is subject to an intense and ongoing debate, as some researchers and clinicians consider them to be one in the same disease.

Symptom Presentation

As previously noted, cognitive dysfunction in PD can present across a continuum of mild deficits to global dementia. Symptoms can vary in degree as well as nature, meaning that one or more cognitive domains can be involved. These basic cognitive domains include executive function, attention, memory, visuospatial perception, and language (Emre, 2003).

Disturbance of executive abilities constitutes the core feature of cognitive dysfunction in PD. Executive deficits present as difficulty with concept formation and rule finding, problem solving, set elaboration and planning, set shifting, and set maintenance (Pillon, Boller, Levy, & Dubois, 2001). Patients and caregivers will typically report problems balancing the checkbook, formulating a grocery list, driving, and generating new ideas. As cognitive deficits progress into dementia, the patient will become increasingly inflexible in his or her thinking and require concrete versus abstract tasks, with regular cuing from the caregiver. PDD is widely recognized as a dysexecutive syndrome.

Problems with attention can present early in PD and can be measured by cognitive reaction time and vigilance. Patients and caregivers will often describe an inability to handle complex tasks that require mental calculation and concentration. Fluctuations in attention are known to occur in PDD and are a core feature of DLB (Bronnick et al., 2006).

Memory deficits are common in PD, though different in severity and pattern as compared with AD. PD patients generally complain of difficulty with recall, suggesting that new information is stored but not easily accessed (i.e., retrieval deficit as opposed to encoding deficit). There is speculation that this disability is related to executive dysfunction due to the patient's inability to encode and retrieve stored memories (Emre, 2003).

Visuospatial dysfunction has been reported in PD, affecting visuospatial analysis, visuospatial orientation, visuoperception, and visuomotor tasks. Patients and caregivers often depict these problems with reports of visual misperceptions, such as missing the plate with the fork, thereby spearing the table. Visuospatial impairment has been linked with executive dysfunction and tends to be greatest in patients with severe motor symptoms (Emre, 2003).

Verbal fluency is the primary language abnormality seen with PD and is generally more severe than in AD. Other language deficits, such as naming difficulties, decreased information content of spontaneous speech, and impaired sentence comprehension, are known to occur but to a lesser degree than in AD (Cahn-Weiner et al., 2002). PD patients will often complain of word-finding problems or the so-called tip-of-the-tongue phenomenon, even in early disease.

As PDD progresses, related behavioral consequences quickly supersede the underlying symptoms and become the primary focus of the caregiver and clinician. Demented patients are prone to becoming agitated, psychotic, argumentative, and impulsive, resulting from frontal disinhibition, fear, and confusion. Moreover, these behaviors can be exacerbated by their increased susceptibility of developing psychosis and sleep disturbances (Weintraub & Stern, 2005).

Assessment and Diagnostic Considerations

The assessment of cognition and memory is a key element of standard clinical care and should be introduced at the time of diagnosis. It is often helpful to obtain baseline neuropsychological testing in early PD to monitor cognitive changes over the course of disease. As with all potential psychiatric complications in PD, problem-focused questions should be asked of the patient and caregiver at each examination. Reported changes should be thoroughly discussed to reveal the duration and nature of presenting symptoms. A comprehensive diagnostic investigation is also advised following the onset of symptoms. Common laboratory, neuroimaging, and electroencephalographic studies are typically ordered as part of a routine dementia workup. These tests will assist the clinician in ruling out other etiologies of cognitive dysfunction, such as normal pressure hydrocephalus, vitamin B_{12} deficiency, hypothyroidism, urinary tract infection, medication toxicity, metabolic disorders, dehydration, vascular dementia, and pneumonia. A systematic neurological examination will also reveal unexpected clinical features of PD, such as aphasia and apraxia, suggesting alternative or concomitant diagnoses like AD (Rabinstein & Shulman, 2000). Furthermore, the presentation of cognitive fluctuations and psychosis at the onset of motor dysfunction supports the diagnosis of dementia with Lewy bodies (McKeith et al., 2005).

AAN recently recommended use of the Mini-Mental State Examination and the Cambridge Cognitive Examination as appropriate screening tools for PDD (Miyasaki et al., 2006). These screens can be especially valuable in a clinical setting as they are brief and easy to administer in the context of routine care. Anecdotally, other instruments have been applied, including the Hopkins Verbal Learning Test–Revised, the Clock Draw Test, and simple bedside screens, such as verbal fluency tests and Luria's manual sequencing (Weintraub & Stern, 2005). Neuropsychological testing is the most valuable approach to assessing PDD. It offers the greatest sensitivity, can detect early deficits, can differentiate cortical and subcortical symptoms, can distinguish domain-specific deficits, and may diagnosis behavioral disorders, such as depression and anxiety (Rabinstein & Shulman, 2000). If cognitive dysfunction is suspected, it is advisable to consult a neuropsychologist for formal testing.

Management and Treatment

When cognitive dysfunction is detected, it is prudent to review the patient's medication profile to determine if potentially offensive medications can be reduced or discontinued. Anticholinergics, benzodiazepines, muscle relaxants, and anxiolytics can aggravate dementia and psychosis and should be initially targeted for reduction and discontinuation (Rabinstein & Shulman, 2000). All antiparkinsonian drugs are known to potentially exacerbate psychotic symptoms and confusion (Burn & McKeith, 2003). If warranted, the clinician should taper and discontinue the least potent, and therefore least therapeutic, dopaminergic agents. This may include selegiline (Eldepryl) and amantadine (Symmetrel). Next, dopamine agonists should be slowly tapered and discontinued, relying instead on levodopa monotherapy. In late-stage dementia the clinician may choose to reduce or, in rare cases, discontinue carbidopa/levodopa (Sinemet). If these adjustments result in motor deterioration with suboptimal improvement of cognition, in the absence of psychosis the clinician may choose to restore the original PD pharmacological regimen (Rabinstein & Shulman, 2000).

Cholinesterase inhibitors, commonly used for AD, have been found to be efficacious in the treatment of PDD. Rivastigmine (Exelon), which was approved by the U.S. Food and Drug Administration for this indication in 2006, was endorsed by a large, multisite, placebo-controlled study (Emre et al., 2004). Additionally, two smaller studies reported significant improvement in global cognitive functioning with donepezil (Aricept; Aarsland, Laake, Larsen, & Janvin, 2002; Leroi et al., 2004). Clinically, these medications have been widely adopted, despite reports of worsening of parkinsonism in some patients (Aarsland, Mosimann, & McKeith, 2004). Galantamine (Reminyl or Razadyne) is a third agent used clinically without strong empirical reference. All cholinesterase inhibitors should be slowly tapered as abrupt discontinuation can result in acute cognitive and behavioral decline (Minett et al., 2003).

Nonpharmacological approaches for PDD are centered on patient and family education and safety. Though the topic of dementia is often alarming, education on this potential complication should be introduced early in disease to ensure prompt detection and treatment. As the syndrome progresses, family members will require ongoing education regarding home safety and environmental measures, community resources, and long-term care options. Caregivers often become overwhelmed by the complex nature of dementia, especially in the presence of psychosis, falls, and behavioral disturbances (e.g., sundowning, wandering). *Sundowning* is a term referring to an increase in confusion, agitation, and disorientation as evening appears. It is thought that as patients loose the cues of lighting, shadowing and distortions combined with fatigue and dementia become problematic. For those residing in residential facilities, and even for some at home, activity level changes in the late afternoon, perhaps a flurry of activity as people come and go at change of shift, or young children come home from school. This can be disorienting and cause behavioral problems.

Caregiver burden is extremely prevalent when dealing with PDD, and it is not uncommon for the caregiver to assume the role of primary patient. Orientation, memory prompts, and attention cues should be introduced as techniques for preserving the highest level of self-care and awareness. Caregivers should be encouraged to utilize all available resources, including family assistance, to promote their own quality of life. Support groups are invaluable avenues for peer support and guidance. See Table 4.4 for a quick reference guide to PD with dementia.

PSYCHOSIS

Background

Thus far, we have discussed psychiatric conditions that are directly associated with the extensive neurodegenerative pathology of PD. In addition to these intrinsic complications, PD patients are commonly faced with drug-induced psychiatric syndromes, such as psychosis. Hallucinations and delusions define the term *psychosis*. Prevalence rates in PD vary, with an estimation of 15% to 40% for visual hallucinations and illusions and 5% for delusions co-occurring with hallucinations (Aarsland, Larsen, Cummins, & Laake, 1999). Psychosis can present at any point of illness but more commonly presents as the disease progresses. Risk factors include

TABLE 4.4 Quick Reference Guide: Parkinson's Disease With Dementia

Key assessment questions[a]	• How is your memory?
	• Do you find it difficult to express yourself (e.g., language skills)?
	• Are you able to organize your thoughts and feelings as you did in the past?
	• Do you find it difficult to concentrate and complete tasks?
	• Is there anything that you cannot do now because of problems with your memory?
	• What is today's date (and other orientation questions)?
Applicable assessment tools	• Mini-Mental State Examination (MMSE)
	• Cambridge Cognitive Examination (CAMCog)
	• Hopkins Verbal Learning Test–Revised (HVLT–R)
	• Clock Draw Test (CDT)
	• Simple bedside screens, such as verbal fluency tests and Luria's manual sequencing
Differential diagnoses	• Dementia with Lewy bodies
	• Alzheimer's disease
	• Drug-induced delirium
	• Other medical etiologies
	• Depression
	• Anxiety
	• Sleep disorder
Nonpharmacological approaches	• Orientation, memory prompts, and attention cues
	• Patient and family education and supportive therapy
	• Support group participation

(continued)

TABLE 4.4 *(continued)*

Pharmacological approaches	• Consider reducing and/or discontinuing potentially offensive agents (e.g., anticholinergics, benzodiazepines, muscle relaxants, anxiolytics)
	• Consider reducing and/or discontinuing antiparkinsonian medications as tolerated (e.g., selegiline, amantadine, COMT inhibitors, dopamine agonists, levodopa)
	• Consider introducing cholinesterase inhibitor therapy (e.g., rivastigmine [Exelon], donepezil [Ariecpt], galantamine [Reminyl or Razadyne])
Other considerations	• Initiate education of dementia shortly after PD diagnosis
	• Screen for cognitive changes at every visit
	• Order diagnostic investigation (e.g., "dementia work-up")
	• Consider diagnosis of dementia with Lewy bodies if cognitive fluctuations accompany psychosis and early motor disease
	• Consider psychiatric and social work consultations

[a]Questions can also be directed to the caregiver with the patient's consent.

disease duration, increasing disease severity, use of dopaminergic drugs, older age, cognitive impairment, and comorbid sleep disorder (Ismail & Richard, 2004; Poewe, 2003). For the majority of PD patients, psychosis cannot be explained by premorbid psychiatric illness.

Psychosis in PD is predominantly, though not exclusively, a result of dopaminergic pharmacotherapy. All antiparkinsonian drugs have the ability to produce psychosis; however, there is anecdotal speculation that dopamine agonists carry a slightly higher risk than levodopa (Ismail & Richard, 2004). Psychosis is not always correlated with dopaminergic dosage or duration of use, suggesting a complex interaction of neuropathology and comorbid vulnerabilities that are aggravated by drug exposure (Aarsland et al., 1999). The exact mechanisms responsible for psychosis in PD are poorly understood. Cholinergic deficits and an imbalance of the serotonergic and dopaminergic systems are mostly likely involved, as is widespread neuropathology (Weintraub & Stern, 2005).

Psychosis in PD is a difficult and disturbing issue for patients, caregivers, and providers alike. It is known that psychosis intensifies caregiver burden and represents the greatest risk factor for permanent nursing home placement. Most importantly, psychosis directly influences the morbidity and mortality rates of the PD population (Goetz & Stebbins, 1995).

Symptom Presentation

Visual hallucinations are the most prevalent manifestation of psychosis in PD and can be defined as spontaneously fabricated perceptions when awake. True visual hallucinations are characteristically well formed, rich in detail and color, and consist of familiar or unfamiliar people, animals, and objects (Molho & Factor, 2005). Patients with clear sensorium will typically retain insight into the nonreality of their perceptions and describe the hallucinations as benign or even pleasant. However, cognitive impairment and delirium can allow for frightening, threatening, and disturbing hallucinations with limited insight, impacting up to one-third of cases (Moskovitz, Moses, & Klawans, 1978). This variation of hallucinosis is most concerning as patients are likely to respond with behavioral disturbances and can be difficult to orient and redirect.

The continuum hypothesis of hallucinosis in PD suggests that visual hallucinations contribute to a progressive pattern of psychiatric dysfunction (Moskovitz et al., 1978). Vivid dreaming precedes visual hallucinations to be followed by delusions and delirium, according to this theory. Researchers have also correlated the progression of hallucinations to the earlier development of visual illusions. These types of false perceptions are triggered by visual misinterpretation of fixed stimuli. For example, a patient may wrongly perceive a garden hose as a snake. The connections between vivid dreaming, visual illusions, and visual hallucinations suggest possible markers in the progression of psychosis in PD (Poewe, 2003).

In addition to visual hallucinations, auditory hallucinations can present with PD. Inzelberg, Kipervasser, and Korczyn (1998) found that 8% of patients experienced auditory hallucinations accompanied by visual hallucinations, which were described as "nonimperative, nonparanoid, and often incomprehensible" (p. 533). Auditory hallucinations in the absence of visual hallucinations are extremely rare in this population. Unlike schizophrenia, auditory hallucinations in PD are seldom command in nature, though they can become part of a paranoid syndrome when experienced with delusions and delirium (Poewe, 2003). Tactile hallucinations, such as a sensation of crawling bugs on the skin, are much less common but can occur with PD-related psychosis. Additionally, gustatory hallucinations, involving false perceptions of smell, have been reported in isolated cases (Molho & Factor, 2005).

Delusions are not as common as visual hallucinations in PD, affecting up to 10% of patients, but generally constitute a much greater challenge and typically reflect advanced disease (Aarsland et al., 1999). Delusions can be defined as false and fixed beliefs that are based on incorrect inference (Molho & Factor, 2005). Delusional patients embrace these ideas, despite evidence to the contrary. In PD, delusions tend to be paranoid in nature, making treatment and care difficult. Chou et al. (2005) found that the most common delusional themes reported by PD patients included stealing, spousal infidelity, abandonment, and ideas that their spouses were imposters or that they were not in their own homes.

According to Weintraub and Stern (2005), psychotic syndromes in PD can be roughly categorized by two phenomenological groups. The first group is generally limited to visual illusions and hallucinations with no obvious delusions or advanced psychotic symptoms. These patients typically retain insight into the nature of hallucinations, are not troubled by the symptoms, and may not require treatment. The second group experiences a more complex psychotic syndrome that progresses to include threatening hallucinations, paranoid delusions, and related behavioral disturbances. Goetz, Fan, Leurgans, Bernard, and Stebbins (2006) recently argued that psychosis, specifically visual hallucinations, will progress in the vast majority of affected PD patients. It was recommended that the term *benign* be exchanged for *mild* when describing hallucinations experienced by the first phenomenological group, implying that these symptoms are at the beginning of a continuum.

Assessment and Diagnostic Considerations

Patients and family members are often hesitant to discuss symptoms of psychosis due to social stigmas and embarrassment. It is therefore important for the clinician to introduce these issues during routine evaluation and ask poignant but unstructured questions that will encourage discussion. It is helpful to be in a private and comfortable environment when broaching this subject. Unfortunately, a uniformly accepted rating scale does not yet exist to guide this interaction (Miyasaki et al., 2006). The Parkinsonian Psychosis Rating Scale was developed for use in one 6-week open-label study but has not been widely adopted in clinical practice (Ismail & Richard, 2004). If psychosis is suspected on interview, the clinician must attempt to uncover the nature, duration, and extent of disability associated with the presenting symptoms.

A complete diagnostic investigation, including laboratory tests, urinalysis, and other appropriate screens, should be considered to rule out an underlying pathology that may result in delirium. These conditions can include urinary tract infection, stroke, metabolic disturbances, dehydration, and pneumonia. The patient's medication profile should also be reviewed for consideration of drug-induced delirium. This is especially prudent given geriatric sensitivity to medications like anticholinergics, antihistamines, and pain suppressants. Presenting symptoms of psychosis and delirium can be indistinct and are difficult to differentiate without clinical delineation. Abrupt psychotic episodes without prior history commonly represent acute medical events that require immediate evaluation. Psychosis that presents early in disease accompanied by marked cognitive fluctuations and parkinsonian motor symptoms suggests the alternative diagnosis of DLB (McKeith et al., 2005). DLB is associated with a more rapid disease progression and limited levodopa benefit as compared to PD. Furthermore, the clinician must validate the presence of symptoms during wakefulness versus sleep. Hallucinations are often confused with vivid dreams, verbalizations, or movements during sleep, which typically represent a sleep disturbance like REM behavior disorder.

Management and Treatment

The treatment of psychosis in PD is complicated by the competing nature of neurotransmitter dysregulation. The clinician must be cognizant of the delicate balance between optimal motor control and management of psychosis. Traditionally, the first step of the treatment process is to simplify polypharmacy and eliminate potentially offensive agents. Anticholinergics, benzodiazepines, muscle relaxants, and anxiolytics can aggravate dementia and psychosis and should be reduced and discontinued, if possible (Rabinstein & Shulman, 2000). If symptoms persist, it may be necessary to target antiparkinsonian medications for discontinuation, starting with selegiline (Eldepryl) and amantadine (Symmetrel). Catechol-O-methyltransferase inhibitors and dopamine agonists should then be reduced or discontinued. Reduction of carbidopa/levodopa (Sinemet) should be reserved as a final measure (Poewe, 2003). During this process the clinician must monitor for motor exacerbation and the extent of disability produced by such adjustments.

The treatment of psychosis has sparked professional debate as not all clinicians apply medication reduction as the first-line approach. The basis for this argument surrounds the progressive pattern of psychosis in PD and the ultimate need for antipsychotic therapy. The alternative strategy is to initiate low-dose antipsychotic treatment immediately following symptom presentation. Conversely, some clinicians choose to monitor symptoms without intervention if they are rare and benign, deferring treatment until symptoms become problematic.

If antipsychotic therapy is necessary, typical antipsychotics are not recommended for the PD population given their significant extrapyramidal side effect profile (i.e., worsening of motor symptoms) (Weintraub & Stern, 2005). Unfortunately for PD patients, haloperidol (Haldol) and similar agents are still commonly used to treat agitation during hospitalization, which often results in marked motor deterioration. Atypical antipsychotics must also be used with caution due to the same risk of motor worsening and other adverse effects (i.e., weight gain, sedation, endocrine abnormalities, and increased mortality and strokes in elderly patients with dementia) (Friedman & Factor, 2000). The only atypical antipsychotic agent tested in large-scale, placebo-controlled clinical trials with favorable outcomes for psychosis in PD is clozapine (Clozaril; French Clozapine Study Group, 1999). Unfortunately, clozapine is associated with a slight (1% to 2%) risk of agranulocytosis and is therefore subject to regular blood monitoring and national pharmacy regulations. Thus the associated expense and impracticality of clozapine make it a second-line agent that is typically reserved for treatment-refractory patients. Quetiapine (Seroquel) has become the most commonly used antipsychotic in PD care based on clinical experience and several positive open-label trials. Quetiapine carries a lesser risk of parkinsonian exacerbation as compared to other atypical antipsychotics, with the exception of clozapine (Juncos et al., 2004). For these reasons, antipsychotic therapy is generally limited to quetiapine and clozapine, though some clinicians do employ other atypical antipsychotics. Additionally, some studies have suggested that cholinesterase inhibitors may also possess antipsychotic qualities and may be appropriate when treating PD with dementia and psychosis (Emre et al., 2004).

Nonpharmacological management of psychosis in PD focuses on the fundamental needs of patient and family education. Social stigmas and misconceptions must be addressed early to heed adjustment barriers. The general public does not have a proper understanding of psychosis and reverts to false, threatening ideas presented by multimedia. It is for these reasons that clear and accurate information is critical. Additionally, the clinician should teach the caregiver strategies that can be used in the home to minimize psychotic episodes and problematic behaviors. Regulating the environment may help prevent escalation of psychotic episodes and related behavioral disturbances. For example, increasing the lighting during the day and lowering the lighting at night may improve orientation and minimize excessive stimulation. Caregivers should also be reminded that confronting delusions can result in agitation and aggression. Instead, distraction and communication can promote a safe and therapeutic environment. Of greatest importance, caregivers must be prepared to deal with episodes that threaten their safety or the safety of the patient. It must be made known to the caregiver that calling 911 is an appropriate response and that emergency services are prepared to address such situations. Families dealing with psychosis in PD typically require greater professional and social guidance when considering available treatments, hospitalizations, and long-term care placement. Peer support is quite effective and can be encouraged via support group participation. See Table 4.5 for a quick reference guide to psychosis in PD.

TABLE 4.5 Quick Reference Guide: Psychosis in Parkinson's Disease

Key assessment questions	• Do you ever see, hear, feel, or smell things that may not be real? If so, are you bothered by these symptoms? When and how often do they occur?
	• Do you ever look at an object and see something different?
	• Does your loved one ever appear to be staring or talking into space? *(directed to the caregiver)*
	• Does your loved one convey unusual or bizarre ideas? *(directed to the caregiver)*
Applicable assessment tools	• Parkinson's Psychosis Rating Scale (PPRS)

(continued)

TABLE 4.5 *(continued)*

Differential diagnoses	• Delirium from an underlying medical condition
	• Drug-induced delirium
	• Dementia with Lewy bodies
	• REM behavior disorder
	• Idiopathic psychiatric disorder
Nonpharmacological approaches	• Patient and family education and supportive therapy
	• Educate caregivers on personal and environmental strategies that can minimize agitation surrounding the psychotic event
	• Support group participation
Pharmacological approaches	• Consider reducing and/or discontinuing offensive agents (e.g., anticholinergics, benzodiazepines, muscle relaxants, anxiolytics)
	• Consider reducing and/or discontinuing antiparkinsonian medications as tolerated (e.g., selegiline, amantadine, COMT inhibitors, dopamine agonists, levodopa)
	• Consider quetiapine (Seroquel) as first line agent
	• Consider starting clozapine (Clozaril) for refractory psychosis
	• Consider cholinesterase inhibitors for psychosis accompanied by dementia (e.g., donepezil [Aricept], rivastigmine [Exelon], galantamine [Reminyl or Razadyne])
Other considerations	• Initiate education of psychosis shortly after PD diagnosis
	• Screen for psychosis at every visit
	• Order diagnostic investigation
	• Assess patient and caregiver safety concerns
	• If using clozapine (Clozaril), follow guidelines for agranulocytosis monitoring
	• Consider psychiatric and social work consultations

IMPULSE CONTROL DISORDERS

Background

Impulse control disorders (ICDs) have most recently been recognized as a psychiatric phenomenon affecting the PD community. An ICD can be defined as the inability to resist an impulse, drive, or temptation that is potentially harmful to the individual or others. Over the last decade, ICDs have been associated with the use of dopaminergic medications, almost always dopamine agonists (Weintraub et al., 2006b). Current research estimates that 0.5% to 4.9% of PD patients develop ICDs, with greatest impact on men and young-onset patients (Driver-Dunckley, Samanta, & Stacy, 2003; Molina et al., 2000). ICDs can present as one primary fixation (e.g., gambling) or as multiple, coexisting fixations (e.g., gambling and hypersexuality).

The pathophysiology of ICDs in PD can be explained by the wide-reaching effects of dopamine replacement therapy. Dopaminergic agents, especially dopamine agonists, are known to stimulate areas beyond the targeted substantia nigra, including central dopaminergic pathways. These pathways regulate the brain's reward circuit and mediate aspects of impulsivity. When these areas are overstimulated, they can trigger a hedonistic homeostatic dysregulation similar to basic addiction (Giovannoni, O'Sullivan, Turner, Manson, & Lees, 2000).

Symptom Presentation

ICDs can include, but are not limited to, pathological gambling; pathological eating; pathological shopping; hypersexuality; and repetitive, purposeless motor tasks known as *punding* (Evans et al., 2004; Weintraub & Potenza, 2006). Consequently, patients may exhibit signs of social withdrawal, embarrassment, agitation, weight loss or gain, appetite changes, depression, and anxiety. Many times, there are no signs but only symptoms of the ICD, which the patient may be hesitant to reveal and discuss due to confusion and embarrassment.

Assessment and Diagnostic Considerations

Many patients and families remain uneducated about the risk of ICDs and therefore do not consider a possible relationship to PD therapy. Furthermore, many clinicians underestimate the prevalence of ICDs in the PD community and fail to assess this issue in the context of routine clinical care. Combined, these factors cultivate the progression of ICDs and result in catastrophic social impact. It is not uncommon for affected PD patients to report losing their life or retirement savings as a result of pathological gambling.

The most critical element in the assessment of ICDs is problem-focused questions. Do you currently gamble? Do you find it difficult to overcome insensible urges? Is there anything about your behavior that is concerning to you or your caregiver? Often, family members will intervene with specific examples, observations, and concerns. If there is suspicion of an ICD, the clinician should further inquire about the history and duration of symptoms, the nature of the fixation, and social consequences. Screening instruments for one or more of these disorders can also be valuable, such as the Minnesota Impulsive Disorders Interview, the South Oaks Gambling Screen, and the Early Intervention Gambling Health Test (Weintraub et al., 2006a).

Management and Treatment

Management of ICDs requires a multifaceted and individualized approach with a strong educational component. Owing to the novelty of ICDs in PD, there is no current research to guide treatment recommendations. Anecdotally, it is suggested that the offending drug be reduced or discontinued. If the patient is treated with a dopamine agonist, it is routinely effective to lower the dosage, switch to another agonist, or revert to levodopa monotherapy. In rare cases when levodopa is the suspected offender, the clinician may choose to reduce the dose, while aiming to preserve motor control. At times, it may be necessary to sacrifice slight motor exacerbation for resolution of problematic behaviors. SSRIs and atypical antipsychotics have been proposed for mood stabilization associated with ICDs, however, there are no empirical data to support these interventions in PD (Weintraub et al., 2006a).

In addition to pharmacological strategies, behavioral modification should be discussed with patients and families. For example, exposure to casinos and lotteries should be restricted for patients with gambling fixations. Families may also choose to restrict access to banking accounts, credit cards, stock market and retirement accounts, and cash until the syndrome has fully resolved. It is especially important to appreciate the position of family members, who often require a great deal of professional guidance and support in dealing with these socially sensitive behavioral

TABLE 4.6 Quick Reference Guide: Impulse Control Disorders in Parkinson's Disease

Key assessment questions[a]	• Do you find it difficult to overcome an impulse or temptation?
	• Do you currently gamble? If so, do you find it difficult to control the urge to gamble?
	• Do you experience sexually preoccupied thoughts or urges?
	• Do you find yourself performing repetitive actions?
Applicable assessment tools	• Minnesota Impulsive Disorders Interview (MIDI)
	• South Oaks Gambling Screen
	• Early Intervention Gambling Health Test
Differential diagnoses	• Bipolar disorder/mania
	• Substance abuse
	• Obsessive–compulsive disorder
Nonpharmacological approaches	• Patient and family education and supportive therapy
	• Psychotherapy
	• Support group participation
	• Community resources (e.g., Gamblers Anonymous)
Pharmacological approaches	• Reduce dopaminergic exposure as tolerated
	• Consider use of SSRIs or antipsychotics for mood stabilization
Other considerations	• Initiate education of ICDs when dopaminergic treatment is introduced
	• Screen for ICDs at every visit
	• Consider psychiatric consultation

[a]Questions can also be directed to the caregiver with the patient's consent.

issues. This is especially true for caregivers dealing with verbal and physical abuse from sexually inappropriate patients. Clinicians can suggest psychotherapy, community resources (e.g., Gamblers Anonymous), and support group participation as additional measures to cope with ICDs. See Table 4.6 for a quick reference guide to ICDs in PD.

IN SUMMARY—THE ROLE OF THE NURSE IN THE PSYCHIATRIC REALM OF PD: EDUCATOR, CLINICIAN, ADVOCATE

Educator

Historically, patients and families turn to nurses for education and guidance infused with compassion and practicality. This is especially true of the Parkinson community, with education serving as a primary nursing responsibility due to the many facets of this chronic disease. It is generally nurses who bridge the gap between medical complexities and lay comprehension.

Psychoeducation should be introduced in the early stages of PD. Educated patients and families will be prepared when and if psychiatric illness presents and will ease the task of exclusive clinical detection. Comprehensive education will also lessen the force of psychiatric stigmas that create barriers for discussion, diagnosis, and treatment. It is crucial that the patient and family recognize the biological influences of psychiatric illness and challenge labels such as *crazy* or *mad*. The nurse may choose to share the metaphor that depression is like diabetes, both resulting from chemical imbalances that cannot be willfully controlled by the patient. It is also important to reinforce the relationship between mental health complications and PD versus the emergence of an idiopathic psychiatric condition. Individuals and families affected by dementia commonly assume that the patient suffers from AD in addition to PD, which is inaccurate for most cases. The nurse must be cognizant of personal, ethical, cultural, and religious beliefs surrounding mental health issues and should introduce this discussion in a meaningful and individualized manner.

Nurses can refer to nonprofit PD organizations for materials and resources to augment the education process. The National Parkinson Foundation offers a comprehensive handbook on the neuropsychiatric issues of PD titled *Parkinson's Disease: Mind, Mood, and Memory* that is designed for the lay community (Martine & Duda, 2004). These types of materials can serve as valuable take-home references for patients and families. In summary, nurses will find that disease education, practical advice, and family involvement are critical in the treatment of psychiatric illness in PD.

Clinician

As clinicians, nurses share the duty of evaluating, treating, and managing the neuropsychiatric complications of PD. The nurse–patient relationship, often centered on trust and rapport, allows the nurse to explore and uncover these sensitive areas of disease. Empathy, acceptance, and honesty will facilitate comprehensive assessment and successful treatment.

The nurse should conceptualize each unique case based on psychiatric history, psychosocial factors, and personality profile. By gaining an understanding of the person, the nurse can see beyond the patient role and appreciate the universal impact of psychiatric illness. The nurse may find that simple conversation will naturally disclose the presenting issues and eliminate the need for a forced interview.

The process of formal psychiatric assessment is often unnerving for PD patients, many of whom have no prior experience with this area of health care. The nurse should fully explain the purpose of all inquiries and tests prior to initiating evaluation. Time must also be allowed for patients and families to discuss their own concerns and questions. Additionally, the nurse can facilitate referrals to multidisciplinary providers, such as a psychiatrist, psychotherapist, neuropsychologist, and social worker.

In addition to collaborating with physician colleagues on treatment strategies, the nurse should encourage incorporation of nonpharmacological modalities. These unconventional management strategies typically require strong endorsement and education before they are accepted by patients and families. Physical exercise, relaxation techniques, massage, yoga, acupuncture, tai chi, support group participation, and psychotherapy can be powerful influences in the stabilization of mental health. As PD progresses and psychiatric symptoms become less responsive to medication, the nurse should institute palliative care. This model focuses on comfort, pain relief, and enhancement of quality of life. Interventions surrounding advanced psychiatric illness include home health assistance, hospice services, home safety services (e.g., Lifeline), guidance on long-term care options, and caregiver counseling.

Advocate

Owing to the novelty of psychiatric complications in PD, the nurse must ensure that these issues are properly acknowledged and addressed for each and every patient. Unfortunately, research continues to validate the need for better recognition and understanding of psychiatric illness associated with parkinsonism. As suggested by Shulman et al. (2002), even movement disorder specialists struggle to incorporate this aspect of disease into routine clinical care. By educating patients, families, and fellow providers, nurses can accelerate the rate at which mental health awareness is embraced by the global health care community.

The psychiatric complications of PD quickly become the primary concern of affected patients and families, overshadowing the effects of motor disease. Disability stemming from mental illness is often severe, resulting in marital and family distress, social isolation, impaired safety, poor hygiene and self-care, and exacerbation of motor disease. These issues significantly impact quality of life and the overall burden afflicted by PD.

The greatest role a nurse can serve is that of patient advocate. This is achieved by appreciating the patient experience, discussing the patient's health care wishes, protecting the patient's rights and dignity, and serving as a liaison between the patient, family, and health care team. Mental illness, whether exclusive or in conjunction with neurological disease, warrants a strong nursing presence and partnership.

REFERENCES

Aarsland, D., Andersen, K., Larsen, J. P., Lolk, A., & Kragh-Sorensen, P. (2003). Prevalence and characteristics of dementia in Parkinson disease: An 8-year prospective study. *Archives of Neurology, 60,* 387–392.

Aarsland, D., Andersen, K., Larsen, J. P., Lolk, A., Nielsen, H., & Kragh-Sorensen, P. (2001). Risk of dementia in Parkinson's disease: A community-based, prospective study. *Neurology, 56,* 730–736.

Aarsland, D., Laake, K., Larsen, J. P., & Janvin, C. (2002). Donepezil for cognitive impairment in Parkinson's disease: A randomised controlled study. *Journal of Neurology, Neurosurgery, and Psychiatry, 72,* 708–712.

Aarsland, D., Larsen, J. P., Cummins, J. L., & Laake, K. (1999). Prevalence and clinical correlates of psychotic symptoms in Parkinson disease: A community-based study. *Archives of Neurology, 56,* 595–601.

Aarsland, D., Mosimann, U. P., & McKeith, I. G. (2004). Role of cholinesterase inhibitors in Parkinson's disease and dementia with Lewy bodies. *Journal of Geriatric Psychiatry and Neurology, 17,* 164–171.

Allott, R., Wells, A., Morrison, A. P., & Walker, R. (2005). Distress in Parkinson's disease: Contributions of disease factors and metacognitive style. *British Journal of Psychiatry, 187,* 182–183.

American Psychiatric Association. (1994a). Anxiety disorders. In *Diagnostic and statistical manual of mental disorders* (4th ed., pp. 393–444). Washington, DC: Author.

American Psychiatric Association. (1994b). *Diagnostic and statistical manual of mental disorders* (4th ed.). Washington, DC: Author.

Anderson, K. E., & Weiner, W. J. (2002). Psychiatric symptoms in Parkinson's disease. *Current Neurology and Neuroscience Report, 2,* 303–309.

Bower, J., Grossardt, B., Maraganore, M., Ahlskog, J., de Andrade, M., & Rocca, W. (2005). The Mayo Clinic Cohort Study of Personality and Aging: Results for Parkinson's disease. *Neurology, 64*(Suppl. 1), A282–A283.

Bronnick, K., Ehrt, U., Emre, M., De Deyn, P. P., Wesnes, K., Tekin, S., et al. (2006). Attentional deficits affect activities of daily living in dementia associated with PD. *Journal of Neurology, Neurosurgery, and Psychiatry, 77,* 1136–1142.

Burn, D. J., & McKeith, I. G. (2003). Current treatment of dementia with Lewy bodies and dementia associated with Parkinson's disease. *Movement Disorders, 18*(Suppl. 6), 72–79.

Cahn-Weiner, D. A., Grace, J., Ott, B. R., Fernandez, H. H., & Friedman, J. H. (2002). Cognitive and behavioral features discriminate between Alzheimer's and Parkinson's disease. *Neuropsychiatry, Neuropsychology, and Behavioral Neurology, 15,* 79–87.

Chou, K. L., Messing, S., Oakes, D., Feldman, P. D., Breier, A., Friedman, J. H. (2005). Drug induced psychosis in Parkinson disease: Phenomenology and correlations among psychosis rating instruments. *Clinical Neuropharmacology, 28,* 215–219.

Cole, K., & Vaughn, F. L. (2005). The feasibility of using cognitive behaviour therapy for depression associated with Parkinson's disease: A literature review. *Parkinsonism and Related Disorders, 11,* 269–276.

Driver-Dunckley, E., Samanta, J., & Stacy, M. (2003). Pathological gambling associated with dopamine agonist therapy in Parkinson's disease. *Neurology, 61,* 422–423.

Emre, M. (2003). What causes mental dysfunction in Parkinson's disease? *Movement Disorders, 18*(Suppl. 6), 63–71.

Emre, M., Aarsland, D., Albanese, A., Byrne, E. J., Deuschl, G., De Deyn, P. P., et al. (2004). Rivastigmine for dementia associated with Parkinson's disease. *New England Journal of Medicine, 351,* 2509–2518.

Evans, A. H., Katzenschlager, R., Paviour, D., O'Sullivan, J. D., Appel, S., Lawrence, A. D., et al. (2004). Punding in Parkinson's disease: Its relation to the dopamine dysregulation syndrome. *Movement Disorders, 19,* 397–405.

French Clozapine Study Group. (1999). Clozapine in drug-induced psychosis in Parkinson's disease: The French Clozapine Parkinson Study Group. *Lancet, 353,* 2041–2042.

Friedman, J. H., & Factor, S. A. (2000). Atypical antipsychotics in the treatment of drug-induced psychosis in Parkinson's disease. *Movement Disorders, 15,* 201–211.

Giovannoni, G., O'Sullivan, J. D., Turner, K., Manson, A. J., & Lees, A. J. (2000). Hedonistic homeostatic dysregulation in patients with Parkinson's disease on dopamine replacement therapies. *Journal of Neurology, Neurosurgery, and Psychiatry, 68,* 423–428.

Goetz, C. G., Fan, W., Leurgans, S., Bernard, B., & Stebbins, G. T. (2006). The malignant course of "benign hallucinations" in Parkinson disease. *Archives of Neurology, 63,* 713–716.

Goetz, C. G., & Stebbins, G. T. (1995). Mortality and hallucinations in nursing home patients with advanced Parkinson's disease. *Neurology, 45,* 669–671.

Henderson, R., Kurlan, R., Kersun, J. M., & Como, P. (1992). Preliminary examination of the comorbidity of anxiety and depression in Parkinson's disease. *Journal of Neuropsychiatry and Clinical Neuroscience, 4,* 257–264.

Inzelberg, R., Kipervasser, S., & Korczyn, A. D. (1998). Auditory hallucinations in Parkinson's disease. *Journal of Neurology, Neurosurgery, and Psychiatry, 64,* 533–535.

Isella, V., Melzi, P., Grimaldi, M., Iurlaro, S., Piolti, R., Ferrarese, C., et al. (2002). Clinical, neuropsychological, and morphometric correlates of apathy in Parkinson's disease. *Movement Disorders, 17,* 366–371.

Ishihara, L., & Brayne, C. (2006). What is the evidence for a premorbid parkinsonian personality: A systematic review. *Movement Disorders, 21,* 1066–1072.

Ismail, M. S., & Richard, I. H. (2004). A reality test: How well do we understand psychosis in Parkinson's disease? *Journal of Neuropsychiatry and Clinical Neuroscience, 16,* 8–18.

Jetty, P. V., Charney, D. S., & Goddard, A. W. (2001). Neurobiology of generalized anxiety disorder. *Psychiatry Clinics of North America, 24,* 75–97.

Juncos, J. L., Roberts, V. J., Evatt, M. L., Jewart, R. D., Wood, C. D., Potter, L. S., et al. (2004). Quetiapine improves psychotic symptoms and cognition in Parkinson's disease. *Movement Disorders, 19,* 29–35.

Kirsch-Darrow, L., Fernandez, H. F., Marsiske, M., Okun, M. S., & Bowers, D. (2006). Dissociating apathy and depression in Parkinson disease. *Neurology, 67,* 33–38.

Krupp, B. H. (1997). Ethical considerations in apathy syndromes. *Psychiatric Annals, 27,* 50–54.

Lauterbach, E. C., & Duvoisin, R. C. (1991). Anxiety disorders in familial parkinsonism. *American Journal of Psychiatry, 148,* 274.

Leroi, I., Brandt, J., Reich, S. G., Lyketsos, C. G., Grill, S., Thompson, R., et al. (2004). Randomized placebo-controlled trial of donepezil in cognitive impairment in Parkinson's disease. *International Journal of Geriatric Psychiatry, 19,* 1–8.

Marin, R. S., Biedrzycki, R. C., & Firinciogullari, S. (1991). Reliability and validity of the Apathy Evaluation Scale. *Psychiatry Research, 38,* 143–162.

Marin, R. S., Fogel, B. S., Hawkins, J., Duffy, J., & Krupp, B. (1995). Apathy: A treatable syndrome. *Journal of Neuropsychiatry and Clinical Neuroscience, 7,* 23–30.

Marsh, L. (2000a). Anxiety disorders in Parkinson's disease. *International Review of Psychiatry, 12,* 307–319.

Marsh, L. (2000b). Neuropsychiatric aspects of Parkinson's disease. *Psychosomatics, 41,*15–23.

Marsh, L., Williams, J. R., Rocco, M., Grill, S., Munro, C., & Dawson, T. M. (2004). Psychiatric comorbidities in patients with Parkinson disease and psychosis. *Neurology, 63,* 293–300.

Martine, R., & Duda, J. E. (Eds.). (2004). *Parkinson's disease: Mind, mood, and memory.* Miami, FL: National Parkinson Foundation.

McKeith, I. G., Dickson, D. W., Lowe, J., Emre, M., O'Brien, J. T., Feldman, H., et al. (2005). Diagnosis and management of dementia with Lewy bodies: Third report of the DLB Consortium. *Neurology, 65,* 1863–1872.

Menza, M. A., Robertson-Hoffman, D. E., & Bonapace, A. S. (1993). Parkinson's disease and anxiety: Comorbidity with depression. *Biological Psychiatry, 34,* 465–470.

Merschdorf, U., Berg, D., Csoti, I., Fornadi, F., Merz, B., Naumann, M., et al. (2003). Psychopathological symptoms of depression in Parkinson's disease compared to major depression. *Psychopathology, 36,* 221–225.

Minett, T. S., Thomas, A., Wilkinson, L. M., Daniel, S. L., Sanders, J., Richardson, J., et al. (2003). What happens when donepezil is suddenly withdrawn? An open label trial in dementia with Lewy bodies and Parkinson's disease with dementia. *International Journal of Geriatric Psychiatry, 18,* 988–993.

Miyasaki, J. M., Shannon, K., Voon, V., Ravina, B., Kleiner-Fisman, G., Anderson, K., et al. (2006). Practice Parameter: Evaluation and treatment of depression, psychosis, and dementia in Parkinson disease (an evidence-based review): Report of the Quality Standards Subcommittee of the American Academy of Neurology. *Neurology, 66,* 996–1002.

Moellentine, C., Rummans, T., Ahlskog, J. E., Harmsen, W. S., Suman, V. J., O'Connor, M. K., et al. (1998). Effectiveness of ECT in patients with parkinsonism. *Journal of Neuropsychiatry and Clinical Neuroscience, 10,* 187–193.

Molho, E., & Factor, S. (2005). Psychosis. In R. Pfeiffer & I. Bodis-Wollner (Eds.), *Parkinson's disease and nonmotor dysfunction* (pp. 49–74). Totowa, NJ: Humana Press.

Molina, J. A., Sainz-Artiga, M. J., Fraile, A., Jimenez-Jimenez, F. J., Villanueva, C., Orti-Pareja, M., et al. (2000). Pathologic gambling in Parkinson's disease: A behavioral manifestation of pharmacologic treatment? *Movement Disorders, 15,* 869–872.

Moskovitz, C., Moses, H., III, & Klawans, H. L. (1978). Levodopa-induced psychosis: A kindling phenomenon. *American Journal of Psychiatry, 135,* 669–675.

Noe, E., Marder, K., Bell, K. L., Jacobs, D. M., Manly, J. J., & Stern, Y. (2004). Comparison of dementia with Lewy bodies to Alzheimer's disease and Parkinson's disease with dementia. *Movement Disorders, 19,* 60–67.

Parkinson, J. (1817). *An essay on the shaking palsy.* London: Neely and Jones.

Pillon, B., Boller, F., Levy, R., & Dubois, B. (2001). Cognitive deficits and dementia in Parkinson's disease. In F. Boller & S. Cappa (Eds.), *Handbook of neuropsychology* (pp. 311–371). Amsterdam: Elsevier.

Pluck, G. C., & Brown, R. G. (2002). Apathy in Parkinson's disease. *Journal of Neurology, Neurosurgery, and Psychiatry, 73,* 636–642.

Poewe, W. (2003). Psychosis in Parkinson's disease. *Movement Disorders, 18*(Suppl. 6), 80–87.

Poewe, W., Karamat, E., Kemmler, G. W., & Gerstenbrand, F. (1990). The premorbid personality of patients with Parkinson's disease: A comparative study with healthy controls and patients with essential tremor. *Advances in Neurology, 53,* 339–342.

Rabinstein, A. A., & Shulman, L. M. (2000). Management of behavioral and psychiatric problems in Parkinson's disease. *Parkinsonism and Related Disorders, 7,* 41–50.

Rascol, O., Payoux, P., Ferreira, J., & Brefel-Courbon, C. (2002). The management of patients with early Parkinson's disease. *Parkinsonism & Related Disorders, 9(1),* 61–67.

Rektorova, I., Rektor, I., Bares, M., Dostal, V., Ehler, E., Fanfrdlova, Z., et al. (2003). Pramipexole and pergolide in the treatment of depression in Parkinson's disease: A national multicentre prospective randomized study. *European Journal of Neurology, 10,* 399–406.

Richard, I. H. (2006). Apathy does not equal depression in Parkinson disease: Why we should care. *Neurology, 67,* 10–11.

Shulman, L. M., Taback, R. L., Rabinstein, A. A., & Weiner, W. J. (2002). Nonrecognition of depression and other non-motor symptoms in Parkinson's disease. *Parkinsonism and Related Disorders, 8,* 193–197.

Starkstein, S. E., Mayberg, H. S., Preziosi, T. J., Andrezejewski, P., Leiguarda, R., & Robinson, R. G. (1992). Reliability, validity, and clinical correlates of apathy in Parkinson's disease. *Journal of Neuropsychiatry and Clinical Neuroscience, 4,* 134–139.

Stein, M. B., Heuser, I. J., Juncos, J. L., & Uhde, T. W. (1990). Anxiety disorders in patients with Parkinson's disease. *American Journal of Psychiatry, 147,* 217–220.

Thanvi, B. R., Munshi, S. K., Vijaykumar, N., & Lo, T. C. (2003). Neuropsychiatric non-motor aspects of Parkinson's disease. *Postgraduate Medical Journal, 79,* 561–565.

Turvey, C. L., Conwell, Y., Jones, M. P., Phillips, C., Simonsick, E., Pearson, J. L., et al. (2002). Risk factors for late-life suicide: A prospective, community-based study. *American Journal of Geriatric Psychiatry, 10,* 398–406.

Vazquez, A., Jimenez-Jimenez, F. J., Garcia-Ruiz, P., & Garcia-Urra, D. (1993). "Panic attacks" in Parkinson's disease: A long-term complication of levodopa therapy. *ACTA Neurologica Scandinavica, 87,* 14–18.

Weintraub, D., Moberg, P. J., Duda, J. E., Katz, I. R., & Stern, M. B. (2003). Recognition and treatment of depression in Parkinson's disease. *Journal of Geriatric Psychiatry and Neurology, 16,* 178–183.

Weintraub, D., Moberg, P. J., Duda, J. E., Katz, I. R., & Stern, M. B. (2004). Effect of psychiatric and other nonmotor symptoms on disability in Parkinson's disease. *Journal of the American Geriatric Society, 52,* 784–788.

Weintraub, D., Oehlberg, K. A., Katz, I. R., & Stern, M. B. (2006a). Test characteristics of the 15-item geriatric depression scale and Hamilton depression rating scale in Parkinson disease. *American Journal of Geriatric Psychiatry, 14,* 169–175.

Weintraub, D., & Potenza, M. N. (2006). Impulse control disorders in Parkinson's disease. *Current Neurology and Neuroscience Report, 6,* 302–306.

Weintraub, D., Siderowf, A. D., Potenza, M. N., Goveas, J., Morales, K. H., Duda, J. E., et al. (2006b). Association of dopamine agonist use with impulse control disorders in Parkinson disease. *Archives of Neurology, 63,* 969–973.

Weintraub, D., & Stern, M. B. (2005). Psychiatric complications in Parkinson disease. *American Journal of Geriatric Psychiatry, 13,* 844–851.

5

Nonmotor Complications in Parkinson's Disease

Constance Ward, MSN, RN, BC, CNRN
Lisette Bunting-Perry, MScN, RN
Julia E. Howard, CCC-SLP
Rebecca Martine, APRN, CS, BC
Jacqueline H. Rick, PhD

HISTORICAL OVERVIEW AND SIGNIFICANCE OF NONMOTOR SYMPTOMS

Parkinson's disease (PD) is a chronic, progressive, neurodegenerative loss of neurons and the neurotransmitter dopamine, which is housed within the substantia nigra of the basal ganglia. The disease is characterized by a combination of tremor, rigidity, bradykinesia, and postural instability (motor symptoms); however, nonmotor symptoms also accompany PD. The clinical features of PD can be categorized as motor, nonmotor, and neuropsychiatric. In 1817, a British physician, Dr. James Parkinson, reported on the symptoms of several of his patients in his monograph *An Essay on the Shaking Palsy* and touched on symptoms that extended beyond the prominent motor presentation of parkinsonism. Dr. J. M. Charcot later expanded on this description by elaborating on the more subtle emotional and physical nuances of the disease and named the disease Parkinson's (Duvoisin, 1987). Some hundred years after Charcot's work, these secondary manifestations have been properly classified as the nonmotor phenomenology of PD. As suggested by its title, the nonmotor subset includes all symptoms that are not regulated by the motor system. This encompasses a wide spectrum of psychiatric, sensory, autonomic, sleep, gastrointestinal, visual, and olfactory dysfunction.

PD is primarily recognized as a motor disease. However, PD has very prominent nonmotor symptoms that can, at times, be more disabling than the motor components of the disease (Shulman, Taback, Rabinstein, & Weiner, 2002). Unfortunately, nonmotor symptoms are both underrecognized and undertreated during routine neurology visits (Shulman et al., 2002). Nonmotor symptoms significantly contribute to the patient's overall disability and are negatively associated with patient and caregiver quality of life (Thanvi, Munshi, Vijaykumar, & Lo, 2003; Willson, Bunting-Perry, Arzbaecher, Vernon, & Moskowitz, 2004). It is now understood that nonmotor symptoms occur early in the disease and can fluctuate with the dopaminergic medication cycles (Jankovic, 2002). Nonmotor symptoms of PD have received limited attention from a clinical and research standpoint but have been identified as a leading cause of impairment and poor quality of life for the Parkinson community. In fact, patients often describe nonmotor complications as more disruptive and problematic than motor symptoms. It has taken experts some time to fully appreciate the impact of nonmotor symptoms, however, notable strides have been taken over the past decade to acknowledge, diagnose, and manage these complex aspects of PD.

Nonmotor complications span across many biological systems and can result from pathological changes as well as adverse effects of pharmacology. The progressive neuronal pathology occurring in PD imparts global normal function, thereby disregulating other neurological functions and regulatory systems. This diffuse neurodegenerative process has the potential to cause nondopaminergic disruptions and manifestations. For example, while dopamine depletion remains the precursor for neurotransmitter dysregulation in PD, acetylcholine, serotonin, and norepinephrine levels can be subsequently affected. Additionally, dopaminergic medications can improve but also exacerbate nonmotor symptoms. Conventional PD treatment may stimulate nondopaminergic pathways that do not respond predictably to dopaminergic therapy (Weintraub & Stern, 2005). It is for all these reasons that the understanding of nonmotor complications of PD therapy have evolved.

Like motor symptoms, nonmotor symptoms can fluctuate according to sustained levodopa levels. Pain, confusion, sadness, and lower urinary tract symptoms can come and go throughout the day relative to dopaminergic medication dosing. Again, these nonmotor symptoms are often reported by patients as more distressing and embarrassing when compared to motor symptoms and are especially problematic when nonmotor symptoms are intermittent and unpredictable (Jankovic, 2002).

In this chapter we will further examine nonmotor complications, discuss their etiology and pathology, and most importantly, acknowledge how nurses can intervene and directly impact quality of life for PD patients. Nonmotor symptoms of PD require poignant discussion and education with persons living with PD (PLWP) and their family members. Nurses are often first-line providers who are in a unique position to uncover and address these obscure yet significant symptoms.

AUTONOMIC NERVOUS SYSTEM (ANS) CHANGES IN PARKINSON'S DISEASE (PD)

Nonmotor symptoms in PD fall under three categories:

- Nonmotor symptoms *with* autonomic nervous system involvement
- Nonmotor symptoms *without* autonomic nervous system involvement
- Neuropsychiatric symptoms (see chapter 4)

Autonomic dysfunction impacts 90% of PLWP and may lead to considerable disability and poor quality of life (Stern, Horn, Kleiner-Fisman, & Weintraub, 2006). Parkinson-related abnormalities of the ANS involve abnormal activation of the parasympathetic and sympathetic systems, producing constipation, delayed gastric emptying, urinary retention, erectile dysfunction, orthostasis, and heat and cold intolerance (Hanak, 1992).

The pathophysiology of PD produces degenerative changes in the ANS, motor, and neuropsychiatric systems. The autonomic nervous system regulates the following:

- Respiration
- Heart rate
- Contraction and dilation of blood vessels
- Body temperature
- Gastrointestinal function
- Sexual function
- Internal organ function.

ANS dysfunction can result in the following symptoms:

- Constipation
- Dysphagia
- Orthostatic hypotension
- Sialorrhea (drooling)
- Sexual dysfunction
- Sweating and thermoregulation
- Syncope and presyncope
- Urinary and bladder dysfunction

Dysregulation of the ANS can result in troublesome symptoms for many PLWP. Rarely occurring in early PD, ANS symptoms are seen early in the Parkinson's plus population. Unfortunately, many of the medications used to treat PD also have autonomic side effects and can confound ANS dysfunction in PLWP.

In Parkinson's plus syndromes, ANS dysfunction symptoms are frequently more severe than ANS symptoms seen in PD. For example, progressive supranuclear palsy (PSP) is differentiated from PD by ataxic gait, frequent and early falls, and paralysis of the eye's downward gaze (Ward, 2006a). Many of the Parkinson's plus syndromes initially are diagnosed as PD, However, symptoms progress with ANS dysregulation, and another diagnosis evolves such as PSP, multiple system atrophy (MSA), or corticobasal degeneration (CBD).

In CBD, there is asymmetrical limb rigidity, postural imbalance, apraxia, and cortical dementia early in the disease course, unlike PD. This disorder is also called the *alien limb phenomenon* because the limb, such as the arm, can act completely independently and levitate rigidly, holding itself extended for long periods of time. Approximately 50% of all CBD patients exhibit this levitation phenomenon at some point in their disease process (Kumar, Bergeron, & Lang, 2002).

MSA includes syndromes in which the symptoms are progressive and have severe autonomic dysfunction, unlike PD. These syndromes include Shy-Drager syndrome, olivopontocerebellar atrophy, and striatonigral degeneration, which display bowel and bladder incontinence, severe hypotension that necessitates treatment to maintain an organ-perfusable blood pressure, sexual dysfunction, and an overall rapid decline in the ability to perform activities of daily living and quality of life (Ward, 2006a).

Parkinson's plus syndromes are accompanied by significant morbidity and mortality. Patients diagnosed with Parkinson's plus syndromes have a trajectory of approximately 10 years from diagnosis to death. However, Parkinson's plus syndromes are amenable to palliative care.

Constipation

Constipation is a complaint of many PLWP. The National Parkinson Foundation (NPF) reports that approximately 70% of PLWP suffer from constipation (NPF, 2003a). PD can cause the nerves in the colon to degenerate, slowing the passage of stool through the large intestine, creating gastric hypokinesis. This results in delayed gastric motility, emptying and reflux with difficult defecation. This can be a chronic problem for PLWP. Likewise, dystonias in the pelvis may contribute to fecal impactions (NPF, 2003a). Motor activities of the intestine are regulated by the ANS, and adequate management of constipation is must be based on prevention. The etiology of constipation is multifactorial due to disease, lack of dietary fiber, inadequate fluid intake, lack of exercise, aging, antiparkinsonian medications, and in many cases other comorbidities.

Likewise, numerous medications used to treat PD can contribute to constipation. For most people, the anticholinergics are the most likely to cause constipation. Stopping medication such as anticholinergics, amantadine, carbidopa/levodopa, and dopamine agonists to prevent constipation may not be realistic. Therefore lifestyle changes should include ways to prevent the occurrence of constipation.

A high-fiber diet, hydration, exercise, and regular toileting schedules can aid in preventing constipation. Bulk agents and laxatives may be prescribed, along with stool softeners. Psyllium and docusates are effective within 1–3 days; diphylmethane cathartics work within 8 hours; and milk of magnesia is generally effective on the day of administration. Enemas may be required for severe constipation. However, enemas should be used judiciously (NPF, 2003a).

The National Parkinson Foundation (2003b) recommends a proven prune juice cocktail:

Mix ½ cup applesauce, 2 tablespoons Millers' wheat bran and 4–6 ounces prune juice. Drink each day to prevent constipation. (p. 18)

There are many variations on the quantities of the above ingredients that patients use to thicken the cocktail to a oatmeal-like consistency. This, too, works to prevent constipation.

Dysphagia

Swallowing disturbances may impact up to 95% of PLWP. PD produces changes in the oropharyngeal musculature and reduces sensory awareness, which impacts the safety and effectiveness of swallowing. Decreased sensory awareness in PLWP can result in lower appreciation of difficulty swallowing as compared to older adults without PD. Moreover, PLWP are more likely to experience silent aspiration or aspiration without triggering a spontaneous protective cough response.

Swallowing occurs in three phases, namely the oral phase, the pharyngeal phase, and the esophageal phase. *Dysphagia* is a term that refers to abnormality anywhere during the process of swallowing. Swallowing disturbances in PD may occur at any one swallowing phase or during a combination of phases. Some common oral phase symptoms include drooling or anterior spillage of a bolus. Other common oral symptoms are reduced oral transit time and reduced initiation of lingual movement. PLWP may demonstrate a very characteristic tongue pumping and repetitive anterior–posterior tongue-rolling pattern. Pharyngeal disturbances may include a delay in the swallow trigger, pharyngeal residue, and incomplete airway closure. These disturbances put the PLWP at risk for aspiration and potentially life-threatening pneumonia. The person with PD may also demonstrate reduced esophageal peristalsis, which may cause a sensation of food sticking in the esophagus or throat (Yorkston, Miller, & Strand, 2004).

A speech language pathologist may evaluate the swallowing function using a variety of methods. First, a thorough interview should help identify the patient's complaints and establish any patterns of swallowing difficulty. A clinical swallow examination consists of feeding the person a variety of food and liquid consistencies while palpating the swallow mechanism and listening carefully for any subtle clinical signs of aspiration. A modified barium swallow study, synonymous with video fluoroscopic swallowing evaluation, consists of feeding the patient a variety of foods and liquids while watching the function under video fluoroscopy. Video fluoroscopy helps not only to identify definitively the presence or absence of dysphagia, but also to identify more accurately the exact point during the swallowing process at which dysfunction occurs; thus results from fluoroscopy testing can be used in planning appropriate treatment. If a patient has severe postural changes, a fiber-optic endoscopic evaluation of swallowing (FEES) may be appropriate. A FEES consists of passing a fiber-optic scope through the patient's nostril to directly visualize the upper airway. This test is especially useful in patients with stooped posture who cannot sit upright for a modified barium swallow or who are too large to fit into the video fluoroscopy machine (Logemann, 1998).

Treatment of swallowing disturbances in PLWP relies largely on dietary alterations and compensatory strategies. A certified speech language pathologist will be able to establish specific modifications based on the type and severity of dysphagia. Examples of dietary modifications include using thickened liquids, which are more cohesive than regular liquids to compensate for reduced airway closure. Also, PLWP may need to eat soft or pureed foods to facilitate mastication and posterior propulsion of the bolus. Examples of compensatory techniques include volitionally coughing to clear any aspirate or volitionally completing a double swallow to clear any pharyngeal residue. Specific postures while feeding can also help to improve swallowing safety. In patients with very severe dysphagia, eventually, a percutaneous endoscopic gastrostomy tube may be needed to provide primary or supplementary nutrition and hydration (Logemann, 1998).

Some areas of ongoing and future research into the treatment of swallowing disorders in PLWP include examining the use of electrical stimulation to improve function and examining if improvements in respiratory support from Lee Silverman Voice Treatment (LSVT) can translate into improvements in swallowing. LSVT is a voice treatment that was developed using elements of neurology, physiology, motor learning, muscle training, and neuropsychology to assist with speech, swallowing, and voice volume (Trail et al., 2005).

Nurses can assist and educate the patient and family in managing swallowing difficulties by providing them with the following guidelines:

1. Position the patient upright at 90° during mealtimes; the patient should remain upright for at least 30 min after eating.
2. The patient should take small sips (5 mL) of liquid and small bites of food, alternating food and liquid swallows. The patient should avoid taking large swallows of thin liquids; a thickener

can be added to liquids, which makes them easier to swallow, and the patient should avoid tough foods that require excessive chewing.

3. The patient should eat slowly, with pauses between swallows.
4. The patient should be monitored for overt coughing, choking, and audible fluids in the chest; if evident, notify the patient's primary care provider.
5. The patient should be monitored for medical signs of aspiration (e.g., unexplained fever, coughing, and congestion); if evident, notify the patient's primary care provider.
6. Caloric intake or weight should be monitored and a dietician consulted as needed.

Orthostatic Hypotension

Orthostatic hypotension occurs in 20% to 50% of PLWP (Stern et al., 2006). A number of neurodegenerative disorders, such as PD and Shy-Drager syndrome, are accompanied by ANS dysfunction; thus blood pressure does not accommodate to rising from a supine or sitting position. The sluggishness of the ANS may cause the PD patient to complain of dizziness or lightheadedness, indicating low blood pressure and decreased blood flow to the brain. Orthostatic hypotension is defined as a decrease in blood pressure by 20 mm Hg systolic or 10 mm Hg diastolic after lying supine for 10 min and standing for 5 min (Stern et al., 2006). In addition, carbidopa/levodopa and dopamine agonists have a hypotensive effect and may need to be evaluated if hypotensive episodes are persistent.

Presyncope and syncope can occur in PLWP related to symptomatic orthostatic hypotension. The pathophysiological basis for syncope is decreased cerebral blood flow secondary to limitation of the cardiac output (CO). Neurological disorders that involve the ANS interrupt the sympathetic flexes and impair normal adrenergic responses when standing. Two of the primary neuropathic disorders are Shy-Drager syndrome and idiopathic orthostatic hypotension. For Shy-Drager syndrome, there seems to be a depletion of plasma norepinephrine on standing. In idiopathic hypotension, there is a decrease in norepinephrine from the sympathetic nerve endings (Wenning, Shepard, Magalhaes, Hawkes, & Quinn, 1993). With these conditions, there is widespread ANS dysfunction.

When a patient experiences faintness, lightheadedness, dizziness, or mental or visual blurring, there is probably a reduction in cerebral blood flow. If the patient has a more severe form of restricted cerebral blood flow, fainting can occur.

Treatment depends on the underlying cause of syncope. If orthostatic hypotension is due to hypovolemia, then fluid resuscitation should be instituted. Pharmacological treatment may need to be directed toward peripheral vasoconstriction to increase CO, thereby increasing blood pressure. In Shy-Drager syndrome and idiopathic orthostatic hypotension, pharmacotherapy may not be enough to correct the problem, and other measures may be necessary (Ward, 2006b).

There are a few approaches that mediate orthostatic hypotension:

1. PLWP should rise slowly and stand in place for a few minutes before attempting to ambulate. This will allow the ANS to adjust blood pressure and blood flow.
2. Support stockings can help to prevent the blood from pooling in the legs, which could cause a venous stasis and place the patient at risk of developing phlebitis. Support stockings should be donned before arising from bed and with the legs elevated so that blood is not trapped in the calves.
3. Medications are available to treat orthostatic hypotension, such as fludrocortisone (Florinef), which is a mineralocorticoid replacement, and midodrine (ProAmatine), which is a vasopressor or antihypotensive.
4. Proper hydration to promote total blood volume by drinking six 8-ounce glasses of fluid per day will help to maintain a higher blood pressure.
5. Caffeinated drinks may act as a diuretic, depleting circulating blood volume, and may need to be avoided.
6. The use of table salt (sodium chloride) will assist in maintaining a higher circulating blood volume. The function of sodium chloride when reabsorbed by the body is to increase the amount of water held by the body, thereby causing an increase in the extracellular fluid volume and creating a higher circulating blood volume, helping to prevent the blood pressure from falling.
7. The use of diuretic medications, such as furosemide, is common in older adults with PD. Careful monitoring for the development of

orthostatic hypotension in PLWP on diuretics is essential (Weiner, Shulman, & Lang, 2001).

8. Elevating the head of the bed 30° will maintain kidney pressure and reduce nocturnal diuresis.
9. Evaluation of medications for treatment of hypertension should be routinely reviewed. Hypotension related to the physiology of PD and the use of dopaminergic medications may resolve preexisting hypertension.

Sialorrhea

Sialorrhea is the pooling of excessive saliva in the mouth and drooling. The etiology of sialorrhea is due to the slowness of the swallowing reflex and the subsequent pooling of saliva. Sialorrhea may occur in a milder form during the day and in a heavier form during sleep. Drooling can be embarrassing socially for the PLWP and may lead to perioral dermatitis. Pooling of saliva can be a risk factor for aspiration and subsequent pneumonia.

Sialorrhea may be reduced with PD medications and anticholinergics (Artane or Cogentin). If the PLWP does not have heart disease, atropine ophthalmic 1% solution may be used as a mouth rinse. A few drops of the solution can be placed on a tablespoon, and then tap water may be added for a swish and swallow. Botulinum toxin injections into the salivary glands can be of great relief for severe cases of sialorrhea (Adler, 2002). Botulinum toxin is a protein produced by bacteria called *Clostridium botulinum.* When injected subcutaneously into the salivary glands, the action of this protein binds to the nerve at its points of contact with the muscle and prevents the release of the neurotransmitter acetylcholine, subsequently blocking nerve impulses (David, 2003).

Sexual Dysfunction and Sexuality

Erectile dysfunction (ED) or impotence is defined as difficulty in obtaining or maintaining sufficient penile firmness for intercourse and can be an embarrassing problem for men of all ages. ED occurs in 60% to 80% of men diagnosed with PD (Stern et al., 2006). PD usually begins around 60 years of age, at a time when many men have been diagnosed with chronic diseases, such as vascular disease, diabetes, enlarged prostate, or depression. Thyroid disorders, low testosterone, and alcohol use can also precipitate ED. In PD the main cause of ED is ANS dysfunction. The ANS sends messages to the lower spinal cord and from there to the penis and testes. If the patient can achieve an erection, this reflects adequate blood flow to the penis, however, if the erection cannot be sustained, this reflects a failure of the ANS to vasoconstrict the veins in the penis, resulting in penile softening (Lieberman, 2003).

Psychological barriers that contribute to ED could be masked faces that show no emotion, excessive oiliness of the skin, gait disturbances, loss of independence, and a spouse functioning in a caregiver role. Multiple psychological and physiological changes contribute to PLWP feeling less attractive to their partners and to their partners feeling less attracted to them (Bronner & Royter, 2004).

Sexual encounters present a different set of problems for PLWP related to motor impairment, such as a decrease in dexterity of fine finger movement that may be needed for arousal, rigidity, loss of spontaneous movement, tremors that increase with excitement, and difficulty changing body position during sexual activity. These symptoms usually begin in the moderate stage of PD and become worse in advanced disease as the nerves in the ANS that regulate sexual activity and libido degenerate further (Weiner et al., 2001).

Other factors that can play a role in sexual dysfunction are concomitant diseases like depression, hypertension, diabetes mellitus, ischemic heart disease, prostatectomy, and smoking (Bronner & Royter, 2004). In a study of sexuality in young patients with PD, when compared with healthy controls, the results indicated that the perception of sexual functioning and general health of patients with PD was influenced by depression and the state of unemployment (Jacobs, Vieregge, & Vieregge, 2000). This denotes that health care providers must consider psychological issues rather than somatic intervention in younger patients with PD who are dissatisfied with their sexual lives. Concomitant medications may also have unwanted sexual side effects. In one study, levodopa and dopamine agonists had independent negative effects on libido and ED (Bronner & Royter, 2004) and may have possibly induced low libido and ED. Other medications that may cause sexual dysfunction are antidepressants, neuroleptics, and beta-blockers.

In Bronner and Royter's (2004) study, men with PD reported the following types of sexual problems:

- Erectile dysfunction
- Dissatisfaction with sexual life
- Premature ejaculation

- Difficulties reaching orgasm
- Difficulties ejaculating

Women with PD in the same study reported the following types of sexual problems:

- Difficulties getting aroused
- Difficulties reaching orgasm
- Low sexual desire
- Dissatisfaction with sexual life
- Dyspareunia (painful sex)

Management and treatment of sexual dysfunction should begin with discussion about sexual issues with a health care provider, including a careful sexual history with the PLWP and his or her partner. A patient's sex life in general is not commonly addressed in the clinical setting due to the embarrassing aspects of this problem and possibly due to cultural beliefs or discomfort of both the provider or nurse and the patient or family sharing this information. However, a referral to an appropriate counselor who can assist and offer suggestions to the couple on techniques and other issues in individual or group therapy should be offered. The sharing of feelings concerning sexual intimacy can be beneficial to the couple and allay the fears and loneliness that silence can promote. Hormone levels (testosterone) should be checked and replaced if needed. Pharmacological agents may be prescribed that promote and sustain erection during intercourse, such as sildenafil (Viagra), vardenafil (Levitra), or tadalafil (Cialis). These medications belong to a group called phosphodiesterase-5 (PDE-5) inhibitors. The action of PDE-5 simplified is that during the erection process, smooth muscle cells of the penis produce cyclic guanosine monophosphate (cGMP), which is necessary for an erection. PDE-5, an enzyme, allows the erection to withdraw and breaks down the cGMP. The PDE-5 inhibitors block the PDE-5 (Basson, 1998) so that the erection maintains itself for a longer period of time. Health care providers should not prescribe this class of pharmacological agents if any of the following apply to the patient:

- The patient is taking any medicines called *nitrates*
- The patient is using recreational drugs called *poppers,* like amyl nitrate and butyl nitrate

- The patient has been told by a health care professional not to engage in sexual activity because of health problems

In an alert circulated in July 2005, the U.S. Food and Drug Administration (FDA) reported that after taking Levitra, Viagra, or Cialis, a small number of men lost eyesight in one eye. This type of vision loss is called nonarteritic anterior ischemic optic neuropathy (NAION). NAION causes a sudden loss of eyesight because blood flow to the optic nerve is blocked.

Erectile enhancement methods include vacuum erection devices and self-injection of neuromodulator prostaglandin E^1 through the tunica into the corpus cavernosum of the penis. With these two techniques, erection is obtained instantly, independent of physical or mental arousal (Basson, 1998). Dopaminergic drugs facilitate erections, and this knowledge led to the investigational use of apomorphine, which was given sublingually to 10 men in a small study who had psychogenic impotence.

Vaginal lubrication should be used if the female partner suffers from dryness. Friction of two surfaces without lubrication can cause skin damage and pain, which make intercourse uninviting. The use of a vibrator can facilitate orgasms in women and can encourage sufficient erections in men (Basson, 1996).

Libido is the cognitive component of sexual function. Decreased libido manifests as lack of sexual interest and a decrease in sexual thoughts. For men, libido is sensitive to testosterone levels, nutritional status, health, and drugs. Commonly used drugs that can cause ED and affect libido are antihypertensives, anticholinergics, estrogens, anticancer drugs, amphetamines, monoamine oxidase inhibitors, tricyclic antidepressants, anxiolytics, alcohol, opioids, cocaine, and specific serotonin reuptake inhibitors (SSRIs). For women, libido is linked to factors such as trust, respect, attraction, and emotional intimacy between partners, which is connected to female sexual response and needs. If there are problems within the relationship, referral to counseling may be necessary to work out the problems before libido can return. For PLWP, diminished libido may be tied to disability and low self-confidence. The primary care provider can be of great assistance through inquiry, assessment, and the recommendation of treatment options.

Hypersexuality is a known sexual dysfunction disorder that is not frequently publicized; therefore the prevalence of the disorder cannot be accurately determined (Ivanco & Bohnen, 2005). Symptoms demonstrated may be compulsive masturbation, compulsive use of pornography, promiscuity, and as many as five or more orgasms per week. Sexual disorders are classified in the *DSM–IV* (American Psychiatric Association, 1994) as sexual dysfunctions and warrant treatment, whether pharmacological or counseling. The obsessive–compulsive disorder (OCD) spectrum may include sexual disorder if the symptoms are present. It is common for these two disorders to overlap (Keegan, 2001). The exact etiology or neurobiology of hypersexuality is unknown in the absence of pathology, however, it is believed that brain serotonin (5-HT) may be involved in many neuropsychiatric disorders. In animal studies, low levels of brain 5-HT caused an increase in sexual behavior. When given drugs such as SSRIs, which increase brain levels of 5-HT, sexual behavior decreased (Keegan, 2001).

Treatment of hypersexuality involves the use of SSRIs (fluoxetine or sertraline) initially. It is well known that these drugs cause a reduction in sexual desire. If the SSRIs are unsuccessful in reducing the behavior, the physician may prescribe antiandrogens or hormonal treatments. The most common form of hormone therapy is medroxyprogesterone acetate (MPA; Provera). MPA used in clinical trials has had a significant impact on deviant sexual fantasies, urges, and behaviors (Bradford, 2000). Cyproterone acetate is an antiandrogen that decreases many types of sexual behavior, including fantasies, masturbation, deviant sexual behavior, libido, and sexual intercourse, and it has an impact on erections. Last, luteinizing hormone-releasing hormone (LHRH) agonists (triptorelin) have also been used as a treatment for hypersexuality if the behavior is deviant. LHRH agonist overstimulates the hypothalamus and causes the plasma testosterone level to fall to castration levels (Keegan, 2001).

PD and other chronic or disabling conditions have an impact on sexual desire, function, and ability; self-confidence; and ability to find a partner. Health care providers should inquire about, assess, and treat any sexual concerns. Referrals may be needed for counseling, and sexual dysfunction treatment information should be provided so that PLWP can make informed choices about how to best meet their individual sexual needs. Hypersexuality issues require treatment when those behaviors affect others in a negative way. PLWP can develop OCD, which may be a side effect of some of the dopaminergic agonists. Research is currently being conducted on sexual dysfunction in PD.

Sweating and Thermoregulation

Approximately 60% of PLWP report thermoregulatory disturbances (Swinn et al., 2003). The primary thermoregulation disorders reported by PLWP are disorders of sweating. Disorders of sweating can be classified into three categories:

1. Hyperhidrosis (excessive sweating)
2. Hypohidrosis (decreased sweating)
3. Anhidrosis (absence of sweating)

Hyperhidrosis is generally embarrassing for PLWP in social situations where the clothing becomes drenched. PLWP who experience hyperhidrosis have reported physical, social, and emotional impairment (Swinn et al., 2003). Anhidrosis, on the other hand, does not enable the body to cool itself through sweating and predisposes the PD patient to hyperthermia, which may become a medical emergency.

Sweating disturbances are related to autonomic dysfunction, off periods, levodopa peak dosages, and dyskinesias (Cheshire & Freeman, 2003; Swinn et al., 2003). In PD, there exists a condition of alternating on-medication (asymptomatic) periods with off-medication periods, in which symptoms such as dyskinesias (dance-like involuntary movements) are evident. Dyskinesias are disease- and drug-related movements. Dyskinesias usually occur at the peak dose of carbidopa/levodopa, although they can occur between the off and on responses to the medication (Waters, 2002). Hyperhidrosis is usually experienced by the PLWP in either the off state or while having dyskinesias (Swinn et al., 2003).

Treatment approaches that are associated with off-period sweating may respond to dopamine agonist medication. The sweating associated with dyskinesias should be approached by attempts to reduce dyskinesia activity through antiparkinsonian medication reduction or β-adrenergic blockers to control the sweating (Swinn et al., 2003). Patients experiencing anhidrosis should be encouraged to avoid getting overheated, limit strenuous activity, keep hydrated, and wear well-ventilated clothing.

Urinary and Bladder Dysfunction

Little is known about lower urinary tract symptoms in PLWP. The literature reports urinary tract dysfunction occurring in 27% to 70% of patients with PD (Defreitas et al., 2003).

The current literature on lower urinary tract symptoms and PD is limited by study design, data collection methods, lack of theoretical framework, and subject bias. All published research addresses urinary tract symptoms in PD as an autonomic dysfunction, related to the underlying neurological disease, resulting in overactive bladder (OAB). OAB is defined as "urgency, with or without urge incontinence, usually with frequency and nocturia in the absence of proven infection or other obvious pathology" (Josephson & Ginsberg, 2004, p. 25).

No published study has investigated the impact of immobility or tremor on lower urinary tract symptoms in patients with PD, discounting the effect of bradykinesia, rigidity, and resting tremor on toileting in this population. However, researchers examining gait dysfunction in PD have reported that urinary incontinence is significantly related to diminished mobility and suggest that this correlation should be investigated (Giladi, Kao, & Fahn, 1997). Two studies, examining predictors of nursing home placement in patients with PD, list urinary incontinence as a risk factor. However, both studies have small sample sizes, and the results conflict in key findings (Aarsland, Larsen, Tandberg, & Laake, 2000; Fernandez, Tabamo, David, & Friedman, 2001).

Symptoms of urinary tract problems in PLWP include urgency, frequency, dribbling, and nocturia. Daily incontinence and the use of diapers, condom catheters, and other containment devices are common. In an unpublished study of lower urinary tract symptoms in PD, patients and caregivers reported fluid restriction as a method of reducing urine output. Unfortunately, this technique increases the risk of urinary tract infection, hypotension, and falls (Robinson et al., 2004).

No evidenced-based research has been conducted to guide the clinician in managing urinary problems in PLWP. The impact of comorbid conditions such as prostate disease, normal pressure hydrocephalus, and spinal stenosis complicates the clinical evaluation of an aging population. Currently, most treatments for urinary issues in PD are focused on pharmacotherapy to treat OAB. It is plausible that dietary modification, hydration, and pelvic floor exercises may be beneficial in reducing lower urinary track symptoms in PD. However, this research has not been conducted. In addition, the impact of immobility from gait disorders, freezing of gait, and akinesia has not been examined. Thus the occurrence of functional incontinence is not reflected in the current literature (Robinson et al., 2004).

Spastic bladder or bladder hyperrflexia from deltrusor hyperactivity and involuntary contraction of the bladder is common in PD and produces urgency with incontinence; this is exacerbated in off-medication states (Hely, Morris, Reid, & Trafficante, 2005).

Nursing interventions include the following:

- Referral to a urologist for urodynamics to verify if urinary retention or incontinence are obstructive from prostate hypertrophy or childbearing history (depending on urodynamics, urologist may consider referral to bladder retraining program or incontinence nurse specialist)
- Referral to rehabilitative medicine (physical therapy and occupational therapy) for assistive devices for toileting
- Protective bedding (bedside urinals may be useful)
- Consultation with a neurologist to consider the addition of controlled release carbidopa/levodopa or other medications at bedtime to help control nocturnal urinary frequency.

NONMOTOR CHANGES IN PD WITHOUT ANS INVOLVEMENT

Speech Disturbances

Speech disturbances are estimated to occur in up to 89% of PLWP and may cause changes in personal, social, and occupational interactions (Trail et al., 2005). Speech changes are related to a disorder of the basal ganglia, whose role is to regulate muscle tone and goal-directed muscle movements (Duffy, 1995). Bradykinesia and rigidity are hallmark clinical characteristics of PD and manifest themselves also in the speech system. Speech production requires the coordination of respiration (breathing), phonation (voicing), articulation (pronouncing sounds), and prosody (loudness, pitch, expression). A breakdown in any of the necessary components of speech production can result in dysarthria, by definition, "speech disorders resulting from disturbances in muscular control over the speech mechanism due to damage of the central or peripheral nervous system. It designates problems in oral communication due to paralysis, weakness, or incoordination of the speech musculature" (Darley, Aronson, & Brown, 1969, p. 246). The hallmark dysarthria in Parkinson disease is *hypokinetic dysarthria,* literally meaning "dysarthria characterized by reduced movement."

Typical speech complaints in the Parkinson population include reduced loudness and pitch, rushes of speech, increased speech rate, hoarseness, slurring, and repetition of phonemes (neurogenic stuttering) (Yorkston et al., 2004). Impairments in respiration from muscular rigidity, tremor, and reduced amplitude of chest wall movement may result in reduced loudness, inability to maintain volume, and short speech rushes because their breath support will not be able to sufficiently power the speech mechanism (Yorkston et al., 2004). Phonatory, or vocal, deficits also may be results of muscular rigidity of the vocal folds. PD patients may have incomplete closure of the vocal folds, asymmetrical vocal folds, or bowing of the vocal folds, all of which contribute to a hoarse, weak, or tremulous vocal quality (Yorkston et al., 2004). Rigidity and tremor are also culprits in reduced articulatory accuracy of speech, which gives rise to complaints of slurring. Deficits in speech production can occur in any one or in any combination of the speech subsystems.

Treatment for hypokinetic dysarthria is primarily behavioral in nature. Pharmacologic treatments for speech disturbances in PD are not well understood, and the literature cites variable responses of the speech mechanism to medication. There are no reports of a significant, consistent impact of medications on speech disturbances in PD (Trail et al., 2005). Similarly, results of surgical interventions in PD on the speech mechanism have not been studied extensively but may even make some speech symptoms worse (Yorkston et al., 2004). Since medical and surgical interventions do not appear currently to be realistic management options for patients with PD, behavioral treatments have been the primary focus of intervention.

A widely used speech treatment is the Lee Silverman Voice Treatment (LSVT). LSVT is an intensive treatment that was developed using elements of neurology, physiology, motor learning, muscle training, and neuropsychology (Trail et al., 2005). It varies from other forms of speech therapy in that it focuses on voice, improves sensory perception of effort, and is administered in a high-effort style with a high intensity. LSVT teaches the PLWP to use increased effort when speaking, or to speak loudly. It requires 16 sessions of one hour each within a 1-month period. The treatment sessions are simple, redundant, and intensive, which promotes overlearning and internalization of increased vocal effort.

Other elements of behavioral or compensatory treatments that may be incorporated into a program for the patient with dysarthria include using a pacing board to decrease rate, using a portable speech-generating device, or using voice amplifiers.

Seborrheic Dermatitis

Seborrheic dermatitis is a common skin disorder in PD that causes dandruff to develop on the scalp and eyebrows. When seborrheic dermatitis is present, PLWP also have an oily, reddened face and forehead. This skin disorder has been associated with an overactive parasympathetic system.

Nursing intervention should include education about the prevalence of this skin disorder in PLWP, which is easily treated with medicated shampoos, such as coal-tar shampoos, and with creams, such as Ketoconazole. A referral to a dermatologist is indicated for treatment of this disorder.

Sleep Disorders

Sleep disorders are reported by 90% of PLWP (Stern et al., 2006). These sleep disorders may be related to motor symptoms, as seen with restless legs syndrome (RLS), periodic leg movement disorder (PLMD), and REM behavior disorder (RBD), and may be associated with the degeneration of cholinergic and dopaminergic systems (Stern et al., 2006).

RLS is an idiopathic sensory disorder, unrelated to PD, and is characterized by an urge to move the limbs in the evening when the body is at rest, motor restlessness, and paresthesias. The diagnosis of RLS requires the following four symptom characteristics:

1. An urge to move the legs accompanied by unpleasant sensation in the legs.
2. An urge to move the legs or sensations beginning during periods of rest or inactivity.
3. An urge to move or unpleasant sensations that are relieved by movement, such as walking.
4. Urges to move or unpleasant sensations that are worse in the evening and only occur in the evening or nighttime.

This disorder produces chronic sleep loss and reduced quality of life. RLS symptoms improve with limb movement or walking briefly.

There are theories that RLS has been linked to dopaminergic dysfunction related to antiparkinsonian medications (Adler, 2005). The prevalence of RLS in the general population is 2% to 15%, with a mean age of 40–60. RLS is a primary disorder that can occur secondary to other conditions, such as iron-deficiency anemia, end-stage renal disease, and pregnancy (Allen, 2005). Other risk factors for developing RLS are rheumatoid arthritis and gastric surgery.

Treatment for RLS is a dopamine agonist called ropinirole (Requip), which was approved by the FDA in 2005 for moderate to severe RLS. Other agonists, levodopa, opiates, and other classes of medications have been used with various successes but are considered off-label usages. There have been some reports of worsening of symptoms on ropinirole, necessitating the use of opiates and anticonvulsants in conjunction with ropinirole or in place of it (Allen, 2005).

PLMD occurs while the patient is asleep and unaware of his or her limbs' movements, while the bed partner is awakened by the movements. This condition causes poor quality of sleep in patients and bed partners if awakened and daytime sleepiness and fatigue (Adler, 2005).

In contrast to PLMD, the RLS patient is awake, inactive, or resting when the urge to move the legs is accompanied by uncomfortable sensations, such as electric currents in the legs. The patient must walk to obtain relief from RLS symptoms.

RBD is characterized by vigorous behaviors during REM sleep, in which the patient will act out his or her dreams, many times, intense and violent. These dream-enacting behaviors include talking, yelling, punching, kicking, jumping from the bed, arm flailing, and grabbing. This disorder affects approximately 50% of all iodopathic PD patients. This behavior can injure the bed partner, accounts for 20% to 25% of sleep time, and has been linked with psychosis in PD (Stern et al., 2006).

A polysomnography video recording is the diagnostic test for persons suspected of having RBD. This test is performed at a sleep center to observe behaviors during sleep. The polysomnography shows an increase in muscle tone during REM sleep, whereas in healthy persons, REM sleep is associated with an absence of muscle tone.

Treatment for RBD is geared toward the safety of the sleeping environment and the use of clonazepam (Klonopin), relieving approximately 90% of the symptoms. The bedroom of the patient with RBD should be free of dangerous objects. Some furniture may need to be removed, the bed mattress may need to be placed on the floor, a bed with bedrails should be padded, and the bedmate should sleep in another bed until the symptoms resolve.

Other Sleep Disorders Common in PD

Excessive Daytime Sleepiness

Excessive daytime sleepiness (EDS) occurs in 15% to 50% of PLWP, despite a good night's sleep. Sometimes EDS is referred to as a disorder of wakefulness when sleepiness occurs during the daylight hours. The etiology of EDS is believed to be related to dopamine agonist medications or to the disease itself (Stern et al., 2006).

The recommended treatment for EDS is a central nervous system (CNS) stimulant called modafinil (Provigil), which blocks the release of gamma-aminobutyric acid, the most common inhibitory neurotransmitter or CNS depressant in the brain. Second, modafinil releases glutamate, an excitatory neurotransmitter or CNS stimulant in the thalamus and hippocampus. These two actions improve daytime wakefulness (Weinstock, 2003).

Insomnia

Insomnia occurs in 30% of PLWP and is usually related to sleep fragmentation and early awakenings (Stern et al., 2006). However, sleep complaints also grow more common with age in 16% to 68% of aging persons (Martin, 2005). The recommended treatment is good sleep hygiene:

- Maintain a regular sleep schedule and wake schedule
- avoid daytime naps
- Increase activity or exercise during the day
- avoid alcohol, caffeine, and nicotine in the evening
- Limit fluid intake within 2 hours of bedtime
- Practice a relaxing bedtime routine
- Create a sleep-conducive bedroom environment

If medications are warranted for insomnia, the health care provider may prescribe hypnotics (zolpidem), benzodiazepines (temazepam), or sedating antidepressants (amitriptyline, trazadone) (Stern et al., 2006).

Obstructive Sleep Apnea

Obstructive sleep apnea (OSA) affects nearly 18,000,000 Americans and places them at risk for cardiovascular complications, including hypertension, stroke, arrhythmias, heart failure, and myocardial infarction (Budhiraja & Quan, 2005; Williard & Dreher, 2005). OSA is characterized by a complete cessation of breathing that could last more than 10 s. This apnea or hypopnea may last all night and may awaken the patient several times, robbing him or her of deep sleep. The next day, the patient may experience fatigue and sleepiness.

OSA is found in all age groups and both genders, however, it is most often diagnosed in men 30–60 years of age. There are a few risk factors, such as obesity with a body mass index of 30 or more, large neck circumference of greater than 17 inches, hypertension due to oxygen deprivation, and a physical abnormality of the nose, throat, or upper airway.

When diagnosing OSA, the physician may have the patient fill out the Epworth Sleepiness Scale, on which a score above 10 indicates daytime sleepiness, which warrants further testing. An overnight polysomnogram measures the number of apneic episodes while the patient sleeps. Sensors are attached to the patient during sleep that measure and record brain waves, eye movements, muscle activity, and pulse oximetry. The severity of the OSA is determined in the sleep study.

The treatment for OSA involves a weight reduction program, avoiding CNS depressants before bedtime, and continuous positive airway pressure ventilation during sleep (Williard & Dreher, 2005).

Pain

Historically, pain in PD has been recognized as a distressing sensory non-motor symptom for people living with PD (Ford, 1998). Unfortunately, pain in PD is unrecognized, poorly assessed, and undertreated in the clinical setting. Furthermore, clinical research into the phenomenon of PD pain is not well defined, and there is a paucity of research to support evidence-based evaluation and treatment.

Pain with PD was reported as early as 1817, when James Parkinson, a British physician, published the first clinical description of the disease in a monograph titled *An Essay on the Shaking Palsy*. In this remarkable text Dr. Parkinson describes a patient with PD who suffers from pain. The individual is described as follows:

A. B. subject to rheumatic affection of the deltoid muscle, had felt the usual inconvenience from it for two to three days: but at night found the pain had extended down the arm, along the inside of the fore-arm, and on the other side of the fingers, in which a continual tingling was felt. (p. 48)

Through this historical account of pain with PD, one can appreciate the impact on the individual from an emotional and physical perspective. The case describes sleep alteration and sensory changes, which are described in contemporary reports of PD pain. Despite historical and current descriptions of PD pain, no clear conceptual analysis has been written to guide researchers in measuring the pain experienced by individuals with PD.

Seventy percent of PD patients report experiencing pain as a nonmotor symptom of disease. For a minority of people living with PD, pain is more disabling than the motor symptoms of disease (Djaldetti et al., 2004; Ford, 1998). Unfortunately, pain is underassessed and undertreated in the clinical setting.

Pain associated with PD is complex and is influenced by a variety of factors:

1. The existence of painful comorbid diseases
2. Side effects of therapy
3. Motor and nonmotor fluctuations

These factors magnify the difficulties in defining discreet pain syndromes in PD. The increased occurrence of painful diseases, such as arthritis, diabetes, and osteoporosis, contributes to painful experiences of older adults. Second, pain from dopaminergic medications and surgical therapies, used to treat PD symptoms, can result in painful dyskinesias and dystonia. Third, the motor and nonmotor fluctuations experienced by PLWP produce episodic bouts of pain that are often unpredictable and difficult to treat (Ford, 1998).

Pain associated with PD has been categorized as musculoskeletal, radicular-neuropathic, dystonic, central, or akathisia (Ford, 1998). Other researchers have categorized pain associated with PD according to levels of dopaminergic stimulation. Sage (2004) divided PD pain into three categories: low DOPA, describing dysphasic or end-of-dose pain; high DOPA, defined as painful symptoms occurring at peak levodopa efficacy; and other conditions, defined as painful symptoms experienced by PD patients that are not related to dopaminergic stimulation. The categorization of PD pain related to dopamine levels focused on episodic fluctuations of pain mediated by the administration of antiparkinsonian medications (Sage, 2004).

Fluctuations in motor and nonmotor symptoms of PD are related to the down-regulation of dopamine-producing cells in the substantia nigra and pharmacotherapy used to enhance dopamine levels in the brain. Scherder, Wolters, Polman, Sergeant, and Swabb (2005) proposed that the reduction of dopamine in PD can lower pain thresholds and thereby increase pain complaints in cognitively intact individuals. This hypothesis provides a model for explaining centrally mediated pain with PD, which is pain that originates in the brain without peripheral input.

Measuring Pain in Older Adults With PD

Pain associated with PD is complicated by the difficulty in assessing pain in a population of older adults with cognitive impairment. Valid and reliable measures of pain in older adults are essential for PD pain assessment and treatment (Chibnall & Tait, 2001). The growing literature on pain in older adults illustrates the complexities of measurement in a population that has cognitive impairments and sensory changes. Unfortunately, there is no standardized assessment for pain in older adults (Herr et al., 2004).

Current literature is further limited in the use of pain measures, which are not standardized in older adult populations. Also, the definition of older adult populations has not been consistently utilized in validation studies of pain measurement (Gagliese & Melzack, 2006). Thus the clinical standard of a complete and systematic approach to measuring pain in PLWP is problematic (Herr, 2002). This paucity of valid and reliable measures to assist in the assessment of pain in older adults with PD should be considered a priority for research.

Nursing interventions that would be helpful for the health care provider managing PD medications and considering a patient's pain include the following:

- Request that patients graph their pain to assess if pain fluctuates with their medication cycles and on and off periods.
- Assist the patient in describing his or her pain syndrome and what makes it better or worse
- Ask the patient to rate their pain on a scale of 0 (no pain) to 10 extreme pain

Visual Dysfunction

Visual complications in PLWP occur because of the reduction or absence of dopamine along the pathways of the brain and in the substantia nigra.

Dopamineric neurons are also found in the retina of the eyes; however, dopamine is greatly reduced in PLWP. The retina transmits visual images into electrical signals that are given to the brain in a feedback mechanism in most people (Hamby, 2006). However, these electrical signals and feedback are dysfunctional in PLWP and affect vision and eye movements.

Bodis-Wollner (2003) identified six changes in the visual fields related to PD:

1. Saccadic eye movements are required for driving, reading, and walking. These saccades allow the eyes to move rapidly from place to place and may become impaired in PD. It is believed that the neuroanatomical pathway may share some of the neuronal circuits of the basal ganglia and frontal cortex. These pathways are part of the saccadic circuit and may contribute to the visual dysfunction seen in PD.

2. Occulomotor dysfunction can manifest with bradykinesias as evidenced by reduced blinking, motor dysfunction of the eyelids, blepharospasms, and difficulty opening the eyelids, which can yield a potential for falls (Biousse et al., 2004).

3. Color and contrast vision are also affected in PD because of decreased motor function. The decline in color perception processing is progressive, and low-contrast acuity is diminished in this population. Color and contrast perception may contribute to a decreased depth perception and miscalculations of distances and surface changes. This may contribute to the risk of falls. Facial recognition may be a problem for PLWP because for the most part, faces are generally low contrast (Hamby, 2006).

4. Upper visual field deficits occur because of the reduction or absence of dopaminergic neurons, which reduces those with PD the ability to use the upper vision fields.

5. Dry eyes were found in two-thirds of untreated PLWP according to Biousse et al. (2004). Additionally, blepharitis (inflamed eyelids) caused eye discomfort. The use of artificial tears can soothe dry eyes, and the PLWP should see an ophthalmologist annually to monitor vision and other discomforts of the eye.

People living with PD also have difficulty with proprioception, which is the awareness of posture, movement, and changes in equilibrium. There is also the knowledge of position, weight, and resistance of objects in relation to the body. When motor deficits are added, attempts to perform functional upper extremity reaching tasks may be imprecise, causing an over- or underreaching for the object. In PD, gait, postural control, balance, and reaching disorders are common and can be confounded by visual deficits as well as proprioception (Hamby, 2006).

According to Suteerawattananon, Morris, Etnyre, Jankovic, and Protas (2004), visual cues, such as colored tape on the floor before the ambulating patient, influence attention and allow more conscious motor control of gait by going directly through the cerebellum and bypassing the basal ganglia, where the problem lies. The tape acts as a nudge to move the feet without freezing of gait. Auditory cues may also be helpful but not used simultaneously with visual cues because together, they decrease ambulation performance.

Another strategy for visual and perceptual deficits is the use of low vision to decrease glare and increase contrast. The PD patient will need ample time to adjust to lighting changes. An ophthalmologist can prescribe prism glasses to adjust for upper visual field deficits.

First and foremost, visual changes must be addressed and recommended strategies followed for the best results with the perceptual-motor system (Hamby, 2006).

Olfactory Dysfunction

It is now well known that olfactory dysfunction is prevalent in PLWP. In fact, these impairments have been observed in early PD and on a wide range of quantitative olfactory tests, including tests of odor identification, detection threshold sensitivity, and discrimination (Mesholam, Moberg, Mahr, & Doty, 1998). In addition, olfactory impairments have been observed in asymptomatic first-degree relatives of patients with PD (Montgomery, Baker, Lyons, & Koller, 1999).

Importantly, among the major motor disorders, this alteration in ability to smell is relatively specific to PD. Thus smell dysfunction is absent, present infrequently, or only to a minor degree in progressive supranuclear palsy (Doty et al., 1993), essential tremor (Doty, 1991), multiple system atrophy (Wenning et al., 1993), amyotrophic lateral sclerosis (Sajjadian et al., 1994), multiple sclerosis (Doty, 1991), and parkinsonism induced by 1-methyl-4-phenyl-1,2,3,6-tetrahydropyridine (Doty, 1991). Additionally, studies have found that subtle differences exist among subtypes of PD. For example, slightly greater dysfunction is present in patients with postural instability and gait-predominant PD than with tremor-predominant PD (Stern et al., 1994).

Olfactory dysfunction, relative to other clinical signs of PD, is unique on several grounds: olfactory dysfunction is sensory rather than motor, is prevalent to a relatively high degree in the earliest stages of the disease process, is unrelated to the use of antiparkinsonian medications, does not differ during the on and off states of patients with severe motor fluctuations who are on levodopa therapy, and appears to be unrelated in magnitude to the degree of motoric or cognitive symptomatology (implying independence from the more dynamic elements of the disease proper) (Doty, Deems, & Stellar, 1988). Although the basis for PD-related olfactory loss is not yet known, a recent study examined postmortem brains of patients with incidental Lewy body pathology and found Lewy neurites and Lewy bodies in the olfactory bulb, olfactory tract, and anterior olfactory nucleus, suggesting that in its earliest stages, PD can present as a disease of olfactory brain regions (Del Tredici, Rub, De Vos, Bohl, & Braak, 2002). In addition, because olfactory impairments present early in the PD disease course, are independent from motor symptomatology, and are present in asymptomatic first-degree relatives, olfactory dysfunction in PD is often thought to support a genetic predisposition for the disease. There is evidence that genetic factors may play a substantial role in PD and that multiple genes contribute to susceptibility. There is also evidence that disturbances in certain domains of olfactory processing may denote a genetic predisposition to PD (Doty, 1991; Liberini, Parola, Franco-Spano, & Antonini, 2000; Wolters et al., 2000). Although olfaction is not yet widely investigated in PD, the aforementioned factor suggests a role for olfactory testing in the early diagnosis of PD. Certainly more studies are needed to further understand the implications for PD diagnosis, treatment, and prevention.

NURSING INTERVENTIONS FOR NONMOTOR SYMPTOMS IN PD

It is now well recognized that the nonmotor symptoms of PD are as important to recognize and treat as the motor symptoms. Though these symptoms can be embarrassing or difficult to discuss, these nonmotor symptoms are best presented as common problems for PLWP. Nonmotor symptoms are recognized to.

- Occur in the early stages of the disease
- Often, but not always, correlate with the off-medication phase
- Impact patient and caregiver quality of life

Nursing management of PD patients starts with sensitive identification of nonmotor problems and brings them to the attention of the health care provider. Nonmotor symptoms can be reported by the patient through an assessment tool called the Unified Parkinson's Disease Rating Scale, which has questions related to nonmotor symptoms the patient could complete while waiting in a busy clinic. This information would give the health care provider a clear indication of what needs to be treated. Given how complex PD management can be, these patients are best managed through a multidisciplinary approach, where the neuroscience nurse is in an excellent position to coordinate the care. Multiple referrals to treat nonmotor symptoms may be requested of other subspecialities and lead to unnecessary medical procedures (Waters, 2002). These interventions can be invasive, expensive, time consuming, and lead to fragmented care and patient, family, and caregiver frustration. Again, the neuroscience nurse can utilize the knowledge of PD motor and nonmotor symptoms to educate and redirect unnecessary referrals.

Neuroscience nurses are in an excellent position to assess and identify these nonmotor symptoms, educate the patient or caregiver on their prevalence in PD, and facilitate a multidisciplinary team approach to help the patient receive comprehensive care for not only the motor symptoms, but also the nonmotor aspects of this disease. Neuroscience nurses should support the patient or caregiver and educate him or her on the importance of compliance with the prescribed medication regimen for optimal motor and nonmotor ease of symptoms.

REFERENCES

Aarsland, D., Larsen, J. P., Tandberg, E., & Laake, K. (2000). Predictors of nursing home placement in Parkinson's disease: A population-based, prospective study. *Journal of the American Geriatric Society, 48,* 938–942.

Adler, C. H. (2002). Botulinum toxin in movement disorders and spasticity. In J. Jankovic & E. Tolosa (Eds.), *Parkinson's disease and movement disorders* (4th ed., pp. 633–639). Philadelphia: Lippincott, Williams, and Wilkins.

Allen, R. P. (2005). An introduction to restless legs syndrome. *Medscape Neurology and Neurosurgery, 7,* 1–5.

American Psychiatric Association. (1994). *Diagnostic and statistical manual of mental disorders* (4th ed.). Washington, DC: Author.

Basson, R. (1996). Sexuality and Parkinson's disease. *Parkinsonism and Related Disorders, 2,* 177–185.

Basson, R. (1998). Integrating new biomedical treatments into the assessment and management of erectile dysfunction. *Canadian Journal of Human Sexuality, 7,* 213–259.

Biousse, V., Skibell, B., Watts, R., Loupe, D., Drews-Botsch, C., & Newman, N. (2004). Ophthalmologic features of Parkinson's disease. *Neurology, 62,* 177–180.

Bodis-Wollner, I. (2003). Neuropsychological and perceptual defects in Parkinson's disease. *Parkinsonism and Related Disorders, 9,* 83–89.

Bradford, J. M. W. (2000). The treatment of sexual deviation using a pharmacological approach. *Journal of Sex Research, 37,* 248–257.

Bronner, G., & Royter, V. (2004). Sexual dysfunction in Parkinson's disease. *Journal of Sex and Marital Therapy, 30,* 95–105.

Budhiraja, R., & Quan, S. F. (2005). Sleep-disordered breathing and cardiovascular health. *Current Opinion in Pulmonary Medicine, 11,* 501–506.

Cheshire, W., & Freeman, R. (2003). Disorders of sweating. *Seminars in Neurology, 23* (4), 399–400

Chibnall, J. T., & Tait, R. C. (2001). Pain assessment in cognitively impaired and unimpaired older adults: A comparison of four scales. *Pain, 92,* 173–186.

Darley, F. L., Aronson, A. E., & Brown, J. R. (1969). Differential diagnostic patterns of dysarthria. *Journal of Speech and Hearing Research, 12,* 246–269.

David, W. S. (2003). Botulinum toxin therapy: Beyond dystonia and spasticity. *Federal Practitioner, 20,* 17–19.

Defreitas, G. A., Lemack, G. E., Zimmern, P. E., Dewey, R. B., Roehrborn, C. G., & O'Suilleabhain, P. E. (2003). Distinguishing neurogenic from non-neurogenic detrusor overactivity: An urodynamic assessment of lower urinary tract symptoms in patients with and without Parkinson's disease. *Urology, 62,* 651–655.

Del Tredici, K., Rub, U., De Vos, R. A. I., Bohl, J. R. E., & Braak, H. (2002). Where does Parkinson disease pathology begin in the brain? *Journal of Neuropathology and Experimental Neurology, 61,* 413–426.

Djaldetti, R., Shifrin, A., Rogowski, Z., Sprecher, E., Melamed, E., & Yarnitsky, D. (2004). Quantitative measurement of pain sensation in patients with Parkinson disease. *Neurology, 62,* 2171–2175.

Doty, R. L. (1991). Olfactory dysfunction in neurodegenerative disorders. In T. V. Getchall, R. L. Doty, L. M. Bartoshuk, & J. B. Snow (Eds.), *Smell and taste in health and disease* (pp. 735–751). New York: Raven.

Doty, R. L., Deems, D., & Stellar, S. (1988). Olfactory dysfunction in Parkinson's disease: A general deficit unrelated to neurologic signs, disease stage, or disease duration. *Neurology, 38,* 1237–1244.

Doty, R. L., Golbe, L. I., McKeown, D. A., Stern, M. B., Lehrach, C. M., & Crawford, D. (1993). Olfactory testing differentiates between progressive supranuclear palsy and idiopathic Parkinson's disease. *Neurology, 43,* 962–965.

Duffy, J. R. (1995). *Motor speech disorders, substrates, differential diagnosis, and management.* St. Louis, MO: Mosby.

Duvoisin, R. (1987). History of parkinsonism. *Pharmacology and Therapeutics, 32,* 1–17.

Fernandez, H. H., Tabamo, R. E., David, R. R., & Friedman, J. H. (2001). Predictors of depressive symptoms among spouse caregivers in Parkinson's disease. *Movement Disorders, 16,* 1123–1125.

Ford, B. (1998). Pain in Parkinson's disease. *Clinical Neuroscience, 5,* 63–72.

Gagliese, L., & Melzack, R. (2006). Pain in the elderly. In S. B. McMahon & M. Koltzenburg (Eds.), *Wall and Melzack's textbook of pain* (pp. 1169–1178). Philadelphia: Elsevier.

Giladi, N., Kao, R., & Fahn, S. (1997). Freezing phenomenon in patients with parkinsonian syndromes. *Movement Disorders, 12,* 302–305.

Hamby, J. R. (2006). Visual and perceptual changes in Parkinson's disease: Impact on motor control and implications for treatment. *Physical Disabilities, 29,* 1–4.

Hanak, M. (1992). *Rehabilitation nursing for the neurological patient.* New York: Springer.

Hely, M. A., Morris, J. G., Reid, W. G., Trafficante, R. (2005). Sydney multicenter study of Parkinson's disease: Non L-dopa responsive problems dominate at 15 years. *Movement Disorders, 20,* 190–199.

Herr, K. (2002). Chronic pain: Challenges and assessment strategies. *Journal of Gerontological Nursing, 28,* 20–27.

Herr, K., Titler, M., Schilling, M., Marsh, J., Xie, X., Ardery, G., et al. (2004). Evidenced-based assessment of acute pain in older adults: Current nursing practices and perceived barriers. *Clinical Journal of Pain, 20,* 331–340.

Ivanco, L. S., & Bohnen, N. I. (2005). Effects of donepezil on compulsive hypersexual behavior in Parkinson disease: A single case study. *American Journal of Therapeutics, 12,* 467–468.

Jacobs, H., Vieregge, A., & Vieregge, P. (2000). Sexuality in young patients with Parkinson's disease: A population based comparison with healthy controls. *Journal of Neurology, Neurosurgery, and Psychiatry, 69,* 550–552.

Jankovic, J. (2002). Therapeutic strategies in Parkinson's disease. In J. Jankovic & E. Tolosa (Eds.), *Parkinson's disease and movement disorders* (4th ed., pp. 116–151). Philadelphia: Lippincott, Williams, and Wilkins.

Josephson, K., & Ginsberg, D. (2004). Key considerations when treating the older patient with symptoms of urinary frequency and urgency. *Annals of Long-Term Care, 12,* 25–32.

Keegan, J. (2001). The neurobiology, neuropharmacology, and pharmacological treatment of the paraphilias and compulsive sexual behavior. *Journal of Psychiatry, 46,* 1–14.

Kumar, R., Bergeron, C., & Lang, A. (2002). Corticobasal degeneration. In J. Jankovic & E. Tolosa (Eds.), *Parkinson's disease and movement disorders* (4th ed., pp. 116–151). Philadelphia: Lippincott, Williams, and Wilkins.

Liberini, P., Parola, S., Franco-Spano, P., & Antonini, L. (2000). Olfaction in Parkinson's disease: Methods of assessment and clinical relevance. *Journal of Neurology, 247,* 88–96.

Lieberman, A. (2003). *About Parkinson disease.* Sudbury, MA: Jones and Bartlett.

Logemann, J. A. (1998). *Evaluation and treatment of swallowing disorders* (2nd ed.). Austin, TX: Pro-Ed.

Martin, J. (2005). *Expert column—Sleep disorders in older adults and their impact.* Retrieved February 23, 2006, from http://www.medscape.com/viewarticle/519856

Mesholam, R. I., Moberg, P. J., Mahr, R. N., & Doty, R. L. (1998). Olfaction in neurodegenerative disease: A meta-analysis of olfactory functioning in Alzheimer's and Parkinson's diseases. *Archives of Neurology, 55,* 84–90.

Montgomery, E. B., Baker, K. B., Lyons, K., & Koller, W. C. (1999). Abnormal performance on the PD test battery by asymptomatic first-degree relatives. *Neurology, 52,* 757–762.

National Parkinson Foundation. (2003a). *Constipation.* Retrieved December 24, 2003, from http://www.parkinson.org/constipation.htm

National Parkinson Foundation. (2003b). *Nutrition matters* (Vol. 5). Miami, FL: Author.

Parkinson, J. (1817). *An essay on the shaking palsy.* London: Neely and Jones.

Robinson, J., Bunting-Perry, L., McHale, D., Leary, A., O'Neill, A., & Avi-Itzhak, T. (2004, October). *Urinary incontinence in males with Parkinson's disease.* Poster presented at the National Congress on the State of the Science in Nursing Research, Washington, DC.

Sage, J. I. (2004). Pain in Parkinson's disease. *Current Treatment Options in Neurology, 6,* 191–200.

Sajjadian, A., Doty, R. L., Gutnick, D. N., Shirugi, R. J., Sivak, M., & Perl, D. (1994). Olfactory dysfunction in amyotrophic lateral sclerosis. *Neurodegeneration, 3,* 1–5.

Scherder, E., Wolters, E., Polman, C., Sergeant, J., & Swabb, D. (2005). Pain in Parkinson's disease and multiple sclerosis: Its relation to the medial and lateral pain systems. *Neuroscience and Biobehavioral Reviews, 29,* 1047–1056.

Shulman, L. M., Taback, R. L., Rabinstein, A. A., & Weiner, W. J. (2002). Non-recognition of depression and other nonmotor symptoms in Parkinson's disease. *Parkinsonism Related Disorders, 8,* 193–197.

Stern, M. B., Doty, R. L., Dotti, M., Corcoran, P., Crawford, D., McKeown, D. A., et al. (1994). Olfactory function in Parkinson's disease subtypes. *Neurology, 44,* 266–268.

Stern, M. B., Horn, S., Kleiner-Fisman, G., & Weintraub, D. (2006). *Nonmotor symptoms of Parkinson's disease: Recognition, diagnosis, and treatment.* Retrieved May 2, 2006, from http://www.medscape.com/viewprogram/5187

Suteerawattananon, M., Morris, G., Etnyre, B., Jankovic, J., & Protas, E. (2004). Effects of visual and auditory cues on gait in individuals with Parkinson's disease. *Journal of Neurological Sciences, 219,* 63–69.

Swinn, L., Schrag, A., Viswanathan, R., Bloem, B., Lees, A., Quinn, N., et al. (2003). Sweating dysfunction in Parkinson's disease. *Movement Disorders, 18,* 1459–1463.

Thanvi, B. R., Munshi, S. K., Vijaykumar, N., & Lo, T. C. (2003). Neuropsychiatric non-motor aspects of Parkinson's disease. *Postgraduate Medical Journal, 79,* 561–565.

Trail, M., Fox, C., Ramig, L. O., Sapir, S., Howard, J., & Lai, E. C. (2005). Speech treatment for Parkinson's disease. *NeuroRehabilitation, 20,* 205–221.

Ward, C. (2006a). Characteristics and symptom management in progressive supranuclear palsy: A multidiscipline approach. *Journal of Neuroscience Nursing, 38,* 240–245.

Ward, C. (2006b). An ethical dilemma in a Shy–Drager patient: A case study. *Journal of Neuroscience Nursing, 38,* 400–402.

Waters, C. (2002). *Diagnosis and management of Parkinson's disease* (3rd ed.). Caddo, OK: Professional Communications.

Weiner, W., Shulman, L., & Lang, A. (2001). *Parkinson's disease.* Baltimore: Johns Hopkins University Press.

Weinstock, D. (Ed.). (2003). *Nurses' drug handbook.* Philadelphia: Blanchard and Loeb.

Weintraub, D., & Stern, M. B. (2005). Psychiatric complications in Parkinson disease. *American Journal of Geriatric Psychiatry, 13,* 844–851.

Wenning, G. K., Shepard, B., Magalhaes, M., Hawkes, C. H., & Quinn, N. P. (1993). Olfactory function in multiple system atrophy. *Neurodegeneration, 2,* 169–171.

Williard, R. M., & Dreher, H. M. (2005). Wake-up call for sleep apnea. *Nursing, 35,* 46–49.

Willson, P., Bunting-Perry, L., Arzbaecher, J., Vernon, G., & Moskowitz, C. (2004). Movement disorders. In *AANN core curriculum for neuroscience nursing* (4th ed., pp. 701–756). St. Louis, MO: Elsevier.

Wolters, E., Francot, C., Bergmans, P., Winogrodzka, A., Booij, J., Berendse, H., et al. (2000). Preclinical (premotor) Parkinson's disease. *Journal of Neurology, 247,* 103–109.

Yorkston, K. M., Miller, R. M., & Strand, E. A. (2004). *Management of speech and swallowing in degenerative diseases* (2nd ed.). Austin, TX: Pro-Ed.

6

Deep Brain Stimulation Management

Susan Heath, MS, RN, CNRN
Constance Ward, MSN, RN, BC, CNRN
With contributions by Gwyn M. Vernon,
MSN, CRNP

DEFINITION OF DEEP BRAIN STIMULATION (DBS)

Deep brain stimulation (DBS) is an established surgical therapy for treatment of the motor symptoms of Parkinson's disease (PD). DBS is also an established procedure for the treatment of essential tremor and is emerging as a technology to manage a variety of other movement disorders, psychiatric illnesses, and chronic pain. This chapter will focus on DBS therapy as the procedure relates to the care and treatment of patients with PD in regard to patient selection, preoperative care, postoperative care, and the nurse's role in patient and family education for persons living with PD (PLWP).

HISTORY OF DBS

Pallidotomy and thalamotomy were introduced in the 1940s as the first surgical techniques established for the treatment of PD. These early surgical techniques included permanent, destructive surgical procedures that involved lesioning of the brain tissue in the area of the globus pallidus interna (GPi; pallidotomy) and thalamus (thalamotomy). Pallidotomy and thalamotomy, as destructive lesions, were performed prior to DBS surgery to improve symptoms of tremor of PD through permanent destruction of regions in the brain using electrode cautery. Though these surgeries were sometimes effective, the results were permanent and irreversible and often induced cognitive decline, speech disorders, and swallowing difficulties (Ghika et al., 1999). Additionally, though some lesions were safely circumscribed to a small region, after time, the patient's condition progressed, and the small lesion would lose its effectiveness in managing the motor symptoms of disease. Throughout the 1960s, pallidotomy and thalamotomy were the primary surgical treatments for PD. These surgeries, with their high morbidity and mortality, were essentially replaced with the discovery of levodopa in 1967. In the 1980s, DBS surgery became a more effective treatment due to both its reversibility and its adjustability.

In 1995, the first global DBS study was conducted with 160 patients recruited from the United States, Canada, Europe, and Australia who had received DBS implantation in the GPi or subthalamic nucleus (STN) for symptom control in advanced PD. The GPi is an almond-sized nucleus located in the basal ganglia, and when stimulated, it reduces tremor, rigidity, bradykinesia, dystonia, dopamine-induced dyskinesias, and infrequently, gait dysfunction. The STN is a pea-sized nucleus, also located in the basal ganglia, and when stimulated, it reduces tremor, rigidity, bradykinesia, gait dysfunction, and postural instability. Kleiner-Fisman et al. (2006) published an extensive meta-analysis of DBS outcomes and illustrated the effect of DBS on dyskinesia, quality of life, motor fluctuations, and adverse events.

DBS OVERVIEW AND MECHANISM OF ACTION

Though the clinical benefits of DBS have been shown to improve the cardinal symptoms of PD, the mechanisms of action remain unproven and are currently under active investigation (McIntyre, Savasta, Kerkerian-Le Goff, & Vitek, 2004b). The explanation given to laypersons about DBS's beneficial effects is that DBS is similar to delivering "electrical Sinemet" through a type of brain pacemaker. Although this explanation is technically inaccurate, as cerebral dopaminergic levels are not changed with stimulation (Hilker et al., 2003), it is a clarifying description when a brief and nontechnical account is needed for social or general public encounters.

DBS delivers an electrical current that can be shaped, refined, and tuned to produce relief of many symptoms of PD (Lozano & Eltahawy, 2004; McIntyre, Grill, Sherman, & Thakor, 2004a; Volkmann, Herzog, Kopper, & Deuschl, 2002; Volkmann, Moro, & Pahwa, 2006). One theory of the effect of DBS is that high-frequency stimulation produces a local jamming or inactivation of cell bodies in a stimulated nucleus (Grill, Snyder, & Miocinovic, 2004). However, seemingly paradoxically, DBS has been found to produce a simultaneous increase in output or activation in the descending pathways from these same nuclei (Hashimoto, Elder, Okun, Patrick, & Vitek, 2003; McIntyre et al., 2004a). Though DBS may override or suppress abnormal cell body activity, it is unclear how this produces a modulation of abnormal axonal outputs leading to a near-normal return of motor function (McIntyre et al., 2004b). The duality of action (excitatory and inhibitory) and latency of benefit is still unexplained and under active investigation. Lozano and Eltahawy (2004) explain how the properties of electrical current from stimulation are thought to first excite axons before cell bodies, large axons, before small axons, and myelinated before unmyelinated fibers. STN stimulation has been shown in animal models to increase the levels of excitatory glutamate in the ipsilateral globus pallidus, which then increases glutamate levels in the substantia nigra pars compacta (Grill et al., 2004.) Some hypothesize that this increase in glutamate may result in a neuroprotective effect (Lozano & Eltahawy, 2004). Current research in understanding the exact mechanism of DBS action is rapidly advancing, but despite the lack of scientific evidence on how DBS produces its effect, the clinical outcomes are significant and dependent on patient selection, surgical placement of hardware, and postoperative management through programming of the electrodes.

SUCCESSFUL OUTCOMES

The success of DBS depends on (a) selection of an appropriate candidate, (b) surgical accuracy of lead placement within the desired target, (c) skill in selecting the appropriate contact or in programming the device, and (d) postimplant symptom management, including medication adjustment and patient education. If the above process is accomplished and acceptable, the benefit is significant and sustained for many years. Success of DBS therapy includes improvement of the following symptoms: tremor, rigidity, bradykinesias, and control of dyskinesias. There is also relief of muscular pain related to reduction in dystonia and rigidity. Often, neck, shoulder, and low back pain syndromes significantly improve and, for some, completely resolve after DBS surgery. Some patients experience a significant decrease in daytime sleepiness as nocturnal sleep patterns improve.

Moreover, many PLWP are able to taper off or considerably reduce preoperative levels of dopamine agonist medications, which have sleepiness as a major side effect (Lyons & Pahwa, 2006). In addition, improvement in sleep may result from a reduction of nocturnal wearing off symptoms, increased ability to turn over in bed, or improvement of tremor, rigidity, and dystonia. Patients frequently report improved sleep patterns related to decreased vivid dreams and hallucinations (Chang & Chou, 2006; Lyons & Pahwa, 2006).

DBS SYMPTOM MANAGEMENT

DBS surgery and therapy do not disrupt or change the normal course of the progression of the disease. The cardinal motor symptoms of PD are well controlled with DBS technology for a considerable period of time, however, the disease continues to progress, and many patients develop nonmotor symptoms. Nonmotor symptoms do not generally improve with DBS because the leads are placed within the motor subterritory of the brain, which specifically improves limb motor function.

Other Parkinson symptoms refractory to DBS are hypophonic speech, micrographia, and medication on-period freezing. Refractory on-period freezing is also referred to as freezing of gait (FOG), which occurs at peak medication doses. It is important to stress that only symptoms that respond to carbidopa/levodopa (Sinemet) respond to DBS. Symptoms that are refractory to carbidopa/levodopa are typically refractory to DBS. For the majority of PLWP, the long-term effects from DBS are well tolerated. Postmortem studies have found minimal focal gliosis around the implanted lead and no focal tissue damage at the site of the leads (Moss, Ryder, Aziz, Graeber, & Bain, 2004).

DBS PATIENT SELECTION

DBS is a complicated therapy and should be reserved for patients who tolerate ambiguity and are not opposed to frequent follow-up visits. DBS is a function of an implanted device in the brain and chest and is subject to the possibility of hardware failure, infection, and the need for periodic battery replacement surgery. Additionally, frequent postoperative visits are needed to program the device and adjust medication therapy. Therefore

DBS therapy is not recommended for those who are reluctant to return for multiple follow-up and programming sessions. The following are *exclusion criteria* for potential DBS candidates:

- Atypical or secondary parkinsonism
- Advanced disease (Hoehn and Yahr score of 4 or greater)
- Cognitive dysfunction (dementia, Mini-Mental State Exam score < 24, Mattis Dementia Rating Scale scores below 1.5–2 SD from age-controlled norm)
- Severe postural instability
- Untreated depression or untreated psychiatric disease
- Uncontrolled hypertension or bleeding diathesis
- Need for repeated magnetic resonance imaging (MRI)
- Unwillingness or inability to cooperate during surgical procedure
- Unrealistic expectations (wanting relief of symptoms that are not improved with levodopa)

The medication management goal for the potential DBS candidate is to evaluate if additional medications or adjustment in the current schedule will qualitatively reduce the patient's off time and disabling dyskinesias. Those who are advanced in disease trajectory may be unable to walk, confined to a wheelchair, bed bound, posturally unstable, have difficulty with swallowing, or experience cognitive changes with minimal response to medication. Ideally, patients should be referred for DBS while they have robust response to dopaminergic medications, but have started to develop motor fluctuations, dyskinesias, or disabling tremor. It is important to consider DBS surgical therapy before patients become too deconditioned or disabled and are forced to retire from gainful employment. Individuals who persist in seeking DBS surgery early in the disease should be carefully evaluated for atypical parkinsonism syndromes and dopaminergic responsiveness (Lang & Widner, 2002).

PATIENT EDUCATION

Teaching patients a vocabulary to use in assessing and labeling their individual Parkinson's symptoms is key to a successful communication pattern throughout the trajectory of disease. Often, patients are unfamiliar with the medical terminology of PD, the symptoms' relationships to their medications, and how to monitor and report symptoms to the treatment team. Nurses should help the patient develop a vocabulary to describe symptoms when they observe them clinically at each visit. If a patient is having tremor, then the nurse should explain that "this is a tremor" or "this is dyskinesia." By learning the clinical terms used in PD evaluations the patient and family will be able to communicate effectively with the health care team.

Preoperative Evaluation and Patient Education

The patient undergoing DBS implantation should be educated during the preoperative phase regarding the benefits and risks of surgery. The patient and immediate family members should all be present for educational sessions and be encouraged to verbalize expected benefits from the procedure in relation to PD medications and symptom improvement. Misconceptions the patient and family may have about the surgical outcome should be discussed openly to reinforce realistic expectations of the procedure (Okun & Foote, 2004). The following section lists steps the treatment team should take with patients and their families during the preoperative phase.

Prior to surgery, a list of all prescription and over-the-counter medications, supplements, and herbals should be reviewed. The patient should be instructed not to take medications that may delay clotting 7–10 days before surgery. Examples of such drugs include aspirin, antiplatelet medications, warfarin (Coumadin), tramadol (Ultracet), nonsteroidal anti-inflammatory drugs and over-the-counter supplements such as vitamin E, gingko, and ginseng. Anticoagulants should be stopped in concordance with recommended guidelines such as the American Association of Clinical Pathologists or other reputable evidence-based guidelines. If the patient is prescribed selegeline (Eldepryl), this should also be stopped 7–10 days prior to surgery to prevent postoperative hypertension, which could be serious if selegeline is combined with meperieine (Demerol) given for pain (Sanghera, Desaloms, & Stewart, 2004).

A preoperative anesthesia assessment should be conducted for surgical risk and risk for anesthesia. Although the patient is typically awake for the first part of the DBS procedure (the insertion of the microelectrodes), the patient will undergo general anesthesia and intubation for placement of the connective wire and the implantable pulse generator (IPG). Part of the anesthesia preoperative clearance includes assessment for any current infections (including respiratory infections) due to risk of postoperative coughing during the intraoperative period which could increase intracranial pressure and upwardly herniate the brain through the burr hole. The anesthesia preoperative clearance also reviews the patient comorbidities for control, such as diabetes, heart disease, and HIV, and requests that any disease such as prostate cancer be in remission. The patient will have laboratory tests before surgery to assess hemoglobin, electrolytes, and clotting factors. A chest X-ray and electrocardiogram (EKG) will be performed as part of the routine preoperative phase (Watson, Bunting-Perry, & Heath, 2007).

Another very important part of the presurgical evaluation assesses for any psychiatric comorbidity such as anxiety, cognitive deficits, and obsessive–compulsive traits. If a patient is extremely anxious in the "off" state, this could cause surgery to be aborted, as the patient's medications are held beginning the evening prior to surgery. The nurse should communicate any noted anxiety to the neurosurgeon so that antianxiety medication can be administered if needed during the lengthy procedure.

All patients seeking DBS should have baseline neuropsychiatric and cognitive testing performed. Any baseline cognitive dysfunction is important to define. Bifrontal approach surgery carries the risk of transient or, for some, permanent decline in cognition. Therefore, with older adults with PD who have mild cognitive impairment, the potential for developing significant decline from DBS surgery may outweigh the potential benefit to motor function (Machado et al, 2006; Sanghera et al, 2004).

A frank discussion of possible addictive or obsessive–compulsive behaviors should be part of the presurgical assessment for the patient seeking DBS. These behaviors have been noted in PD patients taking dopamine agonists. Patients with addictive or compulsive behaviors such as gambling, pornography, or illicit drug use need to be identified in order to ascertain if these behaviors are related to PD medication and are not a result of the surgical procedure. The presence of known compulsive behaviors will also assist the treatment team in making decisions regarding postoperative medication changes.

Patients should be advised that dopaminergic medications will be stopped at midnight prior to the day of surgery to prevent medication-induced dyskinesias, which could interfere with the microelectrode recordings during the intraoperative phase. Also, with the patient in the off-medication state, the neurosurgeon is able to observe clinical improvement of the symptoms after the electrode is passed into the targeted area and intraoperative stimulation is applied (Sanghera et al., 2004).

Although some patients choose to have their hair cut short, the patient should be informed that the surgical team will prep his or her head for surgery in the operating room. Most surgeons are able to perform the surgery with limited hair shaving. Patients should be prepared for the neurosurgeon to attach a stereotactic frame to the head, illustrated in Figure 6.1. The frame stabilizes the head during the MRI and surgery to assist the surgical team in targeting coordinates for microelectrode placement. Another purpose of the stereotactic frame is to immobilize the head when it is attached to the operating table. The patient is maintained in a semi-sitting position for approximately 4 hours for the lead placements. The frame holds the head stable as the lead wire is passed down into the brain toward the identified target (Machado et al., 2006; Sanghera et al., 2004).

FIGURE 6.1 Location of the Subthalamic Nucleus (STN) and Globus Pallidus Interna (GPI) with Electrode Placement in the Brain. Patient in Sterotactic Head Frame.

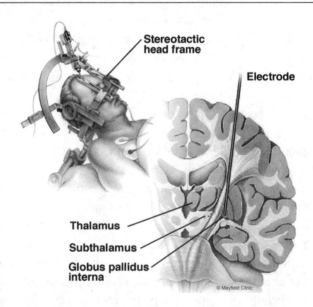

Source: Reprinted with permission of the mayfield clinic.

Educate the patient that the neurosurgeon will drill a burr hole into the top of the skull for the passing of the microelectrode wire. The burr hole may be bilateral or unilateral, depending on the PD treatment ordered by the neurologist or neurosurgeon. The electrodes are carefully placed using anatomical referencing (MRI) and neurophysiological (computer-guided navigation) into the predetermined area. After the microelectrodes are placed, the second phase of the surgery will be conducted to place the IPG device. This portion of the surgery is done under general anesthesia.

The patient and family should be made aware of the possible risks and benefits associated with DBS surgery. The two primary risks are hemorrhage or stroke from the placement of the leads and risk of hardware infection resulting in complete removal of the system. Sometimes the hemorrhages are small and subclinical; other times, they can be devastating, causing coma and death. The risks of hemorrhage or stroke are center-dependent, but the reported rate is 3% to 4%, and the rate of infection is 5% to 8% (Lyons & Pahwa, 2004). Other risks of DBS surgery are postoperative headache; skin erosion over connector sites; and memory loss or confusion from bifrontal implants, especially in the frail elderly, who may exhibit postanesthesia delirium. Other changes that could occur are personality changes; pneumonia; pulmonary embolism; seizures; cerebrospinal fluid leak; hardware connection issues, including possible lead fracture; and connector damage. Also, the IPG has a limited battery life and must be replaced within 3–5 years (Benabid, Chabardes, & Seigneuret, 2005; Watson et al., 2007).

Postoperative Teaching

The patient and family should be educated regarding the postoperative phase of DBS surgery and encouraged to verbalize concerns and care needs. Much of postoperative care is managed at home, and the success of the procedure is enhanced with family who are engaged in the care process. The following section lists steps the treatment team should take with patients and their families during the postoperative phase.

Instruct the patient and family to report temperature elevations, which may be signs of surgical wound infection. Some bruising, swelling, and tenderness at the implantation sites is expected. The patient should refrain from lifting anything greater than 20 pounds for at least 30 days. Sutures will be removed 1–2 weeks following surgery. Occasionally, benign periorbital edema can occur following DBS surgery from the local anesthetics injected for the frame placement. This should resolve within a week and can be minimized by applying ice packs over the affected body part for short periods (Watson et al., 2007).

Preserving the patient's body image is paramount in assessing for postoperative adjustment to DBS technology. Surgical scars and skull changes relating to the placement of hardware should be reviewed. On top of the head, the patient will typically have bilaterally placed scars and two small bumps that protrude from the normally shaped skull. The patient will have a scar about 3 in across where the IPG is placed and an inch-long scar behind the ear from the connection wire. Patients and families often find that these changes in body image are tolerable, provided that mobility improves. Women may choose to wear a wig and men often wear a hat until hair growth is achieved to be styled to meet the patients' care preferences (Watson et al., 2007).

Patients should be educated that postimplant, they may experience a significant improvement in PD symptoms and may be tempted to stop or drastically decrease their PD medications. Patients who reduce or stop their PD medications place themselves at risk for developing neuroleptic malignant syndrome (NMS). NMS is a potentially lethal condition that has been described in patients with idiopathic PD after long-term dopaminergic medications are suddenly stopped or moderately decreased. If patients with PD develop severe rigidity, stupor, and hyperthermia, levodopa withdrawal should be suspected, and the patient should be taken to the emergency room of his or her local hospital immediately and the dopaminergic drug restarted as soon as possible to prevent rhabdomyolysis and renal failure (Ward, 2005).

Many patients develop mood complaints, such as apathy, after DBS surgery, and emotional changes can be secondary to large reductions in doses of dopaminergic drugs. Occasionally, patients experience temporary bradyphrenia, or slow, apathetic affect, from bifrontal surgical approaches. Changes in mood and affect should be discussed preoperatively to prepare family members for any potential transient changes (Sanghera et al., 2004).

It is tempting for patients and families to attribute symptom changes after surgery to the implantable device. By providing education in the preoperative stage regarding possible symptom experiences, such as painful limb dystonia or curling of the foot, these symptoms can be effectively identified and managed by the treatment team through programming of the IPG. However, if after DBS surgery there are intermittent problems, it may be a result of PD symptoms, medications, or another unexplained etiology. By using a motor diary the patient can assist the treatment team in identifying and tracking symptoms in relation to medication schedules and daily activities. The provider can then help correlate problems with stimulation, medication, or symptom progression.

Postoperatively, the patient may experience a phenomenon called the *microlesioning effect,* in which the patient may experience a dramatic reduction in PD symptoms for 1–3 weeks. If the patient experiences the microlesioning effect, this is a good indication of the surgery's success (Watson et al., 2007). It must be explained to both the patient and the family that this honeymoon period does not last and that they should not be concerned when the preoperative symptoms return. When the stimulator is turned on and programmed, most PD symptoms should resolve. Over the first 3 months, patients may require up to six visits before final programming is achieved. Postoperatively, the physician or trained neurology nurse will assume the monitoring and programming of the stimulator and establish when the stimulator will be activated. Some teams activate the stimulator immediately after surgery, while others wait several weeks before IPG activation.

DBS SURGERY

Components of the Implanted DBS System

The components of the implanted hardware include Medtronic (Minneapolis, MN) leads approved by the U.S. Food and Drug Administration (FDA), extension wires, and the IPG. The lead wire tip contains four platinum–iridium electrodes, powered by the IPG, that emit the electrical field to the brain tissue. The lead wire is implanted into a specific region of the basal ganglia, usually the motor subterritory in a selected basal ganglia nucleus. The battery is implanted in the subclavian region or abdomen, and extension wires are tunneled to connect with the IPG. When the lead is connected to the pulse generator, it is ready to deliver its concentric or elliptical electrical charge to surrounding brain tissue.

Selection of DBS Surgical Team

DBS surgery is an equipment-intensive, complicated procedure with many nuances that make the accuracy of placement of the electrode challenging. Medical centers with experienced and collaborative teams benefit the patient and family and have higher success rates (Edmondson, Bohmer, & Pisano, 2001). Typically, a neurosurgeon and neurophysiologist lead the DBS team. A neurophysiologist often performs the brain mapping. Brain mapping is the second diagnostic tool for ensuring the correct placement of the lead into the targeted area. The neurophysiologist uses the coordinates calculated from the MRI, and as the neurosurgeon lowers the platinum–iridium microelectrode into the brain, extracellular recordings are mapped to an oscilloscope and played on an audio monitor. Each area of the brain has its own electrophysiological signature that can be seen on the oscilloscope (Sanghera et al., 2004). Large university movement disorder centers and the Veterans Administration PADRECC offer not only the skilled neurosurgeons and neurophysiologists needed to perform the procedure but also multidisciplinary teams to perform the presurgical assessments and postsurgical management in most cases.

Surgical Procedure

The DBS procedure is performed in stages and consists of three parts:

1. The DBS lead wire with four contacts (electrodes) at the end of the lead wire is inserted deep into the target area of the brain.
2. The extension or connecting wire that runs underneath the skin from the DBS lead at the burr hole site is placed behind the ear and down the neck into the chest, where it will connect to the battery pack or IPG.
3. The IPG is placed under the skin in the subclavian region, like a pacemaker. The IPG is about 2 in. in diameter and 0.5 in. thick. There is a battery and computer chip inside the casing. The IPG sends electrical impulses through the connecting wire to the DBS electrodes placed deep within the brain.

On the morning of surgery, the patient's head will be prepped in the operating room suite. Most surgeons are able to perform the task limiting hair removal to a focused area, not a complete shave. A stereotactic head frame will be placed, which is a large, open casing made of metal bars that screw into the patient's skull at several points. Local anesthesia is given at frame contact points for patient comfort. With the frame in place, the patient will undergo MRI, where calibrations on the head frame are merged with brain images to form a computerized map of the targeted area. Merging of the MRI and stereotactic frame gives the coordinates needed for accurate placement of the lead wire into the target area of the basal ganglia. Computerized stereotactic targeting is critical to accurate placement of the lead wire into the selected anatomic location for optimal symptom control. After the coordinates are obtained, the stereotactic frame will be bolted to the operating table to maintain the head in a fixed position throughout the operation (Machado et al., 2006; Medtronic, Inc., 2003).

The lead wire is introduced into the brain tissue 1 mm at a time with concurrent electrophysiological brain mapping using a microelectrode. The electrophysiological brain mapping technique uses tiny electrodes that can record electrical activity from the brain cells. The brain cell activity seen during the mapping procedure is able to identify cells within the thalamus, globus pallidus, and subthalamic nucleus as the cell activity of each has its own signature, which assists the neurosurgeon in guiding the lead wire toward the desired surgical target. Target confirmation is obtained by microelectrode recording in most cases. If the patient is to have bilateral implanted leads, a second burr hole is surgically prepared, and the procedure is repeated (Machado et al., 2006).

After the first lead wire is in place intraoperatively, a sterile alligator clamp and cable are attached to a handheld stimulator to test the effect of stimulation on the patient's symptoms. During intraoperative testing of the DBS electrode the patient is observed for GPi or STN stimulation, voltage thresholds for stimulation-induced side effects, spread to capsular fibers, and assessment of tremor control. Often, the patient's tremor or rigidity will resolve during the intraoperative stimulator test process. Symptom relief is a clear indication of the success of the lead placement. Once symptom relief is observed, the lead wire is then secured into a burr hole ring to prevent it from moving, and a burr hole cap is permanently placed over the burr hole. The stereotactic frame is removed, and the lead wire is attached to an extension wire. At this point the patient is given a general anesthetic, and the physician begins percutaneous tunneling under the skin behind the ear down to the subclavian area where the IPG will be implanted and the extension wire will be connected. Surgical incisions are then closed, and an impedance check of the IPG is performed intra-operatively to ensure that the circuit from the lead wire, extension wire, and IPG stimulator is complete (Machado et al., 2006; Medtronic, Inc., 2003). Figure 6.2 illustrates the typical placement of lead wires into the brain and connective wires running down the neck to the IPG implanted in the upper chest area.

FIGURE 6.2 Placement of Lead Wires into the Brain and Connective Wires Running Down the Neck to the Implantable Pulse Generator (IPG) Implanted in the Upper Chest Area.

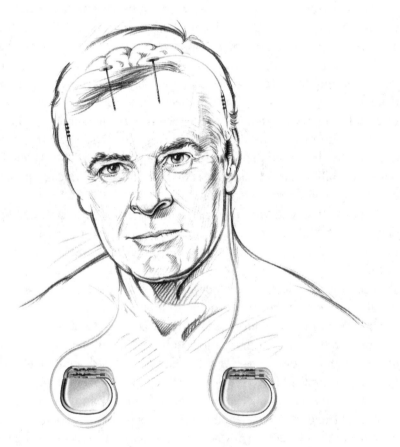

Source: Reprinted with permission of Medtronic, Inc.

The procedure may last from 3 to 6 hours, and the patient is usually discharged 2–3 days postprocedure. Before the patient is discharged, a postoperative MRI or computerized tomography (CT) scan will be completed to confirm proper lead placement within the brain (Mosley, Starr, & Marks, 2003).

Surgical Complications of DBS

DBS therapy has inherent risks and complications that can occur from the surgical procedure or from the implanted hardware (Hariz, 2002; Oh, Abosch, Kim, Lang, & Lozano, 2002). Surgical risks can be minimized if the implanting team is experienced and performs surgical planning techniques that avoid placing the leads through sulci, where small vessels are present, or in the ventricle, where the wall is lined with small vessels. By avoiding these anatomical structures the risk of an intracranial bleed can be reduced. Planned trajectory and ultimate placement of the lead is done using a MRI-based software planning computer program that shows the patient's brain images and larger vessels, but in the end this procedure is done without the ability to directly visualize the trajectory of the lead as it penetrates brain tissue (Machado et al., 2006; Sanghera et al., 2004).

The risk of hemorrhage is 3% to 4% per implanted hemisphere, but not all hemorrhages are clinically significant. The hemorrhage can occur anywhere along the tract of the lead, either superficially or deep within the basal ganglia. The hemorrhage can be either venous or arterial. All hemorrhages produce focal edema around the bleed that generally resolves over 1–3 months. Full recovery can take up to 6 months. The time course of the hemorrhage can be immediate or delayed, but the major risk is within the first 24 hours after surgery (Binder, Rau, & Starr, 2003, 2005).

The risk of an air embolism from venous exposure is another potential complication, especially for those with unknown patent foramen ovalae. Patients with patent foramen ovalae can develop rapid intraoperative stroke symptoms, causing the DBS procedure to be abruptly aborted and the patient rushed to the CT scanner to assess for stroke. Another complication is pneumocephalus, which occurs from the loss of cerebral spinal fluid, which then allows air to enter the cerebral spinal fluid space, causing frontal lobe compression. Some air entering the cerebral spinal fluid space is common and may only produce a mild headache or transient confusion in the postoperative phase. A large amount of air can cause frontal lobe compression with severe headaches and mild frontal lobe compression–related personality changes. To assess for a large pneumocephalus, a postoperative CT scan can readily detect air, and most patients are treated with the usual 100% non-rebreather oxygen mask (Machado et al., 2006; Origitano, Pertuzzelli, Leonetti, & Vandevender, 2006).

It has been reported that some patients who have been implanted with DBS suffer with worsening depression, leading to suicide, postoperative delirium, hypersexuality, or other dopamine dysregulation syndrome personality changes (Saint-Cyr, Trépanier, Kumar, Lozano, & Lang, 2000; Voon, Kubu, Krack, Houeto, & Tröster, 2006). However, there are also reports that there is a high incidence of PD patients who at baseline or predisease manifestation elicit risk-seeking personalities or compulsive behaviors, termed *punding* (Evans, Lawrence, Potts, Appel, & Lees, 2005; Lozano & Eltahawy, 2004). It is not clear if DBS provides patients more functional ability and independence to perform these obsessions or if somehow DBS may contribute to the behavior. Most reports in the literature cite case reports of patients who demonstrate punding activities post-DBS implant without clear understanding of premorbid or baseline behaviors (Benabid et al., 2005).

Hardware device failure or infections are inherent with implantable systems and can be the most disheartening complication if the system must be removed. Most infections occur within the first month of surgery, typically begin asymptomatically, and within 2–3 weeks present with serosanguinous fluid at the incision line, or an incision that is not healing well at the IPG site. Patients are educated to keep the incisions dry and clean in the first week after surgery and to closely monitor the IPG site for puffiness, redness, drainage, or tenderness. Patients are encouraged to report or return to the clinic with any possible sign of infection. If an infection becomes apparent and localized in the IPG site area, the implanted lead wire may be saved and only the IPG removed. The risk for the lead wire becoming infected is significant and requires the entire system removal if the IPG infection contaminates the lead wires. If the entire system is removed, the patient must have 6 weeks of home intravenous antibiotics and wait at least 6 more weeks to verify that the infection is completely resolved before plans to reimplant the DBS system can be undertaken.

POSTOPERATIVE OUTCOMES

The goal of DBS surgery is to improve the quality of life and maintain functioning for PLWP. The motor symptoms of rigidity and tremor control are longer lasting, but bradykinesia tends to be more refractory, especially in the older, more advanced patient. If a patient has freezing of gait that is responsive to levodopa, then stimulation may improve gait abnormalities. However, as the disease progresses, many PLWP develop on-period freezing, which may be refractory to DBS therapy.

Dyskinesias are reduced with DBS stimulation related to the reductions in dopaminergic medication. If the GPi is the implant target, control of dyskinesias is expected despite medication adjustment, as GPi DBS suppresses dyskinesias directly. STN DBS can produce or increase dyskinesias that can be more severe and disabling than preoperative symptoms. STN stimulation–induced dyskinesias often appear in the head and neck region and then may spread to involve the limbs. If dyskinesias occur in the postsurgical state, they are managed using either less stimulation, less medication, or programming techniques (Kleiner-Fisman et al., 2003).

Moderate postural instability often improves with DBS, but severe balance problems do not respond well to DBS. FOG is another symptom seen in more advanced cases of PD, and recent studies show that it is not a result of degeneration from the dopaminergic pathways, but rather from a norephinephrine-mediated pathway localized within the pons of the brain stem nucleus called the predunculopontine nucleus (PPN) (Pahapill and Lozano, 2000). Recently, investigational research studies are underway to implant the PPN with a DBS system to treat FOG and postural instability refractory to medications (Plaha & Gill, 2005).

MEDICATION REDUCTION PLANS

Some patients can safely have PD medications reduced by 25% immediately after bilateral DBS activation. Others delay making changes in the preoperative medication schedule until the microlesioning benefit subsides and the patient has fully recovered from the surgery. It is not always appropriate to reduce levodopa requirements postoperatively. It is important to remind the patient that the goal is not medication reduction, but more on time, fewer fluctuations, smoother days, and a better quality of day. Many patients will have significant changes in medications over the first year. It is important to have the patient follow up with a skilled neurologist and programmer who can work with the DBS and the medications concurrently to gain the best benefit of combined therapy.

IMPLANTABLE PULSE GENERATOR
BATTERY LIFE

Patients with implanted DBS technology should be in regular contact with their managing providers for IPG voltage assessments to determine when the IPG battery life indicates the need for replacement. As partners in their care, patients are frequently provided with a handheld device, called the access controller, that enables the IPG to be switched off or on and voltages increased as needed for symptom management. The access controller does not indicate the IPG battery life status and cannot detect battery end of life. For Parkinson's patients it is recommended that their IPG remain on at all times and batteries be replaced electively before reaching a critically low voltage. Battery life is a reflection of total voltage use, and the typical IPG battery devices require replacement every 3–5 years.

PROGRAMMING THE IPG

Programming the IPG is a skill managed by a variety of members within the interdisciplinary team. Typically, programming is conducted by registered nurses in large movement disorder centers or in teaching hospitals. However, in a health care provider's private practice, programming of the IPG may be performed by a neurologist, neurosurgeon, or neurophysiologist. The device that is used to turn the IPG on is called the clinician's handheld programmer. This programmer provides information about the IPG, such as voltage; pulse width; rate; hours used by the battery; the percent of battery used; impedance numbers; electrodes used; the serial number of the IPG; the limits set that allow the patient to increase his or her voltage at home, if necessary; and unipolar or bipolar setting.

Voltage, pulse width, and rate are three electrical concepts used in the understanding of programming DBS technology. Voltage is the *intensity* of the stimulation that is delivered to the targeted area of the brain. The pulse width is measured in microseconds and is the *duration* of each stimulus. The combination of the voltage and pulse width determines the electrical charge density delivered to the surgical target. The voltage is the strength of the current, and the pulse width is how long the current lingers with each pulse. The rate is measured in hertz and is the number of *pulses* per second delivered to the target. The rate is the least effective parameter in programming, whereas the voltage and pulse width together produce the greatest effect on the patient's symptoms (Stewart, Desaloms, & Sanghera, 2005).

The DBS system delivers electrical therapy through activation of the IPG and to activate contacts on the lead's electrodes. The lead itself has four contacts or electrodes and delivers its electrical charge through a combination of a number of activated electrodes, the voltage, and the pulse width and rate, measured in hertz. The system needs at least one negative and one positive electrode to complete the electrical circuit. The active electrode that produces the focus of therapy is the negative electrode. The negative electrode spreads its current into adjacent tissue and pathways but needs a positive electrode to complete the circuit. The positive electrode should be immediately adjacent to the negative or can be the IPG itself or the case as positive (Stewart et al., 2005).

The electrical field or stimulated area can be shaped, narrowed, or widened by selecting the contact configuration to be unipolar or bipolar. The higher the voltage, the wider the spread of current, and the strongest, or widest spreading, current is produced in a unipolar setting. The unipolar current may stimulate the desired target but also adjacent structures, producing side effects unacceptable to the patient. When adverse side effects are experienced, changing the electrical configuration to a bipolar setting may reduce the spread of current into unwanted structures and still provide the desired benefit. Unipolar settings are stronger and ideal if tolerated and should be used as the initial setting. Bipolar settings generally require 0.5–1.0 V more to produce the same efficacy as unipolar settings, but without spreading to adjacent structures (Stewart et al., 2005).

Tonic muscle contractions are side effects produced from spread of electrical current to the nearby capsular fibers. These fibers contain corticobulbar and corticospinal tracts from the motor cortex down the spinal cord. When these fibers are activated, the patient experiences tightness of various body parts.

Initial programming is typically scheduled 2–4 weeks after surgery, when postoperative edema or transient benefit from the microlesioning effect has diminished and the patient's baseline symptoms have returned. The patient is usually scheduled for initial programming in the morning after medications are withheld overnight (off state) or, at a minimum, for at least 4 hours. Arriving in the relatively off state allows for return of the parkinsonian symptoms and facilitates screening each of the contacts to determine which of the four contacts are most effective in relieving the patient's symptoms. If the patient's microlesioning benefit persists or if he or she arrives for programming in the medication on state, there are no motor symptoms to gauge programming effectiveness. Thus patients must be advised to come to initial programming sessions in the relatively off state to assist the programmer in observing symptoms to target for DBS therapy (Stewart et al., 2005).

Some clinicians successfully gauge programming by using a formal evaluation tool, such as the motor subscale of the Unified Parkinson's Disease Rating Scale (UPDRS). The UPDRS motor scale objectively tests a patient's motor performance by scoring each limb's motor function (Fahn, Elton, & UPDRS Development Committee, 1987). However, some programmers gauge programming sessions based on a single symptom, such as rigidity, bradykinesia, or tremor (Deuschl et al., 2006).

The goal of programming is to identify which one or two electrodes is the most efficacious in improving a specific motor symptom. It is best to use a systematic approach to minimize variables and maximize consistency. The clinician should screen each electrode by increasing the voltage, looking for side effects, tolerability (maximum voltage in each contact), and then efficacy. The objective is to find the amount of voltage that produces the maximum benefit without creating side effects. Specific guidelines in IPG programming and management are beyond the scope of this chapter. However, basic algorithms are published by Volkman et al. (2006) to assist clinicians in DBS programming techniques. The reader should be mindful that DBS programming is a skill that can be learned and that programming is an important tool in managing patients who have undergone DBS surgery. To gain skills in programming, one may take courses offered by the Medtronic corporation or be trained by a skilled, established programmer. Currently there are no criteria designating a health care provider's credentials or minimum training to qualify individuals to perform DBS programming and management. However, the success of DBS surgery is reflected in the programmer's skill at targeting and adjusting DBS technology to treat the cardinal motor symptoms of PD.

SPECIAL CONSIDERATIONS FOR DBS IMPLANTS

Patients with DBS hardware will need information to manage their lives as they will be living with hardware and technology to provide symptomatic relief of Parkinson's symptoms. Patients and families should be educated in the risk and limitations of medical technology that may interfere with their DBS devices. Simple routine activities such as EKGs can be affected by DBS technology. More advanced medical technology that may be contraindicated in patients with implantable devices includes diatheramy, electrocautery, and MRI. The following section will provide a brief overview of medical procedures and technologies to be discussed with patients undergoing DBS surgery.

Patients who need emergency resuscitation with an IPG implanted should be defibrillated to preserve cardiac function. External defibrillation or cardioversion may damage the IPG because of the current these devices produce. It is recommended that if elective cardioversion is warranted for serious arrhythmias, the IPG amplitude should be set to zero and then turned off for the procedure. The defibrillator pads should be placed at least 2 in. away from the IPG. If a patient needs a cardiac pacemaker, the IPG and the pacemaker should be at least 10 in. apart (Lyons & Okun, 2005).

Patients who need an EKG or electroencephalogram should be aware that their IPGs are likely to produce artifacts that can interfere with these procedures. Therefore the IPG should be turned off to prevent this from occurring. Patients may have regular X-rays, such as dental X-rays and mammography, without any special precautions, however, no full-body MRI should be performed on a patient after DBS surgery. MRI uses a radio frequency that can heat up the implanted electrodes and leads, thereby burning the surrounding tissue, which can cause serious injury to the brain or death. Any patient with implanted devices should alert their MRI technician before undergoing an MRI procedure. The recommended maximum displayed head specific absorption rate is 0.1 W/kg, which provides a reasonable thermal safety margin and prevents heating of the internal wires. The MRI must be performed with a head coil and Tesla strength of 1.5 or less (Lange & Malli, 2006; Tremmel, 2005). It is recommended that before a patient is exposed to MRI, the IPG voltage should be programmed to zero. This requires a programming device (Medtronic programmers 7432 and 8840 or the access controller 7438). Persons trained in the use of the programmers are most often found in movement disorder centers or neurology or neurosurgery services. Figure 6.3 illustrates the Medtronic patient access controller, IPG, and lead wire.

Diathermy is contraindicated for all patients with DBS implants. Serious brain injury may be caused by exposure of any part of the IPG device to diathermy. Diathermy is a therapy involving application of a heat coil to the skin or body, which heats the brain electrodes, causing serious brain

FIGURE 6.3 Medtronic Patient Access Controller, IPG, and Lead Wire.

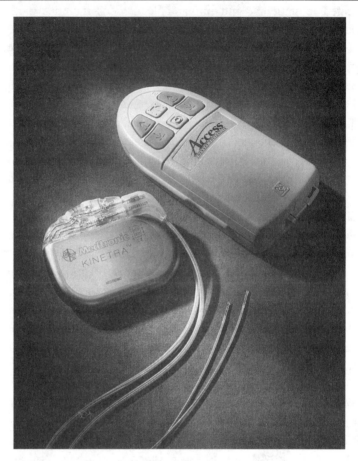

Source: Reprinted with permission of Medtronic, Inc.

injury or death. Diathermy is a procedure used by dentists, pain specialists, and physical therapists to reduce swelling, pain, stiffness, and joint contractures and to promote wound healing (Medtronic, Inc., 2001).

Surgical procedures performed on the DBS patient in which the surgeon must use electrocautery to stop minor bleeding during the procedure are safe if the flow of the electrical current is reduced. The patient should inform the surgeon of the IPG device, and the device should be turned off after the voltage has been programmed to zero. Only a bipolar electrocautery should be used, and a ground lead should be placed on one of the legs of the patient. If any electrical charges from the electrocautery begin to transmit, they will go to the patient's leg instead of the neurostimulator (Rubin, 2002).

Ultrasound is safe; however, the IPG should be programmed to zero and then turned off before the procedure. When a DBS patient must undergo invasive dental work that could cause bleeding, it is recommended that the patient undergo a course of prophylactic antibiotics to prevent the oral bacteria from attacking the implanted hardware (Rubin, 2002).

SUMMARY

The neuroscience nurse plays a pivotal role in the care and education of Parkinson's patients and their families. DBS therapy for PD received FDA approval in 2002, making this treatment a new specialty in the neurological and neurosurgical community. The success of DBS is dependent on careful patient selection and education regarding DBS and preoperative, intraoperative, and postoperative phases of surgery. The patient and family are partners in care and must understand what can be expected from the therapy to avoid disappointments. The neuroscience nurse working with DBS patients plays an important and unique role as consultant and educator for professionals that may have limited understanding and experience with PLWP that have been implanted with DBS technology.

REFERENCES

Avanzi, M., Baratti, M., Cabrini, S., Uber, E., Brighetti, G., & Bonfa. (2006). Prevalence of pathological gambling in patients with Parkinson's disease. *Movement Disorders*, 21(12), 2068–2072.

Benabid, A., Chabardes, S., & Seigneuret, E. (2005). Deep brain stimulation in Parkinson's disease: Long-term efficacy and safety—What happened this year? *Current Opinion in Neurology, 18,* 623–630.

Binder, D. K., Rau, G., & Starr, P. A. (2003). Hemorrhagic complications of microelectrode-guided deep brain stimulation. *Stereotactic and Functional Neurosurgery, 80,* 28–31.

Binder, D. K., Rau, G. M., & Starr, P. A. (2005). Risk factors for hemorrhage during microelectrode-guided deep brain stimulator implantation for movement disorders. *Neurosurgery, 56,* 722–732.

Chang, V. C., & Chou, K. L. (2006). Deep brain stimulation for Parkinson's disease: Patient selection and motor outcomes. *Medicine and Health Rhode Island, 89,* 142–144.

Deuschl, G., Herzog, J., Kleiner-Fisman, G., Kubu, C., Lozano, A. M., Lyons, K. E., et al. (2006). Deep brain stimulation: Postoperative issues. *Movement Disorders, 21*(Suppl. 14), 219–237.

Edmondson, A., Bohmer, R., & Pisano, G. (2001, October). Speeding up team learning. *Harvard Business Review,* 125–132.

Evans, A. H., Lawrence, A. D., Potts, J., Appel, S., Lees, A. J. (2005). Factors influencing susceptibility to compulsive dopaminergic drug use in Parkinson's disease. *Neurology, 65,* 1570–1574.

Fahn, S., Elton, R., & UPDRS Development Committee. (1987). The unified Parkinson's disease rating scale. In S. Fahn, C. D. Marsden, & D. Calne (Eds.), *Recent developments in Parkinson's disease* (pp. 153–163). New York: Macmillan.

Ghika, J., Ghika-Schmid, F., Fankhauser, H., Assal, G., Vingerhoets, A., Albanese, A. et al. (1999). Bilateral contemporaneous posteroventral pallidotomy for the treatment of Parkinson's disease: Neuropsychological and neurological side effects. Report of four cases and review of the literature. *Journal of Neurosurgery, 91,* 313–321.

Grill, W. M., Snyder, A. N., & Miocinovic, S. (2004). Deep brain stimulation creates an informational lesion of the stimulated nucleus. *Neuroreport, 15,* 1137–1140.

Hariz, M. (2002). Complication of deep brain stimulation surgery. *Movement Disorders, 17*(Suppl. 3), 162–166.

Hashimoto, T., Elder, C. M., Okun, M. S., Patrick, S. K., & Vitek, J. L. (2003). Stimulation of the subthalamic nucleus changes the firing pattern of pallidal neurons. *Journal of Neuroscience, 23,* 1916–1923.

Hilker, R., Voges, J., Ghaemi, M., Lehrke, R., Rudolf, J., Koulousakis, A., et al. (2003). Deep brain stimulation of the subthalamic nucleus does not increase the striatal dopamine concentration in parkinsonian humans. *Movement Disorders, 18,* 41–48.

Kleiner-Fisman, G., Herzog, J., Fisman, D. N., Tamma, F., Lyons, K. E., Pahwa, R., et al. (2006). Subthalamic nucleus deep brain stimulation: Summary and meta-analysis of outcomes. *Movement Disorders, 21*(Suppl. 14), 290–304.

Lang, A. E., & Widner, H. (2002). Deep brain stimulation for Parkinson's disease: Patient selection and evaluation. *Movement Disorders, 17*(Suppl. 3), 94–101.

Lange, S., & Malli, S. (2006) Implanted device + MRI = trouble? *Nursing 36,* 75.

Lozano, A. M., & Eltahawy, H. (2004). How does DBS work? *Clinical Neurophysiology, 57,* 733–736.

Lyons, J. M., & Okun, M. S. (2005). *Parkinson disease: Guide to deep brain stimulation therapy.* Miami, FL: National Parkinson Foundation.

Lyons, K. E., & Pahwa, R. (2004). Deep brain stimulation in Parkinson's disease. *Current Neurology and Neuroscience Reports, 4,* 290–295.

Lyons, K. E., & Pahwa, R. (2006). Effects of bilateral subthalamic nucleus stimulation on sleep, daytime sleepiness, and early morning dystonia in patients with Parkinson disease. *Journal of Neurosurgery, 104,* 502–505.

Machado, A., Rexai, A. R., Kopell, B. H., Gross, R. E., Sharan, A. D., & Benabid, A. L. (2006). Deep brain stimulation for Parkinson's disease: Surgical techniques and perioperative management. *Movement Disorders, 21*(Suppl. 14), 247–258.

McIntyre, C. C., Grill, W. M., Sherman, D. L., & Thakor, N. V. (2004a). Cellular effects of deep brain stimulation: Model-based analysis of activation and inhibition. *Journal of Neurophysiology, 91,* 1457–1469.

McIntyre, C. C., Savasta, M., Kerkerian-Le Goff, L., & Vitek, J. L. (2004b). Uncovering the mechanism(s) of action of deep brain stimulation: Activation, inhibition, or both. *Clinical Neurophysiology, 115,* 1239–1248.

Medtronic, Inc. (2001, September). *Safety alert for physicians.* Retrieved April 5, 2006, from http://www.medtronic.com/neuro/diathermy_alert/alert_physicians.html

Medtronic. (2003). *Medtronic DBS implant manual.* Minneapolis: Author.

Mosley, A. D., Starr, P. A., & Marks, W. J., Jr. (2003). Treating Parkinson's disease, part 2—Surgical procedures. *Federal Practitioner, 20,* 66–73.

Moss, J., Ryder, T., Aziz, T. Z., Graeber, M. B., & Bain, P. G. (2004). Electron microscopy of tissue adherent to explanted electrodes in dystonia and Parkinson's disease. *Brain, 127,* 2755–2763.

Oh, M. Y., Abosch, A., Kim, S. H., Lang, A. E., & Lozano, A. M. (2002). Long-term hardware-related complications of deep brain stimulation. *Neurosurgery, 50,* 1268–1274.

Okun, M. S., & Foote, K. D. (2004). A mnemonic for Parkinson disease patients considering DBS: A tool to improve perceived outcome of surgery. *Neurology, 10,* 290.

Origitano, T. C., Pertuzzelli, G. J., Leonetti, J. P., & Vandevender, D. (2006). Combined anterior and anterolateral approaches to the cranial base: Complication analysis, avoidance, and management. *Neurosurgery, 58*(Suppl. 2), 327–336.

Pahapill, P. A., & Loranzo, A. M. (2000). The pedunculopontine nucleus and Parkinson's disease. *Brain, 123,* 1767–1783.

Plaha, P., & Gill, S. S. (2005). Bilateral deep brain stimulation of the pedunculopontine nucleus for Parkinson's disease. *Neuroreport 16,* 1883–1887.

Rubin, R. (2002, December 21). *You need to know this: DBS in the health care environment.* Retrieved April 12, 2005, from http://www.rewiredforlife.org/newsdetail.asp?ID=30

Saint-Cyr, J. A., Trépanier, L. L., Kumar, R., Lozano, A. M., & Lang, A. E. (2000). Neuropsychological consequences of chronic bilateral stimulation of the subthalamic nucleus in Parkinson's disease. *Brain, 123*(Pt. 10), 2091–2108.

Sanghera, M. K., Desaloms, J. M., & Stewart, R. M. (2004). High frequency stimulation of the subthalamic nucleus for the treatment of Parkinson's disease—A team perspective. *Journal of Neuroscience Nursing, 36,* 301–311.

Stewart, R. M., Desaloms, J. M., & Sanghera, M. K. (2005). Stimulation of the subthalamic nucleus for the treatment of Parkinson's disease: Postoperative management, programming, and rehabilitation. *Journal of Neuroscience Nursing, 37,* 108–114.

Tremmel, J. (2005, November). *Urgent device correction—Change of safe limits for MRI procedures used with Medtronic ACTIVA deep brain stimulation systems.* Minneapolis, MN: Medtronic, Inc.

Volkmann, J., Herzog, J., Kopper, F., & Deuschl, G. (2002). Introduction to the programming of deep brain stimulators. *Movement Disorders, 17*(Suppl. 3), 181–187.

Volkmann, J., Moro, E., & Pahwa, R. (2006). Basic algorithms for programming of deep brain stimulation in Parkinson's disease. *Movement Disorders, 21*(Suppl. 14), 284–289.

Voon, V., Kubu, C., Krack, P., Houeto, J. L., & Tröster, A. I. (2006). Deep brain stimulation: Neuropsychological and neuropsychiatric issues. *Movement Disorders, 21*(Suppl. 14), 305–327.

Ward, C. (2005). Neuroleptic malignant syndrome in a patient with Parkinson's disease: A case study. *Journal of Neuroscience Nursing, 37,* 160–162.

Watson, H., Bunting-Perry, L., & Heath, S. (2007). Deep brain stimulation pre-op assessment and teaching. In G. Baltuch & M. B. Stern (Eds.), *Deep brain stimulation for Parkinson's disease.* New York: Taylor and Francis.

7

Palliative Care: Caring for Frail Older Adults With Parkinson's Disease

Lisette Bunting-Perry, MScN, RN

INTRODUCTION

Depending on age of onset, symptom progression, and comorbid diseases, older adults with Parkinson's disease (PD) may be predisposed to poor health. The decline in health for many older adults with PD is a result of disease progression, acute illness, comorbid disease, or serious disease, such as cancer. The reduction of health status in older adults diminishes vitality and resilience, leading to dependence on assistive devices or family members to manage activities of daily life.

The goal of this chapter is to focus on the clinical assessment of the frail older adult with PD and to present a model for palliative clinical care. The goal of care is to maintain the older adult with PD in the community and provide a treatment plan to facilitate transitions across the health care continuum. The definition of an older adult in this chapter is an individual aged 65 years or older.

The need to develop new models of care delivery for frail older adults with PD is influenced by the aging of the global population. In the United States, demographic growth for individuals 65 years and older is projected to increase from 35,000,000 in 2000 to 71,500,000 million by 2030. Thus individuals aged 65 years and older will make up 20% of the total U.S. population by 2030 (Federal Interagency Forum on Aging-Related Statistics, 2004).

PD is typically diagnosed in the sixth decade of life. Young-onset PD cases (with diagnosis prior to the age of 40) represent a small proportion of all people living with Parkinson's (PLWP). Moreover, the global aging of society is resulting in an emergence of PD in developing countries with limited resources for treatment. Furthermore, little research has focused on the frail older adult with PD and the complex needs of this growing population.

Frailty in older adults has been defined as a clinical phenotype and is characterized by the existence of three of the following symptoms: (a) unintentional weight loss of 10 pounds or more in the past year, (b) reports of exhaustion, (c) weakness, (d) slow ambulation, and (e) diminished physical activity. Clinical frailty has been correlated to increased risk of falls, hospitalizations, disability, and death (Fried et al., 2001). Thus the phenotype of frailty is clinically relevant to older adults with PD and may serve as a model to predict poor health outcomes in this population.

It is important to state that not all PLWP will experience frailty related to PD or progress to the advanced stage of disease. This point is illustrated by a newly diagnosed case of PD in a 93-year-old man with good response to levodopa therapy. Such an individual may have minimal complications related to progression of PD or related therapy, however, he may experience greater disability related to cataracts, weight loss, and poor dental health. Likewise, the newly diagnosed 70-year-old woman who presents with tremor-predominant PD and comorbid conditions of osteoporosis, hypertension, and diabetes may have minimal disability from PD. She may go on to develop significant frailty related to comorbid conditions, such as peripheral neuropathy, diminished vision, fractures, and stroke.

PD can be conceptualized in three stages: early, moderate, and advanced. Each stage of PD demonstrates a progression of disability with increasing complexity of care required to manage motor and nonmotor symptoms. Each case of PD presents a unique set of symptoms and disease trajectory. The historical course of disease is often used to provide a future estimate of disease progression. Rapid progression of PD is typically associated with rigid-predominant symptoms with onset in later life. Likewise, the presence of cognitive impairment and depression is also associated with an increased progression of disease. In contrast, PD progresses slowly in patients with tremor-predominant symptoms and early-onset disease (Duda & Stern, 2005). Thus variability of disease progression often leads to a sense of uncertainty for patients and families trying to anticipate what the future will hold with regard to disability and dependence on others (Bunting-Perry, 2006).

PD is a chronic progressive neurological disease with limited therapeutic options in the advanced stages of disease. Thus the precepts of palliative care can provide a framework to guide planning health care for PLWP (Bunting-Perry, 2006). The World Health Organization (2005) defines palliative care as "an approach that improves the quality of life of patients and their families facing the problems associated with life-threatening illness, through the prevention and relief of suffering by means of early identification and impeccable assessment and treatment of pain and other problems, physical, psychosocial and spiritual."

This chapter will focus on palliative care in PD and the physiology of aging related to the treatment of older adults. People living with PD in their 80s and 90s have different physiologic functioning as compared to 65-year-olds with PD and no comorbid diseases. Thus the complexity of care of the older adult with PD is emerging as a clinical concern. Moreover, care of the frail older adult with PD presents ethical issues. Thus nursing should be posed to provide treatment options to care providers, patients, and families across the continuum of care.

PALLIATIVE CARE AND PARKINSON'S DISEASE (PD)

The concept of palliative care in PD has received scant attention in health care literature and research. Historically, palliative care in the United States has been viewed as end-of-life care and has often been synonymous with hospice care. For example, Thomas and MacMahon (2004a, 2004b) discussed palliative care in PD as end-of-life care. Fortunately, the old model of palliative care as restricted to end-of-life is giving way to a new philosophy to support the patient and family throughout the continuum of chronic disease. Palliative care is currently conceptualized as a longitudinal model, encompassing the entire course of chronic disease from diagnosis to bereavement care for families (Bunting-Perry, 2006). Consequently, a qualitative investigation into palliative care and PD was conducted in 2006, concluding that palliative care may be of benefit to patients and families coping with PD. However, the inquiry was limited by small sample size and lack of information on participants' comorbid diseases (Hudson, Toye, & Kristjanson, 2006).

Palliative care is currently viewed as both a philosophy and a model of care (Center to Advance Palliative Care, 2004). By assisting PLWP and their family members to plan for future care, the utilization of emergency medical resources and acute hospitalizations can be moderated at end-of-life. Likewise, patients and families who receive clinical services, guided by the principles of palliative care, can actively engage in advanced care planning (ACP). ACP is a process by which the patient, family, and health care provider collaborate in discussing end-of-life decisions. The documents to support ACP include a living will and durable medical attorney. Incorporating palliative care through the course of PD will assist PLWP in making a successful transition through increasing levels of disability, while maintaining self-efficacy (Bunting-Perry, 2006).

Advanced Care Planning

ACP provides PLWP the ability to achieve autonomy in the context of a chronic progressive neurologic disease. Health care providers often struggle with having conversations regarding ACP out of unrealistic concerns that the patient or family may interpret these discussions as indicating that the end-of-life is near. Through clarifying the intent of ACP and moving the ACP process to the standard of care for patients at diagnosis, the discussions surrounding ACP can provide relief to PLWP who are uncertain of what the future may hold (Bunting-Perry, 2006).

The primary goals of ACP are to establish a communication process that includes the PLWP's care desires and creates contingency plans to achieve the identified goals. The contingency plan will include the identification of a proxy who will act as the surrogate in the event the patient is unable to communicate his or her own treatment needs and desires. A proxy is typically a spouse, adult child, or other family member.

Palliative care is often referred to as family care, and *family focused care* should include family members as well as friends and significant others who are willing to assist in the coordination or provision of care (Levine, 2003). Three steps to ACP include (a) actively listening to patients regarding the quality of their lives, (b) working with patients to develop health care goals, and (c) formulating contingency plans to meet the objectives of palliative care throughout the course of disease (Teno, 2003).

The process of establishing ACP will span the continuum of care for the patient with early, moderate, and advanced PD. Legal documents, such as the living will and durable power of attorney for health care (DPAHC), can be the outcome of developing the ACP. The DPAHC identifies a proxy to make health care decisions in the event that the individual is unable to communicate health care preferences. The living will provides specific instructions for health care and can serve as a guide to the proxy in making decisions regarding resuscitation, pain management, hydration, and artificial nutrition. Living wills and DPAHCs are legal documents and should be developed to meet the legal requirements of the state or jurisdiction where the PLWP resides (Ramsey & Mitty, 2003).

In the advanced stage of PD the patient, family or proxy, and health care provider should review the living will and further discuss the patient's wishes in regard to pain management, fatigue, nausea, vomiting, bowel management, urinary tract disorders, artificial hydration, artificial nutrition, dementia, agitation, and restlessness. Once the PLWP has identified his or her desires for symptom management, there should be a discussion regarding when to withhold and withdraw treatment at the end-of-life. Consultation with a palliative care specialist may be beneficial in educating PLWP in their options for end-of-life care and referral to a hospice program.

Hospice and End-of-Life Care for People Living With PD

Only 15% of Americans have the benefits of hospice services, and 50% of those cases are related to cancer care. Seventy percent of Americans die in the acute care hospital setting, undergoing life-prolonging procedures at the end-of-life. The hospice team is an interdisciplinary group of skilled professionals trained to support PLWP and their families through end-of-life care and bereavement services (Foley & Carver, 2001).

As a frail older adult with PD progresses toward end-of-life, the patient and his or her family should collaborate with the treatment team in making a referral to hospice care services. The ACP will be utilized to transfer care of the PLWP to the hospice team. The patient, family, and proxy should have addressed issues such as artificial nutrition, do-not-resuscitate orders, comfort-care-only orders, do-not-hospitalize orders, and pain management throughout the ACP process.

In the United States, hospice services are paid for by Medicare Part A and are available as home care or inpatient services. Medicare has three eligibility criteria for entering hospice care. The first eligibility requirement asks the physician to determine, to the best of his or her knowledge, that the patient has 6 months or less to live. This requirement is often a roadblock in managing the frail older adult with PD. Fortunately, most hospice program directors will work with referring health care providers in determining hospice eligibility to overcome barriers to care. It is often helpful to ask the primary care provider if it would surprise him or her if the PLWP would die within the next 6 months. The second eligibility criterion requires that the PLWP accept palliative care and not curative care. Last, the patient will need to be treated by a Medicare-approved hospice program (Egan & Labyak, 2001).

Bereavement Care

Family members are often fatigued from years of care provision. Likewise, many caregivers experience social isolation and have few social supports. The death of a loved one is a time when families need support in redefining their roles and grieving for the loss. Bereavement counseling is essential to assist the family and caregiver to successfully transition to a non-caregiving role (Levine, 2003).

PD MODEL OF CARE

The PD Model of Care (PDMC), presented in Figure 7.1, is designed to provide a clinical model for PLWP throughout the course of disease. The model incorporates traditional life-prolonging treatment, palliative care, hospice care, and bereavement services over the trajectory of disease. The PDMC utilizes the Hoehn and Yahr score along the vertical axis to demonstrate stage of disease and the Schwab and England Activity of Daily Living (ADL) score along the horizontal axis to reflect activities of daily living (Fahn, Elton, & Members of the UPDRS Development Committee, 1987; Hoehn & Yahr, 1967; Schwab, England, & Peterson, 1959). The Schwab and England ADL score is represented by a line moving through the three stages of PD, demonstrating the slow decline in functioning over the course of disease. In the advanced stage of disease the dark line, representing the Schwab and England ADL score, fluctuates to demonstrate acute episodes of disability followed by partial recovery. From the advanced stage of disease the model flows into traditional hospice care at end-of-life and incorporates bereavement care for families and caregivers (Bunting-Perry, 2006).

FRAIL OLDER ADULTS WITH PD

Planning care for a frail older adult with PD encompasses many of the nonmotor symptoms, discussed in chapters 4 and 5, such as cognitive impairment, behavioral problems, psychosis, and diminished swallowing. In addition, older adults with PD will need assessments for fall risk, nutrition, hydration, infections, comorbid disease, skin care, and polypharmacy. Designing a treatment plan to provide comfort to the frail older adult with PD encompasses assessment for signs and symptoms that, if untreated, can result in increased morbidity and mortality.

FIGURE 7.1   Model of care for Parkinson's disease.

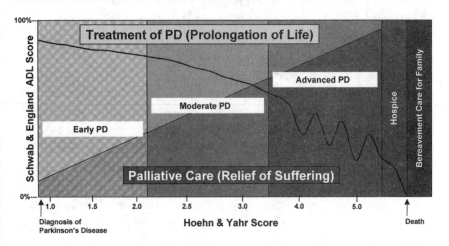

Bunting-Perry, L. (2006). Palliative care in Parkinson's disease: Implications for neuroscience nursing. *Journal of Neuroscience Nursing, 38*(2), 108. Reprinted with permission of the author.

Swallowing difficulty is common in advanced disease and can predispose the older adult with PD to aspiration pneumonia. Routine assessment for choking and swallowing are important in clinical evaluations of the frail older adult with PD. Referral to a speech and swallowing specialist to assess for the risk of aspiration and provide therapeutic techniques to improve swallowing mechanics is recommended. Thickening fluids to a honey-like consistency often improves swallowing and reduces the risk of aspiration (Ramig, Countryman, Fox, & Sapir, 2002). Detailed information on speech and swallowing as nonmotor features of PD can be found in chapter 5.

Occasionally, the risk of aspiration cannot be mediated by a change in diet or techniques to improve swallowing. Feeding tubes are an option for older adults with PD and can be a lifesaving procedure. Yet it must be noted that the placement of a feeding tube is part of the process of delivering artificial nutrition to the frail older adult. The risk and benefits of artificial nutrition should be discussed with the patient, family, and proxy and be included in the ACP.

Polypharmacy

The use of multiple medications in frail older adults with PD is directly related to treatment of comorbid disease and use of over-the-counter (OTC) pharmaceuticals. Polypharmacy can result in adverse drug reactions and has been linked to numerous hospital admissions in older adults (Saltvedt, Mo, Fayers, Kaasa, & Sletvold, 2002).

A complete drug history is essential in evaluating the older adult with PD. The best approach is to ask patients and families to bring all medications (including vitamins, supplements, and herbals) with them to clinic visits or hospital admissions. Thus an assessment of the type, quantity, and indication of drugs and the number of health care providers prescribing medications can be completed. A history of OTC medications is important as nonsteroidal anti-inflammatory drugs, antihistamines, analgesics, and psychostimulants can have significant behavioral effects on frail older adults.

Managing medication compliance in the frail elder with PD can be particularly challenging. As the medication schedule becomes more complex, the ability of the patient and family to manage medication administration becomes more difficult. One goal of medication management is to simplify the number of medications with the least number of pills necessary to attain a therapeutic response (Boxer & Shorr, 2004). Spending time on patient education and providing clear, written instructions can facilitate medication compliance and improve patient outcomes.

Pharmacokinetics

Older adults with PD are generally vulnerable to adverse side effects of medications related to general health, nutrition, hydration, compliance, and polypharmacy. Unfortunately, there is little information on how the elderly absorb, distribute, metabolize, and eliminate medications. The principles of pharmacokinetics are important to understanding how medications can contribute to adverse effects in frail elders with PD.

The following four pharmacokinetic processes of (a) *absorption,* (b) *distribution,* (c) *metabolism,* and (d) *excretion* can alter the effects of medications in older adults. Absorption of medications in older adults decreases relative to diminished absorptive surface in the GI system, increased gastric pH, decreased gastrointestinal motility, and decreased splanchnic blood flow. Physiological changes in the elderly, such as cardiac output, blood flow, and tissue volume, impact how drugs are distributed into interstitial and intracellular spaces. The elderly have diminished muscle mass and increased fat tissue, which will enhance the uptake of drugs designed to distribute in fat tissue, such as diazepam. Thus drugs that bind to fat will stay in the system longer. Older adults with PD will also have diminished serum albumin, thereby impacting medications that require binding to proteins. Serum protein can be decreased with acute illness, limiting the protein available for drug distribution. Bioavailability of protein for protein-binding drugs can result in increased circulation, leading to drug toxicity. Likewise, decreased total body water will diminish distribution of medications in the system (Boxer & Shorr, 2004). Edema and dehydration are common in PD and result in decreased circulating fluid volume.

The ability of the older adult with PD to metabolize drugs is variable and dependent on factors such as age, alcohol intake, diet, smoking, medications, and disease state. Physiologic changes, such as decreased hepatic enzyme activity, decreased muscle mass, and diminished blood flow, also contribute to changes in metabolism of medications. Older adults may experience a 50% loss of renal function by the age of 85, resulting in a reduction in glomerular and tubular function in the kidney. Thus decreased kidney function results in increased serum levels of medications in older adults (Boxer & Shorr, 2004).

Nutrition and Hydration

Assessment of nutrition and hydration of the older adult with PD is key in determining if nutritional intake is adequate. Poor intake of food and fluids can contribute to weight loss, dehydration, constipation, confusion, orthostasis, and falls (Amella, 2003).

Observing the eating patterns of the older adult with PD can be helpful in determining if assistance is required in opening cartons, cutting food, chewing, or swallowing. The presence of depression may also diminish appetite. Likewise, antidepressant medications, such as selective serotonin reuptake inhibitors, can cause appetite suppression.

Mealtime is a social process that holds significant meaning to older adults with PD. Assessing for the importance of mealtime rituals and cultural norms is important in successful completion of mealtime activities. Preserving religious and cultural meal activities can improve nutritional intake and should be encouraged in all health care settings.

Assessing for Fall Risk

The general geriatric literature reports that falls are the sixth cause of mortality in older adults. In assessing for fall risk, the nurse should consider both the *intrinsic* and *extrinsic* fall risk factors in planning for care of the frail older adult with PD. Intrinsic risk factors refer to the personal attributes of the individual being assessed for falls. The following are examples of intrinsic risk factors for falling: chronic disease, cognitive impairment, physical disability, sensory impairment, exacerbation of chronic disease, side effects of medications, and acute illness. Extrinsic risk factors refer to the risk for falls found in the environment. The following illustrate environmental risk factors: inadequate lighting, thick carpeting, shelves that are difficult to reach, lack of grab bars or handrails, chairs and toilets that are low, and slippery floors (Baum, Capezuti, & Driscoll, 2002).

Seventy percent of PLWP in the community report falling, and 13% fall at least once a week. Many falls result in hip fractures, injuries, hospitalizations, pain, and disability. In addition, falls can precipitate placement in long-term care for the frail older adult with PD. Risk factors associated with falling in PD include longer duration of disease, dyskinesias, freezing of gait, postural instability, increased disability, depression, and weaker proximal lower extremity strength. To date, no randomized clinical trials are available to guide fall prevention in PD. Current fall prevention focuses on rehabilitation medicine and a structured plan of care with an experienced physical therapist to assist in strengthening and gait training. Assistive devices and modifications to the home environment may also assist in prevention of falls (Robinson et al., 2005).

Alcohol Use and Dependence

Alcohol use is often overlooked in the clinical setting and can have a significant impact on mobility, falls, and cognition in older adults with PD. Patients will frequently ask if a cocktail in the evening will interfere with PD medications. For many older adults an evening alcoholic beverage is a social event and does not constitute abuse. However, older adults with PD are at risk of falls, incontinence, and cognitive impairment from the use of alcohol and should be educated concerning the risk of using alcohol in the context of a chronic neurologic disease.

The principles of pharmaconetics discussed earlier are relevant to understanding the effects of alcohol in the older adult. Alcohol is water soluble, and older adults have increased body fat and decreased body water ratios. This physical state produces higher concentrations of circulating alcohol in the bloodstream in comparison to a younger population. The following is a list of symptoms that can serve as clinical indicators that alcohol may be a part of the clinical presentation in older adults: high blood pressure, fractures, sleep impairment, urinary incontinence, congestive heart failure, and sexual dysfunction (Campbell, 2004).

Assessing for Infection

Frail older adults with PD are at risk for developing infections related to immobility, comorbid conditions, poor nutrition, and weakened immune systems. In addition, the inability of the older adult to communicate symptoms of an infection makes the diagnosis a challenge. The most common types of infection in the older adult are urinary tract infections (UTIs), respiratory tract infections, gastroenteritis, and soft tissue infections.

UTIs are the most common infection in the older adult population and can be associated with prostatic hypertrophy, neurogenic bladder, diabetes, incontinence, and the use of internal or external catheters. Older adults with PD may have difficulty reporting symptoms indicating a UTI. The following list can assist in the evaluation: foul-smelling urine, complaint of burning on urination, flank pain, and frequency and urgency of urination. If a UTI is suspected, the following laboratory tests should be ordered: urine analysis and urine culture and sensitivity.

Upper respiratory infections are common in the older adult and contribute to significant mortality. Respiratory tract infections are classified as upper and lower respiratory infections. Upper respiratory infections are usually self-limiting, such as the common cold, sinusitis, and otitis media, but in some cases are precursors to lower respiratory infections. Lower respiratory infections carry a higher morbidity and mortality rate for those with Parkinson's disease. These infections include tuberculosis, bronchitis (viral and bacterial), and pneumonia. In advanced Parkinson's disease, the primary cause of lower respiratory tract infections is aspiration of fluids and the development of pneumonia (Bonomo & Johnson, 2004).

Diarrhea related to infectious gastroenteritis is a significant problem for older adults. Diarrhea can contribute to dehydration and renal and cardiac problems in the elderly. The following is a list of risk factors for developing gastroenteritis: gastric atrophy, surgery, systemic illness, medications that decrease gastric acidity, and antibiotic use. The vast majority of medications used to treat PD carry the side effect of decreased gastric motility. Although constipation is more common in PLWP than diarrhea, it is important to assess for gastroenteritis as a potential problem in frail elders with PD. Entacapone (Comtan) is a catecholamine O-methyltransferase inhibitor medication frequently prescribed for the treatment of PD. Eight percent of PD patients in clinical trials experienced diarrhea as an adverse effect of entacapone. When assessing for new-onset diarrhea in PLWP, a current listing of medications is helpful to rule out pharmacologic causes for gastroenteritis (Poewe, Deuschl, Gordin, Kultalahti, & Leinonen, 2002).

Skin integrity is of particular importance in assessing the older adult with PD. Immobility, falls, thinning of the skin, and loss of muscle mass places the older adult with PD at risk for skin breakdown. Prolonged periods of immobility can contribute to pressure ulcers, and a careful assessment of the skin is an important aspect in preventing infection. Pressure ulcers are chronic wounds that result from prolonged pressure on a bony prominence, resulting in skin necrosis and possible infection. Examining the sacrum and heels of the feet for pressure ulcers routinely will alert the PLWP and his or her care provider to the importance of skin integrity. Education in changing positions and using gel pads to provide cushioning will lessen the occurrence of developing pressure ulcers.

Skin tears are another risk for PLWP. Friction causes skin tears, which result in the separation of the epidermis from the dermis. The high risk of falling in PD leads to significant risk for developing infection from skin tears. Areas for assessment of skin tears include the shins, face, hands, and feet (Ayello, 2003).

Pain Assessment

Seventy percent of PLWP report experiencing pain as a nonmotor symptom, and for a minority of patients, pain can be more disabling than the motor symptoms of disease (Djaldetti et al., 2004). Pain as a nonmotor feature of PD is discussed in chapter 5 and is often an underappreciated symptom. The assessment and treatment of pain in PLWP is an emerging field of research, and there is limited evidence-based practice to guide treatment at this time. Thus the general literature on pain in older adults will guide the assessment and treatment of pain in frail elders with PD. Polomano (2002) provides an excellent overview of pain in older adults from the perspectives of pain epidemiology, physiology, assessment, treatment, and measurement. Further information on tools for the assessment of pain in nonverbal adults can be found in a State of the Science Review by Herr et al. (2006). Typical pain assessment tools include face scales, visual analog scales, and the McGill Pain Questionnaire (Herr et al., 2006; Melzack, 1975).

SURGICAL CONSIDERATIONS

The advent of surgical treatment for PD, discussed in chapter 6, adds a layer of difficulty for caring for frail older adults who are have undergone deep brain stimulation (DBS) implant surgery. The technology used in maintaining DBS implant equipment may not be accessible in long-term care facilities and can present unique care-planning issues for families placing loved ones in nursing homes, assisted living, and life care communities. The onset of dementia in a patient with DBS adds a new level of care for an individual with technology that requires technical assessment and maintenance from a skilled movement disorder team of interdisciplinary specialists. The need for PD Nurse Specialists trained in the management of PLWP throughout the health care continuum will be an increasing focus for care over the next decade.

SUMMARY

Caring for frail older adults with PD can be challenging and rewarding. By identifying family members and caregivers as part of the treatment team, planning for care can be enhanced. The basic principles of geriatric care can assist in managing the patient throughout the trajectory of disease and improve quality of life. The PDMC is presented as a model to guide care and treatment of both traditional therapeutics for symptom control and palliation of pain, constipation, dehydration, and skin breakdown, and prevention of infections.

REFERENCES

Amella, E. J. (2003). Mealtime difficulties. In M. D. Mezey, T. Fulmer, I. Abraham, & D. Zwicker (Eds.), *Geriatric nursing protocols for best practice* (2nd ed., pp. 66–82). New York: Springer.

Ayello, E. A. (2003). Preventing pressure ulcers and skin tears. In M. D. Mezey, T. Fulmer, I. Abraham, & D. Zwicker (Eds.), *Geriatric nursing protocols for best practice* (2nd ed., pp. 165–184). New York: Springer.

Baum, T., Capezuti, E., & Driscoll, G. (2002). Falls. In V. T. Cotter & N. E. Strumpf (Eds.), *Advanced practice nursing with older adults: Clinical guidelines* (pp. 245–269). New York: McGraw-Hill.

Bonomo, R. A., & Johnson, M. A. (2004). Common infections. In C. S. Landefeld, R. M. Palmer, M. A. Johnson, C. B. Johnston, & W. L. Lyons (Eds.), *Current geriatric diagnosis and treatment* (pp. 348–358). New York: McGraw-Hill.

Boxer, P., & Shorr, R. (2004). Principles of drug therapy: Changes with aging, polypharmacy, and drug interaction. In C. S. Landefeld, R. M. Palmer, A. Johnson, C. B. Johnston, & W. L. Lyons (Eds.), *Current geriatric diagnosis and treatment* (pp. 421–435). New York: McGraw-Hill.

Bunting-Perry, L. (2006). Palliative care in Parkinson's disease: Implications for neuroscience nursing. *Journal of Neuroscience Nursing, 38,* 105–112.

Campbell, J. W. (2004). Use of alcohol, tobacco, and nonprescribed drugs. In C. S. Landefeld, R. M. Palmer, M. A. Johnson, C. B. Johnston, & W. L. Lyons (Eds.), *Current geriatric diagnosis and treatment* (pp. 407–413). New York: McGraw-Hill.

Center to Advance Palliative Care. (2004). *The case for hospital-based palliative care.* New York: Author.

Djaldetti, R., Shifrin, A., Rogowski, Z., Sprecher, E., Melamed, E., & Yarnitsky, D. (2004). Quantitative measurement of pain sensation in patients with Parkinson disease. *Neurology, 62,* 2171–2175.

Duda, J. E., & Stern, M. B. (2005). Moderate Parkinson's disease. In M. Ebadi & R. F. Pfeiffer (Eds.), *Parkinson's disease* (pp. 851–857). New York: CRC Press.

Egan, K., & Labyak, M. (2001). Hospice care: A model for quality end-of-life. In B. F. Ferrell & N. Coyle (Eds.), *Textbook of palliative nursing* (pp. 7–26). New York: Oxford University Press.

Fahn, S., Elton, R., & Members of the UPDRS Development Committee. (1987). Unified Parkinson's disease rating scale. In S. Fahn, C. D. Marsden, M. Goldstein, & D. B. Calne (Eds.), *Recent developments in Parkinson's disease* (Vol. 2, pp. 153–163). Florham Park, NJ: Macmillan.

Federal Interagency Forum on Aging-Related Statistics. (2004). *Older Americans 2004: Key indicators of well-being.* Washington, DC: U.S. Government Printing Office.

Foley, K. M., & Carver, A. C. (2001). Palliative care in neurology. *Neurologic Clinics, 19,*789–799.

Fried, L. P., Tangen, C. M., Walston, J., Newman, A. B., Hirsh, C., Gottdiener, J., et al. (2001). Frailty in older adults: Evidence for a phenotype. *Journal of Gerontology: Medical Sciences, 56,* 146–156.

Herr, K., Coyne, P. J., Key, T., Manworren, R., McCaffery, M., Merkel, S., et al. (2006). Pain assessment in the nonverbal patient: Position statement with clinical practice recommendations. *Pain Management Nursing, 7,* 44–52.

Hoehn, M. M., & Yahr, M. D. (1967). Parkinsonism: Onset, progression, and mortality. *Neurology, 17,* 427–441.

Hudson, P. L., Toye, C., & Kristjanson, L. J. (2006). Would people with Parkinson's disease benefit from palliative care? *Palliative Medicine, 20,* 87–94.

Levine, C. (2003). Family caregivers: Burdens and opportunities. In R. S. Morrison & D. E. Meier (Eds.), *Geriatric palliative care* (pp. 376–385). New York: Oxford Press.

Melzack, R. (1975). The McGill Pain Questionnaire: Major properties and scoring methods. *Pain, 1,* 277–299.

Poewe, W. H., Deuschl, G., Gordin, A., Kultalahti, E. R., & Leinonen, M. (2002). Efficacy and safety of entacapone in Parkinson's disease patients with suboptimal levodopa response: A 6-month randomized placebo-controlled double-blind study in Germany and Austria (Celomen study). *ACTA Neurologica Scandinavica, 105,* 245–255.

Polomano, R. C. (2002). Pain. In V. T. Cotter & N. E. Strumpf (Eds.), *Advanced practice nursing with older adults: Clinical guidelines* (pp. 333–360). New York: McGraw-Hill.

Ramig, L. O., Countryman, S., Fox, C., & Sapir, S. (2002). Speech, voice, and swallowing disorders. In S. A. Factor & W. J. Weiner (Eds.), *Parkinson's disease diagnosis and clinical management* (pp. 75–86). New York: Demos.

Ramsey, G., & Mitty, E. L. (2003). Advance directives: Protecting patient's rights. In M. Mezey, T. Fulmer, & I. Abraham (Eds.), *Geriatric nursing protocols for best practice* (2nd ed., pp. 265–291). New York: Springer.

Robinson, K. M., Dennison, A. C., Roalf, D., Noorigian, J., Cianci, H., Bunting-Perry, L., et al. (2005). Falling risk factors in Parkinson's disease: A pilot study and review of the literature. *NeuroRehabilitation, 20,* 169–182.

Saltvedt, I., Mo, E.-S. O., Fayers, P., Kaasa, S., & Sletvold, O. (2002). Reduced mortality in treating acutely sick, frail older patients in a geriatric evaluation and management unit: A prospective randomized trial. *Journal of the American Geriatrics Society, 50,* 792–798.

Schwab, R., England, A., & Peterson, E. (1959). Akinesia in Parkinson's disease. *Neurology, 9,* 65–72.

Teno, J. M. (2003). Advanced care planning for frail, older persons. In R. S. Morrison & D. E. Meier (Eds.), *Geriatric palliative care* (pp. 307–313). New York: Oxford University Press.

Thomas, S., & MacMahon, D. (2004a). Parkinson's disease, palliative care and older people: Part 1. *Nursing Older People, 16*(1), 22–26.

Thomas, S., & MacMahon, D. (2004b). Parkinson's disease, palliative care and older people: Part 2. *Nursing Older People, 16*(2), 22–26.

World Health Organization. (2005). *WHO definition of palliative care.* Retrieved June 5, 2005, from http://www.who.int/cancer/palliative/definition/en/

8

Role of the Nurse in the Care of the Patient With Parkinson's Disease

Heidi Watson, BSN
Lisette Bunting-Perry, MScN, RN
Gwyn M. Vernon, MSN, CRNP

Parkinson's disease (PD) is a chronic neurological disease that can range in symptoms and degree of disability throughout the trajectory of disease. Impairment of mobility, compounded by nonmotor symptoms, can lead to frustration, isolation, and vulnerability for people living with PD (PLWP). Motor and nonmotor symptoms affect activities of daily living and bring a complexity of changing roles with family, friends, and loved ones.

Nursing is recognized as "the diagnosis and treatment of human responses to actual and potential health problems" (American Nursing Association, 2003, p. 5). By definition, nursing plays an essential role in the comprehensive care of PLWP. In the United Kingdom and Australia, there are PD Nurse Specialists who are dedicated to caring for patients with PD and their family members. These specialized nurses in the United Kingdom work collaboratively with primary care providers in the community to support patients and families, increase community awareness, monitor illness progression, and make early referrals to therapists (MacMahon, 1999).

Each case of PD can present with a different symptom complex, making each nursing care plan unique to the individual and family. The care is therefore determined by the symptoms that are affecting independence and self-efficacy. The intricacies of the numerous Parkinson's symptoms require the special attention of an educated nurse to identify, assess, treat, and make appropriate referrals within the interdisciplinary team. The nurse must understand the function of each member of the team and his or her role to provide collaborative, patient-centered, and comprehensive care.

Part of the essence of the nurse's role is helping the patient define the meaning of illness. The diagnosis of PD gives the patient a medical name for the disease, whereas illness refers to the patient's odyssey throughout the personal experience of disease (Borneman & Brown-Saltzman, 2001). Nurses should consider the difference between disease and illness and use the nursing process to care for those with PD. The vast majority of people with PD will experience a long duration of illness with slowly progressing levels of disability. The goal of nursing care is to help individuals manage their illness and maximize their quality of life (MacMahon & Thomas, 1998).

This chapter will discuss the role of the nurse in the care of the patient with PD in the context of the family. Trained in the biopsychosocial model of care, nurses function in a myriad of ways, including acting as translators, researchers, assessors, educators, promoters of self-care and efficacy, and patient advocates. In essence, the nurse follows the patient through the trajectory of disease and illness and across the health care continuum (Bunting-Perry, 2006).

ROLE OF THE NURSE AS TRANSLATOR

A nurse frequently functions in the role of translator, interpreter of meaning, assessor of symptoms, and educator through helping to translate the diagnosis to the patient as the patient develops his or her own meaning of PD as an illness. Patients with PD are often not diagnosed with a definitive diagnosis until years after symptoms develop. Some patients will tolerate a dragging foot or slight upper extremity tremor before seeking a medical diagnosis and treatment. Frequently, a family member may be the initial person to observe decreased facial expression or diminished arm swing. It can be several months to years before a person receives an accurate diagnosis. The initial diagnosis of PD or probable PD is made clinically through history and physical examination (Nutt & Wooten, 2005). Delivery of the diagnosis can be devastating to a patient and his or her family, and the reaction to the illness will range with degree of acceptance. This reaction can be used to assess and evaluate what patients, caregivers, and families need in terms of support and education.

Imagine that as a nurse, you are the first one to interact with a patient after receiving a diagnosis. How would you best serve a newly diagnosed patient with PD? First, assess what the patient knows about PD. Ask if he or she has had a family member or friend with PD. Prior exposure or knowledge of PD may affect the patient's acceptance of illness. Does the patient have any questions about the PD symptoms that the other has experienced? What does the patient and family expect? Using these basic questions will reveal knowledge deficits, bias, and fears that the patient and family have and will guide the focus for education on PD. For example, if their only exposure to a person with PD was someone who was bedridden and unable to speak or swallow within 2 years, it is important to clarify this misconception of PD upfront. Consider that the patient is facing a life-changing event and that he or she will not be able to grasp all information at one time. Many educators say that adult learners can only absorb three new facts at once—keep this in mind, and use the reinforcement technique. Absorbing information may be limited by time, willingness of the patient, and volume of content. Assess for learning barriers present in PD, such as cognition, difficulty hearing, anxiety, depression, or other intrusive symptoms. Ask the patient what best suits his or her type of learning style. Patients may need more than one source of information (i.e., verbal, written, Internet, video) to begin to comprehend what PD will mean to them. If the patient has come for his or her visit alone, on returning home and hearing the reaction of the patient's spouse or family, he or she will naturally have more questions and perhaps even a different emotional reaction. It may be wise to bring the patient back soon to address family questions. Education about the PD diagnosis is an ongoing process that begins with diagnosis and is reassessed and reinforced as the needs of patient and family evolve.

Facilitating the translation of the diagnosis of PD into everyday language will foster trust and lead to discussions about the everyday impact of illness on a person's life. Nurses are in a unique position to address the disease from a biopsychosocial aspect and develop a care plan. Who will be involved in the care of the patient? How will PD affect the patient's role in life with regard to work, family, social life, hobbies, and interests? What are the patient's fears, hopes, and concerns? Does the patient rely on a significant other to help make health care decisions? What resources does the patient have access to: finances, family support, spiritual, or community resources? These questions prompt patients and families to think about how to deal with PD. Use this information in the nursing assessment to deduce the needs of the person dealing with PD and to efficiently utilize resources of a multidisciplinary team and the community.

Delivering and discussing bad news with a patient and family is not easy. However, this is part of the ethical responsibility of a nurse as a health care provider (Clark & Volker, 2003). Preserving hope is important in nursing care, but it is a nurse's responsibility to weigh hope with preparing for the future (Back, Arnold, & Quill, 2003). There is no crystal ball with which to predict outcomes of patients with PD. With careful consideration of a patient's current health state, comorbidities, age, and the potential needs of the PD patient in the future, a nurse can be effective in easing the transition of living with PD.

Assessment of Symptoms

The Parkinson community and health care providers have a language for description of PD symptoms. Some symptoms are referred to as fluctuations, dyskinesias, on and off time, freezing or akinesia, and dystonia. These terms may not be familiar to the newly diagnosed patient or his or her family. However, the patient will be clinically rated on scales to measure these symptoms, such as the Unified Parkinson's Disease Rating Scale. Clinicians will ask the patient questions such as, How much of the day are you experiencing off symptoms? Helping to prepare the patient to answer these questions in the context of a new language will be of great benefit to easing his or her frustration and need to communicate with the treatment team. Focus on the language used by patients and ask for clarification using their language to describe their symptoms. Nurses can then interpret these symptom experiences for the medical team.

Example

During a follow-up visit, Mr. Smith says that he has no problem with dyskinesias, however, later in the exam, he starts to have upper extremity movement and is moving in his chair. The nurse discusses this observation with Mr. Smith: "Tell me about this movement you are experiencing." Mr. Smith replies, "Sometimes I can't sit still. I don't even notice that I am rocking in my chair, but my wife will point it out. It goes away after an hour, so I tend to forget about it. The rocking isn't permanent, so I assume it isn't the Parkinson's disease."

The patient is describing dyskinesia, which is defined as extra movement related to PD medications. Nurses must translate "rocking" as experienced by the patient into the language of PD and include this in the symptoms that need to be addressed in the care plan. Follow-up on symptom management using the patient's language is a useful tool for the nurse in assisting the patient in accurately communicating symptoms that may be related to therapy or symptom progression. Recognize that not all PD symptoms will be noticeable during a short clinical visit. Nurses must ask about other symptoms that are experienced commonly. Ask a patient about his or her most bothersome PD symptoms and how they present during the day. Remember to attend to the key words during the patient's description to use for further assessment.

Table 8.1 presents a sample care plan using the nursing process for nursing diagnosis, interventions, and expected outcomes for PD-related symptoms (Lewis, Heitkemper, & Dirkesen, 2000).

MEDICATION TEACHING

Medication teaching is ongoing through all stages of PD. An individual care plan is devised for medication, taking into account a wide variety of factors, such as age, side effects, and disability of symptoms. Medication care planning is modified frequently due to response of symptoms to surgery,

TABLE 8.1 Example Nursing Care Plan for Symptoms Related to Parkinson's Disease

NANDA diagnosis	Expected outcomes	Nursing interventions
Disturbed sleep pattern	1. Attains maximal sleep functioning	1. Assess for disturbance related to daytime somnolence, insomnia, vivid dreaming, sleep fragmentation, depression, urinary symptoms
	2. Verbalizes understanding of tips for good sleep	2. Review sleep hygiene tips
		3. Review medication side effect profiles
		4. Referral to sleep specialist

(continued)

TABLE 8.1   Example Nursing Care Plan for Symptoms Related to Parkinson's Disease *(continued)*

NANDA diagnosis	Expected outcomes	Nursing interventions
Caregiver role strain	1. Maximum functioning of caregiver of PLWP	1. Assess caregiver stress, emotional and physical abuse, financial status, increase care needs
	2. PLWP in adequate safe care environment	2. Discuss adult day services, in-home support, respite care, hospice; involve family of PLWP in education about disease trajectory and advance care planning
		3. Refer to social worker, elder law attorney, or hospice
Impaired physical mobility (related to postural instability and freezing of gait [FOG])	1. Achieves level of safe mobility and reduces falls	1. Assess for FOG patterns and relationship to medications and falling
	2. Verbalizes effect of medications	2. Assess for multifocal balance problem
	3. Identifies periods of good mobility	3. Teach FOG technique to manage freezing
	4. Understands and utilizes FOG techniques	4. Make referrals for walking aid: cane, walker, wheelchair, scooter
		5. Discuss home environment and safety. Recommend evaluation for safety devices for home: railings, shower bars, etc.
		6. Refer to physical therapy

medications, and progression of disease. As there is no clear medication algorithm that fits each PD patient, a key part of this process is providing medication education for patients and family members. Always treat the patient as an integral member of the treatment team. Often, the patient and family become the experts on what medication regimen works best for symptom management.

Medication Response

Nurses should tell patients what they can expect from Parkinson's medications. By educating the patient on the benefits and possible side effect profiles of pharmacologic agents used in the disease, patients and family members will be able to communicate the effectiveness of the treatment plan. As a nurse, you may tell them what to monitor with medications (e.g., "You might feel looser and tremor or shaking will diminish. But balance problems may not improve."). Inform the patient of possible side effects, and ask him or her to monitor (e.g., "Are you getting nausea, vomiting or diarrhea, or increased confusion?"). In large teaching hospitals and movement disorder centers, there are often pharmacists who are quite knowledgeable on the pharmacology of PD and are willing to meet with patients to discuss medications and provide guidance with side effect profiles and titration schedules when stopping or starting PD medications. Medication compliance is an important point of emphasis in care for PLWP. PD patients become sensitive to their regimens, and medications should be given with precise timing.

Outpatient Settings

Nurses should review the trade and generic names of PD medications and show pictures of medication color, shape, and size. Nurses should provide the patient with a written schedule of medications to improve compliance. It is not sufficient to tell the patient to take medications 3 times a day as Parkinson's medications are time-sensitive related to the targeted symptoms for therapy. In order to achieve maximum benefit from the medications, written medication schedules should be constructed and reviewed. Planning for medication compliance includes the patient and family. Compliance measures, such as pillboxes that are checked daily and watches with alarms, help to encourage a strict medication regimen. Promote the use of symptom diaries. A typical 24-hour diary log keeps track of on and off fluctuations, dyskinesias, and dose times. Nurses can use the diaries to track symptom patterns and to help change care plans.

Example

Mr. Williams is a 62-year-old patient with history of PD who comes into clinic to complain of "bad time." He goes on to say he takes Sinemet immediate release 25/100 tablets, 3 times per day instead of 4 times per day as it is "difficult for him to remember." After asking specifics of his "bad time," he recalls that this occurs in the afternoon, when he feels that it is "hard to move" and he is "not with it." He describes an anxious feeling that he is "going down" and occasionally will take the extra Sinemet dose if he remembers.

How do you deal with this as a nurse? First, focus in on the language ("bad time") and assess what the patient means. Assess what time of day he takes his medications. Is he describing on and off motor fluctuations? Is the anxiety related to his fluctuations, or does he experience this all day? Does the patient need to be evaluated for depression or anxiety? Consult with pharmacy and psychiatry. Devise a compliance plan by developing a medication schedule and suggesting a pill alarm. Evaluate the new plan on a follow-up visit using diaries and asking about "bad time."

Inpatient Settings

Often, when patients are admitted to the hospital, strict medication regimens are not adhered to, and the function of the patient declines. Nurses must understand that PD patients depend on their medications for mobility and independence. Wearing off at end of dose can diminish the ability of a patient with PD to complete basic activities of daily living. Patients may have severe on and off fluctuations, and it is essential for nurses to understand that patients might be able to help with a task, such as turning in bed, when their medications are working, and as soon as 20 min later, may have severe difficulty, becoming rigid and unable to move. The nurse's role in the inpatient setting is to ensure the timely administration of medication to maintain functioning and avoid severe off episodes through maintaining patients on their carefully prescribed schedule of dopaminergic medications.

Example

Mrs. Smith, 71, is hospitalized for intravenous antibiotics for a severe cellulitis on her lower leg. She normally takes sinemet four times a day (QID) at home with good results at 0700, 1100, 1500, and 1900. In the hospital QID is defaulted on the computerized medication system to 0600, 1200, 1800, and midnight. She develops significant wearing off periods in the late morning and late afternoon, cannot feed herself dinner, and cannot get herself ready for bed in the evening. She experiences difficulty sleeping, with vivid dreams and restlessness.

What are the nursing care issues here? This patient has had her medications carefully titrated to every four hours (not every six hours, not four times a day), and is experiencing end-of-dose failure when the interval is stretched beyond four hours. Her ability to perform her Activities of daily living (ADLs) has suffered as a result. She is also experiencing sleep dysfunction due to dopaminergic stimulation from the midnight dosage of medication. The solution is to change her dosage to her preferred schedule, that is, 0700, 1100, 1500, and 1900.

NURSES AS PROMOTERS OF SELF-EFFICACY

While recognizing that PD has disabling symptoms, nurses should still encourage patients to actively participate in their care. Nurses can be enormous facilitators in helping patients develop self-efficacy in caring for themselves and improving their quality of life. This is accomplished by establishing support groups, resource libraries, and activity programs and teaching patients about nutrition and exercise that they are able to participate in at home.

In chapter 2 the theoretical approach of bringing self-efficacy to the treatment of PD as a chronic disease was proposed. To develop self-efficacy, clinical and educational programs for PLWP should include a variety of learning strategies, while providing mutual aid and support for learning that involve significant others or family members. Patients should be supplied with encouragement, persuasion, and direct support for participation in the treatment plan. Self-efficacy can be fostered by using a varied approach to providing information in individual sessions, support groups, and phone calls by promoting collaborative relationships and active participation (Marks, Allegrante, & Lorig, 2005).

Start a Resource Library

Collecting information and setting up a resource library for patients and family members is a useful and significant contribution to the Parkinson's community. Nurses are in an ideal position to review literature from pharmaceutical companies, nonprofit organizations, books, and other print materials for accurate content to be included in the library. Preferably, resource library material should be readable at the 6th to 8th grade level. By assembling a list of Web sites and reviewing the content for accuracy and readability, the nurse can provide online information that is accessible from the World Wide Web. Look for patient-friendly information such as the educational books published by the National Parkinson's Foundation. Include materials about patient experiences and therapies such as physiotherapy, speech therapy, surgery, medication, and psychological therapies as well as information on caregiver roles. Look for activity programs directed to PD patients, a local area agency on aging, exercise groups, transportation alternatives to driving, local support groups, and home health care services.

Establish Support Groups

Support groups provide patients and family members with the opportunity to share their experiences and learn from expert guest speakers. Several national Parkinson's organizations sponsor community support groups, and many regional, independent Parkinson's organizations meet regularly throughout the United States. A listing of local support groups can be constructed by reviewing the local paper, contacting a regional movement disorder center, and looking at Web sites dedicated to PD. By collecting a list of support groups in the area and including this as part of the nursing care plan, patients, caregivers, and family members may have the opportunity to participate in their own local Parkinson's community. If they have early stage PD, or young onset, refer the patients to an appropriate support group. Many support groups are dedicated to the patient with young-onset

PD as his or her needs are different from older adults with PD. Nurses can also play a role in leading support groups with the help of a social worker or other interested members of the multidisciplinary team. Focus in on topics that the participants are interested in, such as sexuality, genetics, surgical options, and complementary alternative medicine. A nurse's role is to organize dates, times, and locations, advertise the group with flyers and other PD providers, invite guest speakers, and preside over the group. Nurses can contribute as support group leaders through their role as expert clinicians and clarify information for patients and families. In support groups it is best to avoid giving specific medical advice or generalizing therapies for all participants. Explain that a support group allows the patient to meet other people who are living with PD and creates the opportunity to benefit from sharing stories, gathering information on the disease, networking with others, discovering local resources, and making friends. Establish rules to prevent one participant from dominating the conversation. Identify participants who are willing to take a leadership role, and allow them to help in organization. Facilitating an effective support group can positively influence the way that people cope with PD.

Develop an Activity Care Plan

Exercise can be effective in keeping a patient mobile, flexible, balanced, and strong. Exercise influences mood and general well-being and gives patients a purpose and sense of accomplishment. Nurses should discuss exercise as part of the care plan and inquire about current exercise habits. Remind patients about the three dimensions of exercise: strength, cardiovascular, and flexibility. Providing patients with examples for methods of exercise is helpful. For flexibility, patients may participate in yoga, qigong, Pilates, or a stretching class. Give practical advice, and incorporate this into the care plan. A physical therapist or trainer may be consulted for method of exercise. Provide information about local community exercise facilities, such as a YMCA or YWCA, community pools, or exercise groups dedicated to activities for older adults with limited mobility. Support groups may come together around the opportunity to provide a trained exercise professional to conduct classes exclusively for patients with PD. Consult with a physical therapist to get a listing of chair exercises or an exercise video for the patient to use at home. Suggest that a patient keep an exercise diary and get a friend to exercise with him or her. Reassess patients during follow-up on the exercise progress, if necessary; help the patient overcome barriers to getting proper exercise. Chapter 10 provides extensive information on rehabilitative interventions for PLWP.

Support a Nutrition Care Plan

Nutrition is instrumental in the health of patients, and nurses must recognize obstacles that may be barriers for patients to maintain balanced nutrition and assess symptoms indicating an alteration in the nutritional state. Quick questionnaires for nutritional assessment are available. General nutrition education should include a review of a healthy diet, a food guide pyramid for older adults, calorie requirements, hydration, basic vitamin supplementation, recipes, and eating plans. Owing to various components of the disease, maintaining a sufficient level of nourishment can be challenging. Issues can be related to:

- Mechanics of eating—difficulty getting food into the mouth due to dyskinesias, tremor, dystonia, bradykinesia, or stiffness.
- Chewing and swallowing—inadequate dentition, dry mouth, compromised swallowing, or risk of or actual aspiration.
- Appetite—lack of interest in food, loss of sense of taste or smell, nausea, social embarrassment, or depression; constipation or delayed gastric emptying of PD can affect appetite.
- Fatigue—exhaustion from effort of preparing and eating; bradykinesia, tremor, and muscular stiffness cause extra effort and energy expenditure for activities of ADLs.

Nurses should work with patients and families to identify a medication schedule that will optimize motor function for intake at mealtime. Often, a referral to a nutritionist, occupational therapist, and speech and swallowing therapist is helpful in assessing barriers to adequate intake. Later stage PD patients may need a feeding tube to provide adequate nutrition. However, the placement of a feeding tube provides the patient with artificial nutrition and if be discussed with the patient with regard to wishes at end of life, and ethical issues surrounding the withdrawal of artificial feedings if the patient becomes unable to communicate his or her wishes should also be discussed. Nurses play a significant role in educating patients and families on the risk and benefits of artificial nutrition in advanced disease (Gillick, 2000). Eating is often permitted with a feeding tube, thus allowing the patient to continue to experience the pleasure of food. The nursing care of the older adult with advanced disease can be challenging in the provision of physical and psychological care (Calne, 2003; Calne & Kumar, 2003).

NURSES' ROLE IN THE RESEARCH PROCESS

Research is essential to developing inquiry and designing new treatment models for PD and is at the center of obtaining knowledge to improve the quality of life of PLWP. This includes inquiry into understanding of symptoms, causes, prevention, treatment, and eventually, the cure. Nurses can assist patients in understanding what the research process entails and help them identify research protocols in which to participate.

Nurses often function as research coordinators and are active in recruiting, consenting, and retaining research participants in clinical studies for pharmaceutical and device trials. Patients may look to their nurses to explain and give advice on participating in complex research protocols, and the nurse should be wary of keeping his or her role of professional caregiver from conflicting with the role of researcher. The nurse's role is to protect the patient and provide him or her with information to make autonomous decisions as a research participant in helping the patient to understand what research entails. Consenting research participants is a process in which the nurse provides ongoing education for the potential participant or family member on the description of the research, the purpose, the details of the participant's involvement, and his or her rights as a research participant. This process does not begin with the presentation of the consent and end with the signature on the dotted line, but rather, it is an ongoing process starting at recruitment and lasting throughout the involvement of the study.

Nurses can also take on the role of an investigator, concentrating on a particular aspect of PD, and can design, receive funding for, implement, and publish research findings. However, designing clinical research involving the participation of older adults with neurodegenerative disease poses several ethical considerations for nurses to consider.

Recruitment

Recruitment of participants from the clinical setting where the nurse is a clinician can present interrole conflicts (Habiba & Evans, 2002).

The bioethical principle of beneficence requires nurses to contribute to the welfare of patients. However, the interrole conflict of researcher and nurse clinician may place the patient in a complex position. Patients see nurses as trustworthy and caring. This is especially true of older adults with neurodegenerative disease, who may be dependent on the nurse clinician for disease management.

The recruitment technique of approaching potential participants in the clinical setting may not be in the best interest of the patients. Patients may feel pressured to participate in an effort not to disappoint or offend the nurse. Furthermore, the vulnerability of older adults with PD may preclude them from acting in their own self-interest when approached by their clinicians to participate in clinical trials. Patients' participation in clinical research should be free of interrole conflicts, and this can be accomplished in venues outside of the clinical setting.

Informed Consent

Autonomy is the bioethical principle that guides the process of informed consent. The overarching goal in developing a consent procedure is respecting and protecting research participants' rights. Unfortunately, older adults with PD are vulnerable in the consent process due to mild and intermittent cognitive impairment. The inability of the research subject to read, comprehend, refuse, or withdraw consent is a potential problem for this population.

Older adults with PD can experience cognitive impairment related to medications, disease progression, and subcortical dementia. Cognitive impairment when present may be subtle and not easily recognized by the researcher inexperienced with the study population. Subcortical dementia preserves social and verbal skills but leaves the patient with poor problem-solving capacity. Thus the standard use of the Mini-Mental State Exam (MMSE) in clinical research for older adults with PD may not detect intermittent or subcortical cognitive deficits that may impact a patient's ability to fully participate in the consent process (Folstein, Folstein, & McHugh, 1975; Janvin, Larsen, Aarsland, & Hugdahl, 2006).

To minimize the risk of enrolling and consenting older adults with PD who have cognitive impairment, protocols should be developed with cognitive measures that assess constructional ability in addition to the MMSE. Constructional ability is the capacity to draw figures or shapes. The clock draw is one measure of constructional ability and is a useful tool to evaluate the participant's ability to integrate high-level nonverbal cognitive function with perceptual motor tasks.

Participant Safety

The safety of the participant in clinical research is maintained through the careful management of data collected during the course of the protocol. The bioethical principles of autonomy and fidelity govern the protection of data to ensure confidentiality.

Collecting data on older adults with PD will include personal identifiers and specific treatment information, such as pain management. Participants may discuss opioid use or other methods of pain management with the researcher, which is protected health information. In addition, the researcher will have access to the patient's medical record, which will contain clinical information on the treatment of PD. Thus the careful management of data collected in the course of the protocol is imperative to protect the patient's privacy.

Patients and their family members are often willing to participate in clinical research as a way of contributing to the understanding of PD in the hope of providing researchers with clues to improve the quality of life for persons with PD. Nurses are in a unique position to educate patients on the risks and benefits of participating in clinical research and should discuss protocols with patients to make sure that they are informed of their rights as research participants. If a new surgical or medication therapy is available only by participating in a research protocol, then a patient may be influenced in agreeing to the research and should be fully informed of the risks and benefits of the procedure. Much clinical research is designed as descriptive observational studies that do not have an intervention. These studies are useful in helping to categorize or gain insight into complex symptoms and can be a good way for patients to participate in clinical research with no direct benefits to the participants, other than providing them with a mechanism to contribute to the future of PD research.

Publishing nursing research is important and can lead to tremendous contributions to patient care, treatment alternatives, and improvements in quality of life. Table 8.2 lists some of the PD research published by nurses (Backer, 2006; Carter et al., 1998; Fleming, Tolson, & Schartau, 2004; Habermann & Davis, 2005).

TABLE 8.2 Examples of Nursing Research in Parkinson's Disease

Nurse researchers	Parkinson's disease study
Fleming et al. (2004)	"Changing Perceptions of Womanhood: Living with Parkinson's Disease"
Habermann and Davis (2000)	"Caring for Families With Alzheimer's Disease and Parkinson's Disease: Needs, Challenges and Satisfaction"
Carter et al. (1998)	"Living With a Person Who Has Parkinson's Disease: The Spouse's Perspective by Stage of Disease"
Backer (2006)	"The Symptom Experience of Patients With Parkinson's Disease"

A nurse's role in research can also include being a member of an institutional review board. Nurses review research proposals using their critical thinking skills and expertise to evaluate research protocols. This is a great way to learn about the research process as well as contribute to the ethical responsibility to protect research participants' rights.

SUMMARY

As PD is a chronic progressive neurologic disease, the nurse's role evolves throughout the trajectory of illness. PD affects the ability to function independently from both motor and nonmotor perspectives. The role of a nurse is to help Parkinson's patients manage their illness by evaluating the disease from a biopsychosocial perspective. In order to manage illness through the theory of self-efficacy, a nurse must understand his or her role within an interdisciplinary care team. A nurse embodies the roles of translator, researcher, assessor, educator, and advocate in an effort to maximize quality of life and promote self-efficacy for patients and families living with PD.

Helpful Web resources for PD nursing and patient information follow:

1. National Parkinson Foundation, http://www.parkinson.org
2. American Parkinson Disease Association, http://www.apdaparkinson.org
3. Michael J. Fox Foundation, http://www.michaeljfox.org

4. We Move, http://www.wemove.org
5. National Institute of Neurological Disorders and Stroke, http://www.
   ninds.nih.gov/disorders/parkinsons_disease/parkinsons_disease.htm
6. European Parkinson's Disease Association, http://www.epda.eu.com
7. Parkinson's Disease Foundation, http://www.pdf.org
8. Parkinson's Action Network, http://www.parkinsonsaction.org

REFERENCES

American Nursing Association. (2003). *Nursing: A social policy statement* (2nd ed.). Kansas City, MO: Author.

Back, A. L., Arnold, R. M., & Quill, T. E. (2003). Hope for the best, and prepare for the worst. *Annals of Internal Medicine, 138,* 439–443.

Backer, J. H. (2006). The symptom experience of patients with Parkinson's disease. *Journal of Neuroscience Nursing, 38,* 51–57.

Borneman, T., & Brown-Saltzman, K. (2001). Meaning of illness. In B. Ferrell & N. Coyle (Eds.), *The textbook of palliative care nursing* (pp. 415–424). New York: Oxford University Press.

Bunting-Perry, L. K. (2006). Palliative care in Parkinson's disease: Implications for neuroscience nursing. *Journal of Neuroscience Nursing, 38,* 106–113.

Calne, S. M. (2003). The psychosocial impact of late-stage Parkinson's disease. *Journal of Neuroscience Nursing, 35,* 306–313.

Calne, S. M., & Kumar, A. (2003). Nursing care of patients with late-stage Parkinson's disease. *Journal of Neuroscience Nursing, 35,* 242–251.

Carter, J. H., Stewart, B. J., Archbold, P. G., Inoue, I., Jaglin, J., Lannon, M., et al. (1998). Living with a person who has Parkinson's disease: The spouse's perspective by stage of disease. Parkinson's Study Group. *Movement Disorders, 13,* 20–28.

Clark, A. P., & Volker, D. L. (2003). Truthfulness. *Clinical Nurse Specialist, 17,* 17–18.

Fleming, V., Tolson, D., & Schartau, E. (2004). Changing perceptions of womanhood: Living with Parkinson's disease. *International Journal of Nursing Studies, 41,* 515–524.

Folstein, M. F., Folstein, S. E., & McHugh, P. R. (1975). "Mini-Mental State": A practical method for grading the cognitive state of patients for the clinician. *Journal of Psychiatric Research, 12,* 189–198.

Gillick, M. R. (2000). Rethinking the role of tube feeding in patients with advanced dementia. *New England Journal of Medicine, 342,* 206–210.

Habermann, B., & Davis, L. L. (2005). Caring for families with Alzheimer's disease and Parkinson's disease: Needs, challenges and satisfaction. *Journal of Gerontology Nursing, 31,* 49–54.

Habiba, M., & Evans, M. (2002). The inter-role confidentiality conflict in recruitment for clinical research. *Journal of Medicine and Philosophy, 27,* 565–587.

Janvin, C. C., Larsen, J. P., Aarsland, D., & Hugdahl, K. (2006). Subtypes of mild cognitive impairment in Parkinson's disease: Progression to dementia. *Movement Disorders, 21,* 1343–1349.

Lewis, S. M., Heitkemper, M. M., & Dirkesen, S. R. (Eds.). (2000). *Medical-surgical nursing: Assessment and management of clinical problems.* St. Louis, MO: Mosby.

MacMahon, D. G. (1999). Parkinson's disease nurse specialists: An important role in disease management. *Neurology, 52*(Suppl. 3), 21–25.

MacMahon, D. G., & Thomas, S. (1998). Practical approach to quality of life in Parkinson's disease: The nurse's role. *Journal of Neurology, 245*(Suppl. 1), 19–22.

Marks, R., Allegrante, J. P., & Lorig, K. (2005). A review and synthesis of research evidence for self-efficacy enhancing interventions for reducing chronic disability: Implications for health education practice (Part II). *Health Promotion Practice, 6,* 148–156.

Nutt, J. G., & Wooten, G. F. (2005). Clinical practice: Diagnosis and initial management of Parkinson's disease. *New England Journal of Medicine, 353,* 1021–1027.

9

Caregiving and Psychosocial Issues in Parkinson's Disease

Gretchen Glenn, LSW

Owing to the chronic and progressive nature of Parkinson's disease (PD), it is likely that a patient with this diagnosis will require the assistance of another at some point during the disease process. The level of assistance the patient will require depends on the age of onset of the disease, the progression of symptoms, and other comorbidities he or she may have in addition to PD. This caregiving task can be both a rewarding and a challenging experience. Therefore it is important to include the caregiver—family member, friend, or professional—in the treatment plan and understand his or her caregiving role as well as what he or she may be experiencing. The caregiver should be viewed as an important and valuable person in the care of the patient with PD. It is the intention of this chapter to focus on the family caregiver, view PD from his or her perspective, and highlight some of the challenges the caregiver may face throughout the disease trajectory. The importance of the nurse's role in addressing caregiver issues will also be emphasized.

THE FAMILY CAREGIVERS: WHO THEY ARE AND WHAT THEY DO

In general, family caregivers are those who provide a wide array of care to chronically ill or disabled relatives or friends, usually in the home. A family caregiver can be a wife, husband, daughter, son, grandchild, close friend, or neighbor. However, the literature reports that the majority of caregivers are women, primarily wives (Rabins, Lyketsos, & Steele, 1999). Since the average age of diagnosis for PD is 60 years, this illustrates that spousal caregivers are also elderly and may have their own medical conditions that must be considered. For the sake of this chapter the caregiver will be referred to as "her" and the patient as "him."

Caregiver responsibilities vary and can include providing assistance or supervision with activities of daily living (ADLs) such as bathing, grooming, dressing, shaving, toileting, brushing teeth, assisting with ambulation, and supervising activities. They may also assist with instrumental activities of daily living (IADLs) such as medication management and administration, household chores, financial management, transportation, emotional support, and medical plan management. In addition, caregivers must cope with a wide range of nonmotor symptoms of PD, which are often more difficult to manage than the motor symptoms. These nonmotor symptoms of PD have been skillfully described for you in chapters 4 and 5.

It is important to recognize that the role of the caregiver is demanding, and responsibilities vary throughout the disease trajectory. One study showed that caregiver activities can range from 11 per day in early PD to 30 per day in late-stage PD (Secker & Brown, 2005). The literature has also suggested that young-onset patients with PD prefer to define those who provide them assistance as *carepartners* rather than as caregivers. Carepartners tend to provide less physical and more emotional support, whereas caregivers provide more extensive physical assistance as well as emotional support (Bunting & Reich, 1995).

The demands and responsibilities of caregiving can place constraints on other areas of the caregiver's life, including her social and family life, employment and financial situation, and care for her own health. In addition, this new role can often lead to isolation and feelings of loss as well as high levels of depression. This tends to reduce the caregiver's quality of life and can ultimately lead to feelings of caregiver burden.

CAREGIVER BURDEN

Most people are not prepared for nor expect a loved one to be diagnosed with a chronic and progressive illness like PD. Likewise, they can be overwhelmed in taking on their new role as a caregiver and the associated responsibilities. Being a caregiver is a 24-hour job, often without breaks, and it can be a very challenging, lonely, frustrating, and stressful experience emotionally, physically, and financially. However, caregiving can be a very rewarding and positive experience for those who are able to recognize their limitations and are able to access and accept support and assistance from others when needed.

Caregiver burden is the degree of the caregiver's awareness that her own health, socialization, and financial situation are being adversely affected because of her caregiving obligations (Edwards & Ruettiger, 2002). Those who experience caregiver burden often undergo a mixture of emotional problems, such as frustration, anger, depression, sadness, guilt, fatigue, and isolation, that tend to fluctuate depending on how things are going in any particular day or week (Rabins et al., 1999).

Burden tends to increase as the disease progresses. Cognitive impairment, depression, anxiety, behavioral disturbances, psychosis, and greater ADL dependence of the patient with PD are predictors of burden. In addition, signs of depression, neglect of her own health, disheveled appearance, anger, and crying on the part of the caregiver are warning signs that she may be experiencing burden. Research has shown that an increase in burden places the caregiver at risk for compromising medical conditions, depression, and even death (Lyons, Stewart, Archbold, Carter, & Perrin, 2004). This may be due in part to lack of coping skills, lack of social support, fatigue, and feelings of guilt. Therefore it is pertinent for clinicians to be aware of caregiver needs and provide ongoing education and support to patients and caregivers.

Conversely, caregivers who are able to access assistance and support from others can have a positive and often rewarding caregiving experience. They may still experience caregiver burden, however, they are able to recognize the challenges and are able to devise a plan of care that assists them in overcoming these challenges in a positive and healthy way for both themselves and the patient. By doing this, the burden they experience is minimal and often temporary. Successful caregivers are willing to access family and community support services to provide them with necessary breaks and assistance in the caregiving process and do not feel guilty about doing so. They attend support groups and are able to achieve goals they set for themselves throughout the caregiving experience. Successful caregivers are able to communicate effectively with the patient, family members, and health care providers regarding what they require in order to sustain their caregiving role and are not ashamed or afraid to ask for this assistance. Spousal caregivers who are able to manage caregiving in this way often find that they develop a closer relationship with their spouse that is filled with love and support, not resentment.

Case Vignette

Mrs. S is an 80-year-old woman who is caring for her 82-year-old husband with advanced-stage PD. Mr. S was a successful businessman who shared in a happy marriage and active lifestyle with his wife. They have three grown children, who live in the area. Over the last 8 years, Mr. S's disease and cognition has progressed to the point that he is now dependent for both ADLs and IADLs. In the beginning, Mrs. S provided total care and did not allow their children to know the extent of Mr. S's decline. It was not until she began attending a local PD caregivers group that she started to realize the toll her caregiving role was taking on her life. She was no longer going out with her friends or doing hobbies she once enjoyed. She and Mr. S rarely left the house as she was afraid she would not be able to manage his care in public. She began having feelings of anger and resentment toward Mr. S for the life they were now living and would often find herself crying over the life they used to have together.

Through the support group, Mrs. S learned about community resources such as respite and home health services. She decided to hire a home health aid a few days a week. This provided such relief to Mrs. S that she decided to increase the home health aid service to 8 hours a day, 7 days a week. Mrs. S also allowed her children to help out and be involved in their father's care. In doing this, Mrs. S was able to enjoy outings with friends and engage in hobbies she once took pleasure in.

Mrs. S continued to provide care for her husband but was able to establish a balance between her role as caregiver and her role as wife, friend, and mother. Mrs. S feels that by accepting support and assistance from others, she is able to better appreciate and enjoy the time she spends with her husband and no longer feels resentment toward him. She also feels that her love for Mr. S has grown stronger, and she has been able to accept his disease and feels at peace with their new life.

CHALLENGES THAT LEAD TO CAREGIVER BURDEN

There are many challenges faced by caregivers that can lead to feelings of caregiver burden. Below are just a few challenges that I often see in the patients and caregivers I work with on a daily basis. It is important for nurses to recognize and acknowledge these challenges and offer education and intervention strategies as well as support to both patients and caregivers.

Medication Management

PD medications are time-sensitive and need to be given at a specific time every day in order to be most effective and give the patient optimal benefit. This can be a challenging task for both the person with PD and his caregiver. It is not unusual for people with PD and their caregivers to plan their days and activities around the medication schedule. This can result in limiting their social outings for fear that PD medications will wear off (stop working), resulting in the person with PD suddenly turning off (symptoms of PD worsen, and the patient may not be able to move) in a public setting.

Another challenge in medication management occurs when people with PD are admitted to the hospital or nursing home. Typically, staff nurses have a window of time in which they can administer medications, usually 30 min before the dose is due or 30 min after. This window can cause a patient to decompensate even further. As a result, this can make the nurse's job more difficult because the patient will require more hands-on care as they move to the off state. Often, it becomes the caregiver's responsibility to ensure that PD medications are administered at the correct time and to educate the medical staff on the importance of this time-sensitive schedule. This adds to the caregiver's stress when she is already worried and concerned about the current hospitalization or adjusting to the new nursing home placement.

In managing the medication schedule, nurses can provide education and encouragement to patients and suggest adjustments to the medication regimen to make it less burdensome. Therefore nurses should discuss with patients and caregivers how they are managing medications and pay attention to signs of distress or confusion. In addition, nurses can be advocates for patients who are hospitalized or in a nursing home by collaborating with providers with regard to medication management, education on the disease, and psychosocial stress. In doing this, the burden experienced by the caregiver can be significantly decreased in an already stressful situation like hospitalization or nursing home placement.

Nonmotor Symptoms of Parkinson's Disease

The nonmotor symptoms of PD, often seen in middle- to late-stage PD, can be the most difficult to manage, both medically and emotionally, and can greatly outweigh the motor symptoms (Secker & Brown, 2005). These symptoms include psychosis, anxiety, depression, sleep disturbances, and cognitive impairment. If these symptoms are left uncontrolled and untreated, eventual placement of the patient in a nursing home may become necessary for the safety of the patient and caregiver.

Dealing with these symptoms on a daily basis can take its toll on the caregiver and can leave her both physically and emotionally drained. Therefore it is imperative that the person with PD and his family be educated on the nonmotor symptoms of PD so that they are better equipped to manage them as well as more willing to discuss these symptoms with their clinician. In turn, it becomes the clinician's responsibility to identify and treat the nonmotor symptoms and provide education on available resources that can help support the person with PD and his caregiver in dealing with these symptoms (Aarsland, Larsen, Karlsen, Lim, & Tandberg, 1999).

Sexual Concerns

The topic of sex remains taboo in our society, and this holds true in the medical profession. However, it is a topic of importance to many people and can be one that causes much distress in a marriage. In general, a patient needs to feel comfortable talking to his clinician about all problems regarding sexual dysfunction.

Couples living with PD can experience sexual difficulties that can be due to both physiological and psychological causes. The patient can often maintain sexual desire, however, physical difficulties prevent him from doing so. In men the physiological problems can include urinary incontinence, decrease in size and firmness of the penis, delay in forming an erection, and premature ejaculation. In women these problems can include urinary incontinence and lack of estrogen (menopausal age), which can result in dryness and thinning of the vaginal walls and labia. Fatigue, rigidity, immobility in bed, and effectiveness of PD medications can also impact the quality of sexual function for the patient with PD. Psychologically, both men and women with PD can experience difficulty in adjusting to the illness, which can cause feelings of anger, anxiety, and grief that can interfere with sexual function. In addition, the person with PD can be dealing with self-esteem issues, limitations to activities, fatigue, depression, and changes in appearance (stiffness, emotionless face, balance and gait problems, etc.), all of which can compound sexual dysfunction (Calne & Basson, 2000).

In turn, a spousal caregiver can face challenges in being intimate with her partner due to many of the above physiological and psychological reasons as well as her own struggles with her loved one's illness. Rigidity can cause the body of a person with PD to feel different, stiffer and colder, which can make the person with PD seem less attractive to his partner. Excessive drooling and sweating can also cause the caregiver to shy away from her spouse (Basson, 1996). Spousal caregivers who provide assistance with personal care, such as bathing, dressing, and toileting, can lose their desire for intimacy as they may no longer see their relationship as spouse to spouse but more as mother to child. Spousal caregivers may also express frustration with their loved ones' aggressive pursuit of intercourse, even though they are not able to form or hold an erection. This aggressive pursuit of intercourse can be medication induced as hypersexuality can be a side effect of some PD medications. It can also be seen in those who have the diagnosis of dementia as well as PD. This aggressive pursuit can cause much distress for the caregiver as she knows that intercourse is not going to be possible, yet she does not want to hurt her spouse's feelings by refusing to try.

In addition, some patients experience *delusional jealousy,* which is the belief that their partners are being unfaithful. The behaviors associated with this type of delusion are jealousy, false accusations, paranoia, aggression, and social withdrawal. Often, these delusions are associated with medication side effects, however, they can also be related to dementia. This type of delusion can be very difficult for spousal caregivers to manage and can be very straining on their relationship as accusations made by the patient can be very hurtful and threatening at times. This type of delusion can further decrease the caregiver's desire and ability to be intimate with her partner.

When addressing sexual issues, it is vital to have both partners involved in the treatment plan and to make the environment as comfortable as possible as couples are often hesitant to discuss this topic honestly for fear of hurting their partner. It is important for the nurse to determine in the beginning what each person in the relationship wants and what the couple's emotional and physical relationship was like before PD. If they are both open to finding an intervention for the problem, such as sexual organ function or difficulty turning in bed, then these problems can be addressed and treated as necessary. The difficulty comes when couples do not desire the same thing. It is then necessary to further explore the presenting issues and consider referrals to social work clinicians or other appropriate counseling disciplines, as necessary. For some, that can mean couples counseling, and for others, it can be exploring alternate ways of being intimate without having intercourse, which can also be a very rewarding experience (Calne & Basson, 2000). Overall, one must keep in mind that like the treatment of PD, couples should be treated based on their individual concerns and needs as no two couples will respond the same to treatment for sexual dysfunction. It is important to remember and respect one's natural need to be physically and sexually desired, even with PD.

Sleep Disturbances

Sleep disturbances are a common problem in people with PD. It has been estimated that approximately 67% to 88% of people with PD suffer from sleep disturbances. The exact causes of sleep disturbances are unknown but may be related to stage of disease, medications, anxiety, depression, and incontinence (Pal et al., 2004). Patients with PD have reported such symptoms as sleep fragmentation, early awakening, cramping, pain, nightmares or vivid dreams, stiffness, and impaired motor function (Happe & Berger, 2002). As a result, caregivers subsequently suffer from sleep disturbances. Smith, Ellgring, and Oertel (1997) conducted a study examining sleep disturbances of PD caregivers and found that they reported sleep disturbances related to the nighttime care of their spouses as well as their own levels of stress and depression associated with their caregiving role. Caregivers often report that they sleep better when the patient with PD sleeps better. This demonstrates the importance of properly treating sleep disturbances and recommending practical interventions (i.e., sleeping in separate beds or using baby monitors if the couple sleep in different rooms) in an effort to lessen the burden experienced by the caregiver and ultimately lead to a better quality of life for not only the caregiver, but the patient with PD as well.

Financial Constraints

Every chronic and progressive illness brings the possibility of financial difficulties. This can be due in part to the person who was the so-called breadwinner now being afflicted by a progressive illness and being unable to work. As a result, the income needed to run the home may suddenly end, and the patient with PD may or may not have quick access to disability income. In addition, the limiting health insurance coverage and prescription plans in our society make paying for chronic medical care very expensive. This often results in families needing to downsize their living situations and the caregiver now assuming both employment and family responsibilities in addition to providing care (Bhatia & Gupta, 2003). Therefore it is important for the nurse to provide the patient and caregiver with education on available community resources that can provide financial support for care or refer them to a clinical social worker who can further assess the situation and assist in making appropriate referrals.

Transitions From Home

Many caregivers and patients struggle with the decision to move to an environment that will make it easier to care for the patient, such as placing the patient in a continuing care community (all three levels of care: independent, assisted living, and nursing home). Not only is the struggle based on the financial cost of moving to one of these facilities, but also on the caregiver's feeling of giving up on the patient and giving in to the disease. It is important to explore these feelings with both the caregiver and the patient in order to make this transition as successful as possible.

Often, the decision of placement is one of last resort. Most people prefer to be cared for at home and to care for their loved ones at home as long as possible. However, there are situations in which placement becomes necessary and is often the safest option for both the caregiver and the patient. When a caregiver is no longer able to provide the level of care required for the patient both physically and emotionally, the issue of safety arises for both the patient and the caregiver. In cases when the caregiver is no longer able to perform the physical tasks of caregiving (lifting, pulling, turning, incontinence care, protecting from falls, and preventing wandering) and is unable to enlist sufficient support in the home, then consideration for placement must be made. This also holds true when the caregiver is no longer able to handle the emotional aspects of PD, such as those associated with dementia, psychosis, and sleep disturbances.

Caregivers tend to struggle with their role change when placement occurs and often feel that they are giving up on their loved ones. When this occurs, it is important to emphasize to the caregiver that she is not giving up but has realized that the level of care required exceeds what she can provide in the safest way possible. Also, it is imperative to reinforce that she is still a caregiver and that only the level and type of care she is providing has changed. Instead of providing hands-on physical care for the patient, the caregiver becomes the patient's biggest advocate, and it becomes her responsibility to ensure that the care the patient receives in the facility is at its most optimal level. In refocusing her role as caregiver, this assists her in continuing to see value in her role and regain her sense of importance in the patient's care.

THE ROLE OF THE NURSE IN ADDRESSING CAREGIVER BURDEN

Owing to the degree of emotional impact caregiving places on a person, it is important to recognize and acknowledge the caregiver as an essential part of the treatment team and be aware of signs and symptoms of caregiver burden early in the disease process in order to intervene and offer help and support when indicated. Nurses are often the most involved members of the medical team in the care of PD patients and tend to have the most direct contact with caregivers. Not only do nurses provide ongoing clinical care to the person with PD, but they also provide support, counseling, education, and advocacy and make appropriate referrals for both the patient with PD and his caregiver.

During a clinic visit, nurses should inquire about how the caregiver is coping at home and pay attention to her response. If a caregiver appears to be distressed, depressed, or in need of support, there are resources available in the community that may help her. A referral should be made to a social worker in the clinical setting who is trained to provide counseling to patients and caregivers as well as connect them to resources in the community that can help lessen the stress and burden they are experiencing. If a social worker is unavailable, it then becomes the nurse's responsibility to offer support and education on services available in the community (Table 9.1) and make appropriate referrals as needed.

In working with caregivers, one must take into consideration that each person has a unique set of problems and issues that must be examined and treated individually. Also, perceptions of burden can differ from person to person (Edwards & Ruettiger, 2002). Therefore it is important to listen to caregivers, assess their situation, recognize their pain, and provide suggestions and recommendations of resources available to help decrease the burden as well as introduce new coping strategies that can decrease frustration. In addition, it is important to provide recognition and support for their role as caregiver. This allows the caregiver to feel validated in her role and may open discussion about her fears and concerns in caring for the patient with PD.

Caregivers should be encouraged to attend PD support groups. Support groups are a wonderful way to increase socialization, form supportive

TABLE 9.1   Description of Commonly Used Community Resources

Term	Description
Adult day health care centers (ADHC)	ADHC provides activities and assistance for people with physical and/or cognitive impairments. This service is for people who do not need 24-hr care in a nursing home but who cannot be left alone for long periods of time.
Assisted living	This is a housing option that provides support to residents who need assistance with such activities as personal care, light medical or nursing care, and supervision. This setting allows more independence than a nursing home unit.
Chore service	Provides assistance in the home to frail older adults with such tasks as light housekeeping, laundry, meal preparation, and grocery shopping.
Emergency response system	This is a device that allows a person who lives at home and is at high risk (e.g., home alone and a fall risk) to get immediate help in the event of an emergency. The person who is using the device wears a button either around the neck or wrist that he or she can push if needed. The button connects to the person's phone, which is programmed to send a signal to a response center. Trained professionals in the response center then assess the situation and carry out a series of actions to help the person in need.
Home modification program	This program pays for modifications to be made in the home of a person with a physical disability. The changes are made to allow the person to move safely around the home more freely. Examples of home modifications are a wheelchair ramp or stair glide. This program is typically for those who cannot afford to make the modifications on their own and meet a financial guideline set by the county.

(continued)

TABLE 9.1 Description of Commonly Used Community Resources *(continued)*

Term	Description
Home-delivered meals	Also known as Meals-on-Wheels in some areas. Provides a nutritious meal that is delivered to the person's home. The meals can be either hot or frozen, depending on the person's needs. To qualify for this program, a person must be considered homebound. A fee may be required.
Home maker/ home health aid	Provides assistance with light housekeeping, meal preparation, and personal care needs (bathing, dressing, etc.) for those who cannot manage alone.
Hospice	Hospice programs provide health care and support services, primarily in the home to people with terminal illness. The goal of hospice is to care for the physical, emotional, and spiritual needs of patients and families. Hospice also provides bereavement care to family members and loved ones of a terminally ill person. Most programs are Medicare certified and are covered by most insurance. Patients with end-stage PD can qualify for hospice.
Respite	Respite care is a program that provides relief to caregivers who provide 24-hour-a-day care to someone in need. Respite care can be for one day or weeks at a time, as needed by the caregiver or family. Respite care is usually provided in a state-approved nursing home but can be provided in a private home for shorter periods of time (i.e., 1 day).
Senior center	Senior centers are community-based programs that provide a variety of services and opportunities for people over the age of 60. These centers can provide opportunities for socialization, exercise, trips, volunteer work, etc. Some also provide a hot meal. Those who attend this type of program need to be fairly independent in everyday activities.
Support groups	A support group is a gathering of people with a common experience (i.e., disease, disorder, caregiving) that provides the opportunity to give and receive mutual support, encouragement, and information. It allows people the opportunity to be active on behalf of themselves and others in their community.
Transportation	Most counties have a transportation program that provides door-to-door service at a fixed cost.

Note. This is a general listing of resources. Resources may differ from location to location; contact your local Area Agency on Aging or the ElderCare Locator (800-677-1116) to learn more about resources available in your specific area.

relationships with people who share in a similar experience, vent frustrations, and exchange resource information and coping strategies. Caregivers should also be encouraged to utilize their families' support if available as well as community services in order to allow them some much-needed rest. It is also important to remind them of, and reinforce, the need for caregivers to take care of their own physical and mental health, which is often left neglected (Calne, 2003).

Education on illness is another important role of the nurse. Patients and caregivers should be educated on the symptoms of PD, the disease progression, and ways to manage symptoms of the disease when they occur. When people are adequately informed about the disease and related symptoms, they are more likely to experience less burden (Edwards & Ruettiger, 2002). In addition, education on long-term care issues, such as advance directives, hospice, and nursing home placement options, can also assist in alleviating burden as people tend to be more prepared and aware of their options ahead of time rather than being faced with them during a crisis.

In conclusion, PD is a complex neurological disorder that contains both neurological and psychosocial concerns. Therefore it is vital that health care teams, in particular, nurses, be aware of the psychosocial impact of PD so that they can assess and address these issues. Alleviating burden will allow for a better quality of life for the caregiver and in turn will assist in keeping the patient with PD at home longer and increase his quality of life.

TIPS FOR CAREGIVERS

1. *Take care of yourself.* This includes addressing your own medical needs, eating well, exercising, and taking time for yourself. Remember, you are no good to your loved one if you are not healthy enough to provide his care.

2. *Value yourself.* Do not allow the disease to become you or the center of your life. Maintain the friendships, activities, and hobbies you had before you became a caregiver.

3. *Be realistic and access help.* Know what you can do and recognize when you have given all that you can. Access community resources to help you, such as adult day health care, home health aid, respite, and companion services. Also, if family members or friends offer to help, let them, and be specific on the ways they can help.

4. *Be aware of signs and symptoms of depression.* Do not delay in seeking support or professional counseling.

5. *Join a caregiver support group.* This is a great way to give and receive mutual support and know that you are not alone.

6. *Educate yourself.* Keep up to date on your loved one's disease, and do not be afraid to ask questions at doctor visits.

Internet Resources

http://www.aarp.org

AARP is a nonprofit organization for people aged 50 and over dedicated to enhancing quality of life during the aging process. The Web site provides information on AARP services and benefits.

http://www.alfa.org

The Assisted Living Federation of America is dedicated to the assisted living industry and the older adult population it serves. It provides information on what assisted living is and checklists of what to look for and ask about when looking into assisted living facilities.

http://www.alz.com

The Alzheimer's Association offers various resources for caregivers of individuals suffering from any form of dementia. Resources are available to assist in selecting respite care services and dealing with caregiver stress. Contacts for support groups are also available.

http://www.aoa.dhhs.gov

The U.S. Department of Health and Human Services Administration on Aging provides information on aging services available in the United States and information on the Older Americans Act and the National Network on Aging.

http://www.caps4caregivers.org

The Children of Aging Parents, a nonprofit charitable organization, provides information, referrals, and support to family caregivers. This Web site has listings for caregiver support groups in several states.

http://www.caregiver.com

This is the Web site for *Today's Caregiver* magazine.

http://www.caregiver.org

The Family Caregiver Alliance focuses on services in California but provides general information useful to all caregivers. This site provides facts and statistics on caregiver burnout and reinforces the importance of self-care.

http://www.eldercare.gov

The U.S. Administration on Aging sponsors this Web site, which allows individuals to find information and referral services for their state and local Area Agencies on Aging. These programs can help caregivers identify appropriate services in their local community.

http://www.medicare.gov

This is the official government Web site for Medicare services. This Web site can answer questions on various programs, including Medicare, Medigap, Medicare Managed Care Plans, and the new Medicare Part D prescription plan. In addition, this Web site offers a listing of Medicare-certified nursing homes and home health care agencies.

http://www.ssa.org

This is the official Web site for the Social Security Administration and provides information on the Social Security Administration as well as information on Social Security retirement and disability benefits, including Medicare and Medicaid programs.

http://www.wellspouse.org

National organization focusing on the needs of well spouses caring for a chronically ill or disabled husband, wife, or partner.

REFERENCES

Aarsland, D., Larsen, J. P., Karlsen, K., Lim, N. G., & Tandberg, E. (1999). Mental symptoms in Parkinson's disease are important contributors to caregiver distress. *International Journal of Geriatric Psychiatry, 14,* 866–874.

Basson, R. (1996). Sexuality and Parkinson's disease. *Parkinsonism and Related Disorders, 2,* 177–185.

Bhatia, S., & Gupta, A. (2003). Impairments in activities of daily living in Parkinson's disease: Implications for management. *NeuroRehabilitation, 18,* 209–214.

Bunting, L., & Reich, S. (1995). Carepartners: Taking care of your loved one and yourself. In A. Johnson (Ed.), *The young Parkinson's handbook.* Retrieved January 27, 2007 from http://neuro.www2mgh.harvard. edu/parkinsonweb/Main/YOPDHandbook/Chapter11/html

Calne, S. M. (2003). The psychosocial impact of late-stage Parkinson's disease. *Journal of Neuroscience Nursing, 35,* 306–313.

Calne, S. M., & Basson, R. (2000). Intimacy, sexuality and idiopathic parkinsonism: The uncharted waters. *Loss, Grief and Care: A Journal of Professional Practice, 8,* 21–29.

Edwards, N. E., & Ruettiger, K. M. (2002). The influence of caregiver burden on patients' management of Parkinson's disease: Implications for rehabilitation nursing. *Rehabilitation Nursing, 27,* 182–187.

Happe, S., & Berger, K. (2002). The association between caregiver burden and sleep disturbances in partners of patients with Parkinson's disease. *Age and Ageing, 31,* 349–354.

Lyons, K. S., Stewart, B. J., Archbold, P. G., Carter, J. H., & Perrin, N. A. (2004). Pessimism and optimism as early warning signs for compromised health for caregivers of patients with Parkinson's disease. *Nursing Research, 53,* 354–362.

Pal, P. K., Thennarasu, K., Fleming, J., Schulzer, M., Brown, T., & Calne, S. M. (2004). Nocturnal sleep disturbances and daytime dysfunction in patients with Parkinson's disease and in their caregivers. *Parkinsonism and Related Disorders, 10,* 157–168.

Rabins, P. V., Lyketsos, C. G., & Steele, C. D. (1999). Supporting the family and the care-provider. In P. V. Rabins, C. G. Lyketsos, & C. D. Steele (Eds.), *Practical dementia care* (pp. 111–113). New York: Oxford University Press.

Secker, D. L., & Brown, R. G. (2005). Cognitive behavioral therapy (CBT) for care of patients with Parkinson's disease: A preliminary randomized controlled trial. *Journal of Neurology, Neurosurgery, and Psychiatry, 76,* 491–497.

Smith, M. C., Ellgring, H., & Oertel, W. H. (1997). Sleep disturbances in Parkinson's disease patients and spouses. *Journal of the American Geriatrics Society, 45,* 194–199.

10

Rehabilitation Interventions in Parkinson's Disease

Heather J. Cianci, PT, MS, GCS

Managing patients with Parkinson's disease (PD) throughout the course of their disease requires the efforts of medical professionals from various disciplines. The interdisciplinary team offers patients a broad spectrum of treatment options and coping strategies from the time of diagnosis through the later stages of the disease. It is the collaboration among team members that helps ensure coordinated care for the patient. The physical therapist plays an essential role in this care team. Physical therapists not only provide direct patient care, but also serve as educators for members of the interdisciplinary team by training them in techniques to ensure patient safety and enhance mobility. Recent research supports that patients derive benefit from physical therapy in conjunction with their medication regimens (de Goede, Keus, Kwakkel, & Wagenaar, 2001; Ellis et al., 2005; Gage & Storey, 2004). Physical therapy assists patients in managing the mobility challenges that occur over the time of disease progression. This can range from changes in flexibility and posture, to difficulties with gait and balance, to rising from a chair and getting out of bed. Exercise programs, education in fall prevention and carepartner safety, and training in compensatory strategies are examples of treatments provided by physical therapy. Ultimately, the goal of physical therapy in working with those with PD is to reduce disability, maximize function, and enhance safety within the home and community. Referring patients to physical therapy soon after the time of diagnosis, and periodically as changes occur with disease progression, will help to ensure that reaching these goals occurs. This chapter will review the physical changes that occur in PD and their effect on mobility, while teaching health professionals how to assist patients in maintaining optimal function.

MUSCULOSKELETAL CHANGES

Musculoskeletal changes are subtle in the early stages of PD but, with disease progression, can become quite evident. Posture is the most obvious change. A slight rounding of the shoulders can often advance to an excessive forward curvature of the spine. This increase in thoracic kyphosis, along with a loss of lumber lordosis, can negatively impact patients' speech, swallowing, and respiration as well as their ability to maintain eye contact. This can cause social outings to become embarrassing, and patients may begin to limit their interaction with others. Changes in the alignment of the spine also lead to changes in surrounding joints and muscles. Forward curvature of the spine pulls the chest wall in, causing tightness in the chest wall musculature. This tightness can then lead to a loss of shoulder range of motion, making activities of daily living (ADL), such as reaching into cabinets and putting on jackets, challenging.

Loss of spinal flexibility, even in the early stages of the disease, along with muscle stiffness also directly influence patients' functional abilities (Bridgewater & Sharpe, 1998; Schenkman et al., 2001). Reduced trunk range of motion compromises activities like rolling in bed and reaching, while also impacting the quality of balance reactions (Carpenter, Allum, Honegger, Adkin, & Bloem, 2004; Schenkman et al., 2001). A complete musculoskeletal evaluation should be performed by a physical therapist as soon as the diagnosis of PD is made. Early identification and treatment of musculoskeletal changes is key to helping prevent or limit functional decline in patients.

Postural Assessments

To promote better alignment of the spine through better attention to posture, patients must first be made aware of what changes are occurring. An appropriate assessment tool can accomplish this by helping clinicians highlight and track posture changes to better educate patients (Table 10.1).

Posture Treatment Options

Once patients learn about their postural deficits, strategies must be employed to correct, reduce, or limit the progression of the deficits (Table 10.2).

TABLE 10.1 Postural Assessment Tools

Assessment tool	Technique	Benefit
Digital or instant camera photographs	Take photographs of patients at initial assessment and at intervals throughout treatment	Patients are able to recognize deficits and track improvements in posture. Photographs can be placed around the home to serve as reminders for posture checks.
Videotaping	Videotape patients performing ADLs at initial assessment and at intervals throughout treatment	Patients are able to recognize how deficits in posture affect their ability to perform ADLs.
Inclinometer	Instrument is placed on spine to measure angle of forward bend at initial assessment and at intervals throughout treatment	Patients are able to recognize deficits and track improvements in posture.

In the earlier stages of PD, these strategies are typically easy to apply. However, with disease advancement, there is a noticeable decrease in patients' self-awareness of posture. This leads to carepartners needing to take on an active role in reminding the patients to correct their posture. In cases where patients are truly unable to correct their posture, reclining wheelchairs with specialized cushions may be required.

GAIT DEFICITS

Early-Stage PD

Gait changes in PD are generally mild in the beginning stage of the disease. Slowness, slight dragging of one leg, and slowed or absent arm swing on one side are the common changes noticed. Patients may describe themselves as feeling less coordinated and report episodes of tripping. In this stage, only minimal gait training may be necessary.

Moderate-Stage PD

With disease progression, gait becomes characterized by shortened stride, slower speed, narrowed base of support, and reduced heel strike (Morris,

TABLE 10.2   Strategies for Correcting Posture Deficits

Strategy	Technique
Exercise	• Stretching neck and hip flexors, chest, hamstrings, and heel cords.
	• Strengthening trunk, neck, and hip extensors, shoulders, scapular muscles, and abdominals.
	• Yoga, tai chi, and Pilates.
Home modification	• Use a lumbar roll in chairs to enhance natural lumbar curve (lumbar rolls can easily be used in cars, planes, and theater seats).
	• Avoid recliner chairs and allowing hips to slide forward in regular chairs.
	• Avoid excessive pillows with sleep. Attempt to use one appropriate height pillow at neck or a cervical roll. If side sleeping, use a pillow between knees.
	• Keep television and computer screens at eye level.
	• Place posture reminder signs in commonly used rooms to encourage frequent posture checks.
	• Ask family and friends to give posture reminders.
	• Prop elbows on table to hold books or magazines up directly in front of the face while reading, or use a book stand.
Office modification	• Use a lumbar roll or chair with lumbar support to enhance natural lumbar curve.
	• Keep computer screen at eye level.
	• Place posture reminder sign on computer.
	• Keep chair and desk at appropriate height to one another.
	• Avoid sitting for longer then 20–30 min. During breaks, stretch arms up over the head.
Braces	• Lumbar braces made of elastic and Velcro can provide tactile reminders to keep spine erect.
	• Rigid braces for the neck and trunk can be used with more advanced disease progression.

Huxham, McGinley, & Iansek, 2001). Together, these produce a shuffling gait, which leads to increased episodes of tripping. Even small changes in the walking surface, such as a threshold between a carpeted and noncarpeted room, can become obstacles due the decreased ground clearance of the feet. Gait changes coupled with environmental risk factors and postural instability can ultimately result in falls. Recent prospective studies investigating fall incidences in people with PD showed that falls are a large problem (Bloem, Grimbergen, Cramer, Willemsen, & Zwinderman, 2001; Gray & Hildebrand, 2000; Wood, Bilclough, Bowron, & Walker, 2002) and often result in injuries and fractures (Genever, Downes, & Medcalf, 2005; Wielinski, Erickson-Davis, Wichmann, Walde-Douglas, & Parashos, 2005). Fear also plays a role in the gait of those with PD. Patients with PD report a greater fear of falling than their healthy peers. This fear of falling is further heightened in patients who test poorly on portions (arising from a chair, posture, gait, postural stability) of the Unified Parkinson's Disease Rating Scale (UPDRS) and on particular standing balance tests (Adkin, Frank, & Jog, 2003).

Freezing is another gait deficit that occurs in the moderate stage of PD. Freezing is a motor block where movement suddenly stops or cannot be started. It can become quite disabling and frequently results in falls. Falls often occur when patients do not " 'accept' the block and wait for spontaneous resolution" (Bloem, Hausdorff, Visser, & Giladi, 2004, p. 873). They instead try to push through the freeze in an attempt to produce movement. This causes either the legs to tremble in place or the body's center of gravity to become so anteriorly displaced that the patient is standing on his or her toes and then loses his or her balance.

Freezing often begins as a hesitation of movement and progresses to an absence of movement (Bloem et al., 2004). It is typically context-dependent, commonly occurring when patients move from an open area through a doorway, through crowds, or from one floor surface to another. Freezing also occurs at gait initiation, when approaching a target such as a chair, and during direction changes, as with moving around obstacles and turning. A patient's emotional state can also play a role in freezing. Stress, anxiety, and fear often lead to freezing episodes.

Executing a turn can prove to be a difficult task for people with PD. The person with PD takes more steps and a longer amount of time to make a 360° turn than someone of the same age without PD (Schenkman, Morey, & Kuchibhatla, 2000). This multistep turn often leads to a freeze or fall if the patient attempts to push himself or herself to move faster. The pivot and crossover turns are other unsafe forms of turning seen in PD. The pivot turn is when the patient turns by quickly twisting the feet and body as one unit. The crossover turn is when the patient steps one foot sideways over the other foot. This technique causes the center of gravity to shift too far to one side without proper support. With the legs crossed, the ability to right an imbalance is unlikely.

Propulsion, also known as festination, and retropulsion are also problematic gait changes in PD. These gait changes are characterized by the inability to terminate movement (Morris, 2000). Festination is a progressive increase in the speed of steps with a shortening of the stride. Patients often describe this as feeling like a "train out of control" or as if they are "trying to catch up" with themselves. This can occur when reaching too far forward, when a shuffling gait is not corrected, or while hurrying or being distracted during walking. Retropulsion is short, quick, backward steps. This can occur with pulling open a door or drawer, reaching too far overhead, or stepping backward.

BALANCE DEFICITS

Postural instability is one of the four hallmark signs of PD and often plays a large role in patients falling. While the exact cause of postural instability in PD is not clearly understood, it seems to result from a combination of several factors (Lieberman, 2002). These factors include muscle rigidity, inflexibility, a narrowed base of support, an anterior shift in the center of gravity, and bradykinesia. Patients with postural instability have slowed or absent righting reactions. During a perturbation or loss of balance in someone with PD, muscles react in an attempt to correct the imbalance, but their activation response is delayed, and the size of the movement is reduced (Jöbges et al., 2004). This is seen during the posterior perturbation testing portion of the UPDRS. A patient with PD will often respond to this pull test either by taking multiple steps backward in an attempt to regain his or her balance or by falling straight back into the arms of the examiner. People without PD will regain their balance by dorsiflexing their ankles and reaching forward with the arms, leaning forward from the hips, or taking a step backward (Morris, 2000).

GAIT AND BALANCE ASSESSMENTS

There are a number of assessment tools for examining gait and balance in those with PD (Table 10.3). These tools can be performed relatively easily and quickly, using very little equipment, with the exception of the GaitRite gait lab system.

TABLE 10.3 Gait and Balance Assessment Tools

Assessment tool	Description
Berg Balance Scale (Qutubuddin et al., 2005)	Patient performs 14 tasks such as single leg stance, transfers, and 360° turn. Tasks are scored 0–4 with 56 the maximum score.
Timed "Up & Go" (Morris, Morris, & Iansek, 2001)	Patient transfers from chair, walks a short distance, turns, and returns to sit in chair.
UPDRS	Patient performs postural stability/retropulsion, gait, freezing when walking, and walking portions of the UPDRS.
Modified Falls Efficacy Scale (Hill, Schwarz, Kalogeropoulos, & Gibson, 1996; Tinetti, Richman, & Powel 1990)	Patients self-rate their fear of falling on 14 tasks such as climbing stairs, crossing the street, and performing housework.
Gait velocity	Measure the time it takes patient to walk a certain distance.
GaitRite (Nelson et al., 2002)	Computerized gait lab.
Skilled observation	Observe patient walking in a variety of situations.

Gait Strategies

To facilitate a more normalized gait pattern and better manage episodes of freezing, patients with PD can use compensatory strategies known as attentional cues (Rubinstein, Giladi, & Hausdorff, 2002). These cues help increase patients' conscious awareness of gait, thereby overriding deficits in automatic movements and timing of movements (Howe, Lovgreen, Cody, Ashton, & Oldham, 2003; Morris, 2000). Training patients to use self-monitoring skills and attentional cues should begin early in the disease. This allows patients to become familiarized with the techniques in an attempt to prevent falls and promote a feeling of self-control over the disease. Carepartners must also receive training so that they may assist patients when needed. This is particularly important for patients with anxiety or memory problems.

Attentional cues can be internal or external. Internal cueing means that the patient self-cues or uses visualization techniques. Examples of internal cues are patients imagining they are stepping over an object to initiate gait or focusing on the feeling of the heel hitting the floor as they are walking. External cueing means that the cues come from the surrounding environment. They can be visual or auditory, with the patient performing alone or with assistance. Rhythmic auditory stimulation is an example of external cueing. This technique of walking to music or to the beat of a certain sound can increase gait velocity and stride length (Fernandez del Olmo & Cudeiro, 2003; Howe et al., 2003; McIntosh, Brown, Rice, & Thaut, 1997). Heel strike and stride can also increase when using visual cues like floor markers or laser beams, thereby limiting or avoiding shuffling (Lewis, Byblow, & Walt, 2000). It is important to note that attentional cues do not work for all patients since gait and balance difficulties can increase when patients try to multitask (Hausdorff, Balash, & Galadi, 2003; O'Shea, Morris, & Iansek, 2002). Some patients may actually experience more shuffling and freezing episodes when performing cognitive or motor tasks while walking. Trying a variety of techniques with patients and their carepartners is the only way to find what works best.

In dealing with freezing episodes, the first task is to determine what causes the freeze and where it is most likely to occur for that individual. A patient may have a pattern of freezing when rushing to answer the phone or when approaching a chair to sit and not be aware of it. Once causes and locations are identified, the next task is to make modifications to the home environment and train the patient to use attentional cues. There are a variety of ways this can be accomplished (Table 10.4). However, before any strategy will work, patients must be trained never to fight through a freeze in an attempt to force movement as this often leads to a fall. Carepartners should also be included in training sessions since some patients are unable to recall strategies without assistance.

Assistive Devices

Many patients with PD will need to use an assistive device to improve the safety of their gait. Four-post standard walkers and quad canes generally do not work well for PD patients as they require multitasking and disrupt fluid movement. Four-wheeled rolling walkers with hand brakes and seats tend to work best. The wide base and front swivel wheels make turning easier, while the brakes add more control and can be helpful for those who festinate. The seat provides a place to rest for those who tire easily or who experience unexpected off periods. The walker itself can serve as an external cue, as the patient can use it as a moving target. All patients in need of

TABLE 10.4 Freeze Reduction Strategies

Freeze "trigger"	Freeze reduction strategy
Answering the phone	• Never rush to answer the phone.
	• Keep a cordless phone within easy reach.
	• Use an answering machine.
	• Keep pathways open by rearranging furniture, and keep floors free of clutter.
Walking onto elevator, crowded train, or bus	• Allow everyone else to get on or off first.
	• Announce that you have PD and ask people to be patient.
	• Walk up to the threshold, stop, and then focus on stepping over it.
Walking through doorway	• Tell yourself not to focus on the doorway, but rather how your feet are hitting the ground.
	• Guess how many steps it will take to walk from where you are through the doorway, then count your steps as you move through to see how close you were to your guess.
	• Look through the doorway at an object inside and focus on stepping to approach the object.
	• Walk up to the threshold, stop, and then focus on stepping over it.
	• Place colored tape on threshold to draw attention to stepping over it.
	• Place colored tape in horizontal stripes in front of and through doorway to step over.
	• Keep areas around doorways open and free of clutter.
	• Keep area well lit.
Walking in crowds	• Try to walk near walls.
	• Take slow, deep breaths and focus only on how your feet are moving, not on the people around you.
	• Cycle between only walking a few feet, stopping yourself, and then starting again.

(continued)

TABLE 10.4 Freeze Reduction Strategies *(continued)*

Freeze "trigger"	Freeze reduction strategy
Turning	• Never pivot.
	• If turning right, step with the right foot first. If turning left, step with the left foot first.
	• Try making a U-turn in open spaces.
	• Try marching to turn.
	• Try to avoid stepping backward to turn.
	• If using a rolling walker,
	▪ in tighter spaces, make a small move with the walker, take two steps, pause, and repeat the process.
	▪ in open spaces, make a wide U-turn, taking care to keep your body inside of the walker at all times.
	• Keep areas where turns commonly occur, like the kitchen and bedroom, open and free of clutter.
	• If there is not enough room to make a safe turn, try sidestepping.
	• Finish one task at a time—do not try to turn while closing the refrigerator.
Gait initiation	• Stop all movement, and take a deep breath.
	• Make sure weight is evenly placed throughout both feet.
	• Visualize stepping over or kicking an object.
	• Shift weight side to side and then step with un-weighted foot.
	• March in place before stepping.
	• Have your care partner place his or her foot ahead of your foot and step to it.

Note. In general, when a freeze begins, patients should first try to stop all movement, take a deep breath and relax, and then get their weight evenly distributed on both feet before trying to move again. "Think before moving" is a great strategy to teach patients. For all strategies, focusing on the task is crucial. Rushing, carrying objects, talking with others, or even looking away for a moment may limit how well the strategy will work.

an assistive device for walking should have an assessment from a physical therapist to ensure that they receive the proper device.

When safe ambulation with a walker is no longer possible, motorized wheelchairs and scooters can provide patients with an alternate means of mobility. Physical therapists can make recommendations concerning the proper type of device and features as well as provide education in using the device correctly. It is important to note that not all patients are able to safely handle motorized wheelchairs or scooters. In this situation a carepartner will need to propel the patient in a manual wheelchair.

Balance Strategies

Training in new movement strategies is vital to those with PD because performing even a simple task like reaching into a cabinet can lead to a loss of balance (Table 10.5).

TABLE 10.5 New Movement Strategies to Reduce Loss of Balance

Activity	New movement strategy
Reaching into a high cabinet in kitchen or bathroom	• Stand as close to the counter or sink as possible (body can touch surface) before reaching. ▪ Keep feet wide apart and one foot slightly forward. ▪ Hold onto counter or sink with one hand while reaching for object with the other. • If you must move up onto your toes to reach an object, it is too high. Bring the object to a lower shelf or keep it on the counter. • Use a reacher for high objects that are light, like cereal boxes. • Avoid step stools. • If possible, slide objects along counter instead of carrying.
Opening and closing a door, oven, microwave, or refrigerator	• Do not stand directly in front of the door. Stand sideways at a right angle to the door. This will keep you from stepping backward. ▪ Keep feet wide apart. ▪ Place one hand on counter or wall (a vertical grab bar can be installed here). ▪ Shift your weight from front to back to help pull the door open. Shift weight from back to front to close.

(continued)

TABLE 10.5 New Movement Strategies to Reduce Loss of Balance *(continued)*

Activity	New movement strategy

Reaching forward into a closet or for an object	• Do not reach forward while walking.
	• Stand as close to the clothing or object as possible before reaching.
	  ▪ Keep feet wide apart and one foot slightly forward.
	  ▪ Steady yourself with one hand on the wall (a vertical grab bar can be installed here). If you have to lean forward or move up onto your toes, you are not close enough and/or the clothing/object is too high.
	• Move commonly needed objects to lower and easier to reach places.
	• Lower the clothing bar and/or move it forward.
	• Keep floor of closet free of clutter.

Picking up objects from the floor or out of low cabinets	• Use a reacher.
	• Move commonly used items to an easy to reach area.
	• Steady yourself with one hand on the counter or steady furniture.
	  ▪ Keep feet wide apart and one foot slightly forward.
	  ▪ Bend at the knees, not the back.
	  ▪ Return to standing very slowly.

Dressing	• Gather all clothing and put it in one place first. • Sit down to dress. • Use adaptive devices like long-handled shoe horns, sock donners, and button hooks.

Note. For all strategies, focusing on the task is crucial. Rushing, carrying objects, talking with others, or even looking away for a moment may limit how well the strategy will work.

FALL PREVENTION

Home Assessments

Patients with PD can reduce and prevent falls not only by following new movement strategies, but also by making their home environments safer.

A home safety assessment by a health professional will ensure that proper changes are made to accomplish this. The assessment should include, but need not be limited to, evaluating (a) the layout of each room's flooring, lighting, furniture, closets and cabinets, appliances, and maneuverability with and without a gait assistive device; (b) all entrances to the home; (c) parking areas; and (d) all hallways and stairways. The patient should then be evaluated walking, transferring, and performing ADLs in all of these areas. After this is accomplished, recommendations for home modifications can be made.

Home Modifications

Simple changes to a home can greatly improve patient safety. Attaching grab bars in hallways and showers and next to toilets and doors provides increased stability. Removing clutter and throw rugs from the floors reduces the chances of tripping. Rearranging furniture to allow for open spaces will increase maneuverability, especially for those using assistive devices for walking. Some modifications are more complex, like widening doorways, adding ramps, and remodeling bathrooms to make them wheelchair accessible.

Adaptive equipment is also used to modify the home environment. Placing a small shower chair in the bathroom not only improves safety, but also patient independence. This type of device is relatively inexpensive and easy to obtain from equipment catalogues and drug stores. Larger devices, however, like motorized lift chairs, are more costly and are generally ordered through specialized medical equipment stores.

Transfers and Bed Mobility

With disease progression, transfers and bed mobility become increasingly challenging. This is due in part to bradykinesia, a lack of trunk flexibility, and difficulty performing fluid sequential motor activities (Morris, 2000). Low nighttime levodopa levels can also make trips from the bed to the bathroom more difficult. Teaching patients to break down complex activities like bed mobility into a series of small steps often makes the task much easier to perform. Below is an example of this technique.

Rolling From Supine to Side Lying

1. Bend knees.
2. Turn head in direction of turn.
3. Gently rock knees side to side for momentum.
4. Allow knees to fall together to the side while reaching upper arm in direction of turn.

The following tips can also be used:

1. Avoid flannel sheets and night clothes.
2. Wear silk or satin night clothes.
3. Tuck a folded silk or satin sheet across the middle of the bed where the buttocks will lie.
4. Use a night-light.
5. Use a bed rail.
6. Avoid heavy blankets and too many pillows.
7. Avoid down or egg crate mattress covers.
8. Avoid soft mattresses.
9. Mentally rehearse the rolling technique prior to performing it.

When transferring to stand, patients with PD tend to not lean forward enough, causing their center of gravity (COG) to fall posterior to their feet. This leads to patients either not being able to lift themselves up or to continually "plop" back down into the chair. The correct technique is highlighted below:

1. Scoot to the edge of the seat.
2. Keep feet wide and posterior to knees.
3. Hold armrests.
4. Lean forward "nose over toes" and push to stand.

The transfer to stand can also be made easier by patients first mentally rehearsing the movement, by rocking back and forth before moving, and by sitting in a chair that has armrests and is the proper height. Chairs should be high enough so that the hips are in line with, or higher than, the knees. Patients should avoid low, soft furniture that sinks in when sat on, as is often the case with sofas. For patients with advanced PD, a motorized lift chair or physical assistance from a carepartner may be necessary.

Patients with PD often land in a side sit position when returning to sit from a standing position. This partial landing on the seat edge occurs when patients reach for the surface they intend to sit on before fully turning around. Reaching forward too soon and too far causes an anterior shift in the COG. This shift leads patients to feel as though they are losing their balance, which they then try to resolve by landing in the chair as quickly as possible. Many falls result from patients tipping over chairs or sliding off the seat edge onto the floor. The correct technique is highlighted below:

1. Turn completely around so backside is facing the chair.
2. Be sure back of legs touch the chair.
3. Reach back with both hands for armrests.
4. Slowly lower to sit.

Getting in and out of a car is difficult for many patients with PD for various reasons. It is not just the physical changes from the disease, but also the layout of cars. Small spaces, low seats, and a lack of armrests can all play a role. Patients should be taught not to step into the car, but rather, to back in slowly to sit first and then swing the legs inside. Using the following tips will also ease the process:

1. Slide the car seat back to allow for maximum leg room.
2. Avoid cloth seats by sitting on a plastic bag.
3. Try using the Handybar, an adaptive device that attaches to the car to provide a sturdy surface from which to push.
4. Use a firm cushion on seat if it is too low.
5. Avoid holding the door as it may move and pinch fingers or cause a loss of balance.

EXERCISE

Exercise is an important tool in helping patients with PD manage their disease. Research shows that exercise can improve PD patients' flexibility, strength, gait, balance, and mobility (Hirsch, Toole, Maitland, & Rider, 2003; Reuter & Engelhardt, 2002; Viliani et al., 1999). In rodent models, researchers are demonstrating that exercise restores motor function and protects against neurodegeneration (Cohen, Tillerson, Smith, Schallert, & Zigmond, 2003; Fisher et al., 2004; Tillerson, Caudle, Reveron, &

Miller, 2003; Tillerson et al., 2001). This type of research illustrates the importance of establishing an exercise routine early on in the disease in an effort to help delay, limit, or possibly prevent musculoskeletal changes and motor decline.

Physical therapists continue to develop new rehabilitation strategies, using exercise to improve the quality of movement in patients with PD. One such strategy is using amplitude-based interventions, where patients perform large movements as they mentally focus on how big the movement is that they are performing. Research is showing that patients using this technique improve the speed of upper and lower limb movements (Farley & Koshland, 2005). Another strategy showing promise in both human and rodent models is treadmill training. Studies show that treadmill exercise is improving gait speed and UPDRS scores in patients with PD (Miyai et al., 2002), while improving both gait speed and endurance in rodents with chemically lesioned basal ganglias (Fisher et al., 2004).

In general, an effective exercise routine for patients with PD is one that includes some components of stretching, strengthening, balance, and aerobic activity. Exercises can vary from performing chair aerobics and dancing to using weights and machines like treadmills. Whatever the exercise, it must appeal to the patient in order to keep him or her motivated. Tai chi, yoga, and qigong are also beneficial forms of exercise that can be explored by patients (Schmitz-Hübsch et al., 2006). Physical and occupational therapists can create more specific exercise routines for patients to address their individual needs.

REHABILITATION AND SPECIAL NEEDS OF INDIVIDUALS WITH YOUNG-ONSET PD

While the young-onset PD patient may present with the same symptoms as the older patient, he or she often must deal with situations concerning jobs, children, and sexual activity that older patients may not. Education in new movement strategies can help patients better manage these situations. Young-onset patients can also benefit from work site evaluations by physical and occupational therapists to make recommendations concerning ergonomics and body mechanics. An exercise program should start immediately on diagnosis because research is showing that it may have neuroprotective and restorative properties. Encouraging an active lifestyle early on also helps patients deal with the normal changes that occur with aging.

REHABILITATION AND SPECIAL NEEDS OF INDIVIDUALS WITH ADVANCED PD

Advancing PD often leads to increased functional decline. Increasing immobility, reduced ADL abilities, and in some, cognitive decline lead to patients requiring more assistance from carepartners. Training carepartners in body mechanics and safe movement strategies for assisting with transfers, mobility, and ADLs becomes increasingly important at this stage of the disease. Training must also occur in proper positioning techniques to prevent skin breakdown and muscle contractures; to deal with increasing postural decline, which can affect eating and breathing; and to help control pain. Carepartner-assisted exercise is important in helping to manage these changes as well.

SUMMARY

Patients with PD have many treatment options to help them deal with their symptoms. Physical therapy is one option that can assist patients throughout the course of the disease. Referring patients to physical and occupational therapy should occur soon after the diagnosis of PD is made. An early physical assessment, along with treatment and education, can help patients feel more in control and may help limit motor decline. With disease progression, therapists can make activities like walking and bathing easier and safer by using strategies such as adaptive equipment and mobility training. Even in the end stages of PD, there are many rehabilitation strategies that can assist both patients and carepartners in improving mobility.

Resources
1. Handybar, http://www.handybar.com
2. American Physical Therapy Association, http://www.apta.org
3. American Occupational Therapy Association, http://www.aota.org
4. Free publications from the National Parkinson Foundation, http://www. parkinson.org or 800-327-4545: *Parkinson Disease: Fitness Counts; Activities of Daily Living: Practical Pointers for Parkinson Disease*

REFERENCES

Adkin, A. L., Frank, J. S., & Jog, M. S. (2003). Fear of falling and postural control in Parkinson's disease. *Movement Disorders, 18,* 496–502.

Bloem, B. R., Grimbergen, Y. A., Cramer, M., Willemsen, M., & Zwinderman, A. H. (2001). Prospective assessment of falls in Parkinson's disease. *Journal of Neurology, 248,* 950–958.

Bloem, B. R., Hausdorff, J. M., Visser, J. E., & Giladi, N. (2004). Falls and freezing of gait in Parkinson's disease: A review of two interconnected, episodic phenomena. *Movement Disorders, 19,* 871–884.

Bridgewater, K. J., & Sharpe, M. H. (1998). Trunk muscle performance in early Parkinson's disease. *Physical Therapy, 78,* 566–576.

Carpenter, M. G., Allum, J. H. J., Honegger, F., Adkin, A. L., & Bloem, B. R. (2004). Postural abnormalities to multidirectional stance perturbations in Parkinson's disease. *Journal of Neurology, Neurosurgery, and Psychiatry, 75,* 1245–1254.

Cohen, A. D., Tillerson, J. L., Smith, A. D., Schallert, T., & Zigmond, M. J. (2003). Neuroprotective effects of prior limb use in 6-hydroxydopamine-treated rats: Possible role of GDNF. *Journal of Neurochemistry, 85,* 299–305.

de Goede, C. J., Keus, S. H., Kwakkel, G., & Wagenaar, R. C. (2001). The effects of physical therapy in Parkinson's disease: A research synthesis. *Archives of Physical Medicine and Rehabilitation, 82,* 509–515.

Ellis, T., de Goede, C. J., Feldman, R. G., Wolters, E. C., Kwakkel, G., & Wagenaar, R. C. (2005). Efficacy of a physical therapy program in patients with Parkinson's disease: A randomized controlled trial. *Archives of Physical Medicine and Rehabilitation, 86,* 626–632.

Farley, B. G., & Koshland, G. F. (2005). Training BIG to move faster: The application of the speed–amplitude relation as a rehabilitation strategy for people with Parkinson's disease. *Experimental Brain Research, 167,* 462–467.

Fernandez del Olmo, M., & Cudeiro, J. (2003). A simple procedure using auditory stimuli to improve movement in Parkinson's disease: A pilot study. *Neurology Clinics and Neurophysiology, 2,* 1–7.

Fisher, B. E., Petzinger, G. M., Nixon, K., Hogg, E., Bremmer, S., Meshul, C. K., et al. (2004). Exercise-induced behavioral recovery and neuroplasticity in the 1-methyl-4-phenyl-1,2,3,6-tetrahydropyridine-lesioned mouse basal ganglia. *Journal of Neuroscience Research, 77,* 378–390.

Gage, H., & Storey, L. (2004). Rehabilitation for Parkinson's disease: A systematic review of available evidence. *Clinical Rehabilitation, 18,* 463–482.

Genever, R. W., Downes, T. W., & Medcalf, P. (2005). Fracture rates in Parkinson's disease compared with age and gender-matched controls: A retrospective cohort study. *Age and Ageing, 34,* 21–24.

Gray, P., & Hildebrand, K. (2000). Fall risk factors in Parkinson's disease. *Journal of Neuroscience Nursing, 32,* 222–228.

Hausdorff, J. M., Balash, J., & Galadi, N. (2003). Effects of cognitive challenge on gait variability in patients with Parkinson's disease. *Journal of Geriatric Psychiatry and Neurology, 16,* 53–58.

Hill, K. D., Schwarz, J. A., Kalogeropoulos, A. J., & Gibson, S. J. (1996). Fear of falling revisited. *Archives of Physical Medicine and Rehabilitaiton, 77*(10), 1025–1029.

Hirsch, M. A., Toole, T., Maitland, C. G., & Rider, R. A. (2003). The effects of balance training and high-intensity resistance training on persons with idiopathic Parkinson's disease. *Archives of Physical Medicine and Rehabilitation, 84,* 1109–1117.

Howe, T. E., Lovgreen, B., Cody, F. W., Ashton, V. J., & Oldham, J. A. (2003). Auditory cues can modify the gait of persons with early-stage Parkinson's disease: A method for enhancing parkinsonian walking performance? *Clinical Rehabilitation, 17,* 363–367.

Jöbges, M., Heuschkel, G., Pretzel, C., Illhardt, C., Renner, C., & Hummelsheim, H. (2004). Repetitive training of compensatory steps: A therapeutic approach for postural instability in Parkinson's disease. *Journal of Neurology, Neurosurgery, and Psychiatry, 75,* 1682–1687.

Lewis, G. N., Byblow, W. D., & Walt, S. E. (2000). Stride length regulation in Parkinson's disease: The use of extrinsic, visual cues. *Brain, 123,* 2077–2090.

Lieberman, A. (2002). *Postural instability, balance, Parkinson disease.* Retrieved November 14, 2005, from http://www.parkinson.org/site/apps/s/content.asp?c=9dJFJLPwB&b=108269&ct=89684

McIntosh, G. C., Brown, S. H., Rice, R. R., & Thaut, M. H. (1997). Rhythmic auditory-motor facilitation of gait patterns in patients with Parkinson's disease. *Journal of Neurology, Neurosurgery, and Psychiatry, 62,* 22–26.

Miyai, I., Fujimoto, Y., Yamamoto, H., Ueda, Y., Saito, T., Nozaki, S., et al. (2002). Long-term effect of body weight–supported treadmill training in Parkinson's disease: A randomized controlled trial. *Archives of Physical Medicine and Rehabilitation, 83,* 1370–1373.

Morris, M. E. (2000). Movement disorders in people with Parkinson disease: A model for physical therapy. *Physical Therapy, 80,* 578–597.

Morris, S., Morris, M. E., & Iansek, R. (2001). Reliability of measurements obtained with the Timed "Up & Go" test in people with Parkinson disease. *Physical Therapy, 81*(2), 810–818.

Morris, M. E., Huxham, F. E., McGinley, J., & Iansek, R. (2001). Gait disorders and gait rehabilitation in Parkinson's disease. *Advanced Neurology, 87,* 347–361.

Nelson, A. J., Zwick, D., Brody, S., Doran, C., Pulver, L., Rooz, G., et al. (2002). The validity of the GaitRite and the Functional Ambulation Performance scoring system in the analysis of Parkinson gait. *NeuroRehabilitation, 17*(3), 255–262.

O'Shea, S., Morris, M., & Iansek, R. (2002). Dual task interference during gait in people with Parkinson disease: Effects of motor versus cognitive secondary tasks. *Physical Therapy, 82,* 888–897.

Qutubuddin, A. A., Pegg, P. O., Cifu, D. X., Brown, R., McNamee, S., & Carne, W. (2005). Validating the Berg Balance Scale for patients with Parkinson's disease: a key to rehabilitation evaluation. *Archives of Physical Medicine and Rehabilitaiton, 86*(4), 789-792.

Reuter, I., & Engelhardt, M. (2002). Exercise training and Parkinson's disease. *Physician and Sportsmedicine, 30,* 43–50.

Rubinstein, T. C., Giladi, N., & Hausdorff, J. M. (2002). The power of cueing to circumvent dopamine deficits: A review of physical therapy treatment of gait disturbances in Parkinson's disease. *Movement Disorders, 17,* 1148–1160.

Schenkman, M. L., Clark, K., Xie, T., Kuchibhatla, M., Shinberg, M., & Ray, L. (2001). Spinal movement and performance of a standing reach task in participants with and without Parkinson disease. *Physical Therapy, 81,* 1400–1411.

Schenkman, M., Morey, M., & Kuchibhatla, M. (2000). Spinal flexibility and balance control among community-dwelling adults with and without Parkinson's disease. *Journal of Gerontology: Medical Sciences, 55,* 441–445.

Schmitz-Hübsch, T., Pyfer, D., Kielwein, K., Fimmers, R., Klockgether, T., & Wullner, U. (2006). Qigong exercise for the symptoms of Parkinson's disease: A randomized, controlled pilot study. *Movement Disorders, 21,* 543–548.

Tillerson, J. L., Caudle, W. M., Reveron, M. E., & Miller, D. W. (2003). Exercise induces behavioral recovery and attenuates neurochemical deficits in rodent models of Parkinson's disease. *Journal of Neuroscience, 119,* 899–911.

Tillerson, J. L., Cohen, A. D., Philhower, J., Miller, G. W., Zigmond, M. J., & Schallert, T. (2001). Forced limb-use effects on the behavioral and neurochemical effects of 6-hydroxydopamine. *Journal of Neuroscience, 21,* 4427–4435.

Tinetti, M. E., Richman, D., & Powell, L. (1990). Falls efficacy as a measure of fear of falling. *Journal of Gerontology, 45*(6), P239–243.

Viliani, T., Pasquetti, P., Magnolfi, S., Lunardelli, M. L., Giorgi, C., Serra, P., et al. (1999). Effects of physical training on straightening-up processes in patients with Parkinson's disease. *Disability Rehabilitation, 21,* 68–73.

Wielinski, C. L., Erickson-Davis, C., Wichmann, R., Walde-Douglas, M., & Parashos, S. A. (2005). Falls and injuries resulting from falls among patients with Parkinson's disease and other parkinsonian syndromes. *Movement Disorders, 20,* 410–415.

Wood, B. H., Bilclough, J. A., Bowron, A., & Walker, R. W. (2002). Incidence and prediction of falls in Parkinson's disease: A prospective multidisciplinary study. *Journal of Neurology, Neurosurgery, and Psychiatry, 72,* 721–725.

11

Complementary and Alternative Medicine for Parkinson's Disease

Constance Ward, MSN, RN, BC, CNRN

Complementary and alternative medicine (CAM) comprises diverse medical and health care systems, practices, and products that are not a part of traditional Western medicine. CAM use in the United States has moved into mainstream medicine, as indicated by the $21,200,000,000 spent in 1997, and the dollars spent on CAM match the dollars spent for traditional Western medicine primary care appointments. The medical model that uses physicians to treat the whole person seems to have undergone a paradigm shift and has moved toward a biopsychosocial-spiritual concept, where the individual is treated as a whole person through a complex interaction of physical, spiritual, mental, emotional, environmental, and social factors. This paradigm shift created attention at the national level, when, in 2005, Congress appropriated $123,100,000 to conduct research to identify, investigate, and validate scientific evidence–based CAM therapies.

The aging population in the United States values its quality of life, which is especially true of people living with a chronic condition such as Parkinson's disease. People living with Parkinson's (PLWP) may benefit from some of the CAM therapies to improve stiffness, bradykinesia, gait and posture, and activities of daily living.

This chapter will briefly delve into the categories and subcategories of CAM. The categories are mind–body interventions, manual healing methods, pharmacological and biological treatments, energy medicine, and diet and nutrition.

According to the National Center for Complementary and Alternative Medicine (NCCAM) at the National Institutes of Health (NIH), CAM is broadly defined as a group of diverse medical and health care systems, therapies, and products that are not currently considered to be part of conventional medicine NCCAM, 2004b). This definition further states that complementary medicine is used in conjunction with conventional medicine and that alternative medicine is used in place of conventional medicine.

Complementary and alternative approaches in therapy are not always based on scientific evidence. However, more and more controlled clinical trials are being conducted and reported in the literature using CAM therapies in order to prove or disprove the evidence base of many ancient and traditional therapies.

The secretary of Health and Human Services signed a memorandum in February 1999 creating NCCAM and making it the 25th independent component of the NIH for the purpose of investigating and evaluating promising unconventional medical practices. NCCAM celebrated its fifth anniversary in February 2004 as 1 of 27 institutes and centers at the NIH. NCCAM has made research funds increasingly available to study the efficacy, evidence base, and safety of CAM therapies. In 2005, Congress appropriated $123,100,000 for NCCAM to conduct CAM clinical research studies; to identify and investigate valid CAM therapies; to train CAM researchers; and to disseminate health information to both professionals and the public (NCCAM, 2006).

Many CAM therapies are evidence based, and although they cannot cure Parkinson's disease, they may help specific symptoms and make it easier to cope with the condition. CAM should be used as an adjunct to conventional medicine, not as a replacement for it.

Evidence from fields such as health psychology and behavioral medicine affirms that there is a need for a biopsychosocial-spiritual patient concept, in lieu of the dominant biomedical paradigm seen in traditional Western medicine (Astin, Shapiro, & Schwartz, 2000). This biopsychosocial-spiritual patient concept is further defined in Betty Neuman's Systems Model, in which the patient is treated in a holistic and multidimensional component of interactions that focus on the patient physiologically, psychologically, developmentally, socioculturally, and spiritually (NurseScribe, 2005). Researchers at Harvard Medical School found that one in three American adults used at least one form of complementary or alternative medicine (Harvard Medical School Office of Public Affairs, 2005). Americans were paying out of pocket for CAM therapy an estimated $14,600,000,000 in 1990 and $21,200,000,000 in 1997 (Decker, 2000). These statistics provide valuable information to medical professionals as to the importance of CAM therapy to the patient

FIGURE 11.1 Diagram of the Biopsychosocial-spiritual Concept.

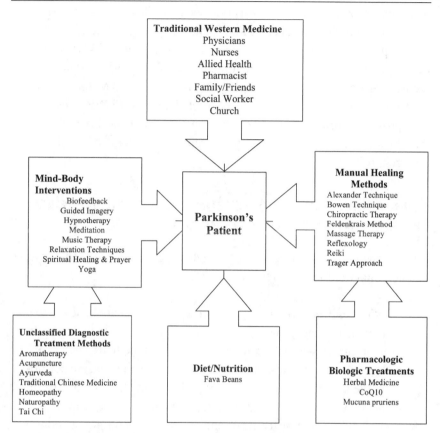

Traditional Western Medicine
Physicians
Nurses
Allied Health
Pharmacist
Family/Friends
Social Worker
Church

Mind-Body Interventions
Biofeedback
Guided Imagery
Hypnotherapy
Meditation
Music Therapy
Relaxation Techniques
Spiritual Healing & Prayer
Yoga

Parkinson's Patient

Manual Healing Methods
Alexander Technique
Bowen Technique
Chiropractic Therapy
Feldenkrais Method
Massage Therapy
Reflexology
Reiki
Trager Approach

Unclassified Diagnostic Treatment Methods
Aromatherapy
Acupuncture
Ayurveda
Traditional Chinese Medicine
Homeopathy
Naturopathy
Tai Chi

Diet/Nutrition
Fava Beans

Pharmacologic Biologic Treatments
Herbal Medicine
CoQ10
Mucuna pruriens

Source: Adapted from "Meditation," by J. Astin, S. Shapiro, and G. Schwartz, 2000, in D. W. Novey (Ed.), Clinician's Complete Reference to Complementary/Alternative Medicine, St. Louis, MO: Mosby, pp. 73–85, and from Betty Neuman's Systems Model.

population and its desire for a biopsychosocial-spiritual concept that needs to be incorporated into health care (Figure 11.1).

Many CAM therapies date as far back as ancient times: Chinese medicine and the yin and yang; the second-century A.D. Greek physician Galen's ideas to study the human body and treat it based on visual and physical objectivity; the peoples of the Indian subcontinent, who 5,000 years ago used Ayurveda to treat the "imbalance" within the body, which they believed was the major cause of disease and illness; the medicine men of the American Indian tribes, who used herbs, roots, and spiritual healing to treat their sick or wounded; and Reiki, which was practiced by Tibetan society over 2,500 years ago to provide balance, harmony, and strength to the body.

The professional medical community must keep up with what the patient is seeking in the line of treatments and therapies. This means that medical professionals must educate themselves on CAM therapy in order to provide informative education and guidance to PLWP. This chapter will provide a brief overview of the most common of CAM therapies, their history, the goal of the specific therapy, and available evidence-based research, if it has been completed.

COMPLEMENTARY AND ALTERNATIVE MEDICINE (CAM) THERAPY BY CATEGORY OF PRACTICE

The following pages will focus on the five categories of CAM therapy and on each intervention within those categories:

1. *Mind–bodyinterventions* focus on strategies that are believed to promote health and reduce the burden of stress on chronic illness. In an environment without distraction, a variety of methods, such as breath therapy, hypnotherapy, imagery, meditation, and yoga, are performed for the purpose of relaxation. The patients limit their focus to a single image or object and must be able to attain a passive attitude (Decker, 2000). Mind–body interventions require multiple sessions and practice for effectiveness. These interventions include biofeedback, guided imagery, hypnotherapy, meditation, music therapy, relaxation techniques, spiritual healing and prayer, and yoga.

2. *Manualhealing methods* are manipulative body practices that focus on the structures and systems of the body. The structures manipulated may include the bones and joints, soft tissues, and circulatory and lymphatic systems. These methods include Alexander Technique, Bowen Technique, chiropractic therapy, Feldenkrais Method, massage therapy, reflexology, Reiki, and the Trager Approach.

3. *Pharmacologicaland biological treatments* include herbal medicine, coenzyme Q_{10} (CoQ_{10}), and mucuna pruriens.

4. *Energy medicine* includes aromatherapy, acupuncture, Ayurveda, traditional Chinese medicine, homeopathy, naturopathy, and tai chi.

These therapies are considered whole medical systems that involve complete systems of theory and practice. For example, Ayurveda medicine uses combinations of herbal medicine, yoga, meditation, and other approaches to restore vital energy (NCCAM, 2004a).

5. *Diet and nutrition* includes fava beans.

Mind–Body Interventions

Biofeedback

This therapeutic technique provides physiologic information to the patient in a meaningful way so that the patient can use the power of the mind to control the body. Biofeedback provides information about skin temperature, muscle tension, blood pressure, heart and respiratory rates, and brain activity. The patient is then trained to self-regulate physiological responses that need modification in order to promote optimal well-being.

At the beginning of the 30-min visit the biofeedback therapist applies sensors to different parts of the body. These sensors monitor the body's physiologic response to stress in the form of beeps or flashing light. For example, during a tension headache, certain muscles contract, and this information is communicated back to the patient through auditory or visual cues. The patient learns to control the pitch of a sound, the rate of a series of beeps, or an image seen on a computer screen, which helps to control the unwanted autonomic or neuromuscular symptom that is being monitored (Schwartz & Olson, 2003). When the patient realizes that the headache is a result of tense muscles, the next step is to learn how to invoke positive physical changes in the body, such as relaxing those muscles when the body is tired or stressed.

There are four types of biofeedback therapy machines that can be used, depending on the health problem and objective:

- *Electromyogram (EMG).* Electrodes are used to measure muscle tension. This therapy is mainly used to promote relaxation of the muscles that induce pain and to treat asthma symptoms, hypertension, incontinence, and muscle and motor rehabilitation.
- *Temperature biofeedback.* Temperature probes are attached to feet and fingers to measure skin temperature. Because temperature usually drops under stress, a low reading can prompt relaxation techniques.

This therapy is used for certain circulatory diseases, for example, Raynaud's disease, hypertension, and migraines.

- *Galvanic skin response training.* Sensors measure activity of sweat glands and perspiration, alerting the patient to early signs of anxiety. This information may be beneficial in treating emotional disorders, for example, phobias, stuttering, and anxiety. Galvanic skin response training can also treat chronic pain and help with stress management.
- *Electroencephalogram (EEG).* This measures brain activity in different mental states, that is, wakefulness, relaxation, calmness, light and deep sleep, epilepsy, learning disabilities, substance abuse, fibromyalgia, and posttraumatic stress disorder (Mayo Clinic, 2004).

Biofeedback teaches how to use the mind to control the body in order to improve health. Through practice, PLWP can learn to control heart rate, skin temperature, blood pressure, muscle tension, and other body functions needing attention.

Scientific Evidence. NCCAM performed a systematic review of literature and found evidence that biofeedback may have an influence on immune, endocrine, and autonomic functioning, which can have an influence on health. Mind–body interventions with some component of stress management, coping skills training, cognitive–behavioral interventions, and relaxation therapy may benefit patients with coronary artery disease and pain-related diagnoses; mind–body approaches when combined with educational information can be effective adjuncts in the management of chronic diseases. Mind–body interventions have proven to have positive effects on psychological functioning and quality of life and may be helpful for patients suffering with chronic illness and in need of palliative care (Andrasik & Lords, 2004).

Guided Imagery

Guided imagery is the use of certain techniques that assist the patient in obtaining a mental image by direct visualization or suggestion through imagery, storytelling, fantasy, exploration, metaphor, game playing, dream interpretation, drawing, or active imagination (Rossman & Bresler, 2000). The imagery practitioner assists the patient in achieving a relaxed state of mind and invites the patient to focus on the confronting issue. In the Parkinson's patient, that issue may be depression. The imagery practitioner may guide the patient to imagine a time and place where the patient experienced happiness and to dialogue that time through. By being guided and returned to a time of happiness, the patient may find a past inner resource and a new and creative solution to the depression.

We know that looking at pictures or images can have a controlling influence on our nervous, endocrine, and immune systems (Freeman, 2004). If we look at a picture of a cake with mouth-watering chocolate dripping off the sides, we may begin to salivate. Viewing an appetizing plate of food on a billboard could induce hunger pangs. Images are powerful and suggestive and can induce a physiologic response that may alleviate symptoms, stimulate motivation, promote relaxation and stress reduction, and find a solution to a mood or situation that is undesirable.

Guided imagery is a relaxation technique that can help reduce stress by creating calm and peaceful images in the mind. It may be helpful with the stress, depression, and anxiety that sometimes accompany Parkinson's disease.

Scientific Evidence. A clinical study examined the effects of imagery on the immune response in patients with leukopenia. Image training resulted in a significant increase in the white blood count, representing a strengthening of the immune system (Donaldson, 2000). In a randomized, controlled, case series study, occupational therapy combined with the practice of imagery was compared with occupational therapy alone in patients who were recovering from stroke. The results showed that the therapy-plus-imagery group improved their motor scores by 13.8 and 16.4 points over the therapy-alone group (Page, Levine, Sisto, & Johnston, 2001).

Hypnotherapy

The goal of hypnotherapy is based on the individual patient's objective. The person being hypnotized should be under his or her own control at all times and not be controlled by someone else. Hypnotherapy can be used for a wide variety of health conditions, too numerous to mention here. PLWP may benefit from hypnotherapy by relieving many of the chronic health conditions the disease presents. Hypnotherapy should be used in conjunction with traditional Western medicine.

Hypnotic-like practices date back to ancient times in many cultures and are referred to in the Bible. Hypnosis comes from the Greek word *hypnos,* meaning "sleep." Hypnosis uses selective attention to induce a specific altered state of consciousness(Wikipedia, 2006).

The three main phases of hypnotherapy involve presuggestion, suggestion, and postsuggestion:

- In the presuggestion phase the goal is to reach an altered state of consciousness so that the participant is susceptible to suggestion by the therapist. Various techniques are used, such as distraction, imagery, or relaxation.
- The suggestion phase introduces questions posed by the hypnotist or goal and memory exploration by the participant.
- Last, the postsuggestion phase returns the participant to the normal state of consciousness. It is in the postsuggestion phase that the goals introduced in the suggestion phase may be practiced by the patient outside of the therapist's office (Green & Lynn, 2000).

Scientific Evidence. Montgomery, Weltz, Seltz, and Bovbjerg (2000) were the first to quantify the magnitude of hypnoanalgesics' effects on pain, regardless of the type of pain. However, hypnosis is commonly used in conjunction with psychodynamic, cognitive–behavioral, or pharmacological therapies.

In a summation review of hypnosis, Lynn, Kirsch, Barabasz, Cardena, and Patterson (2000) found that hypnotic procedures have the ability to reduce or eliminate chronic and acute pain. Fifty-six studies assessing the efficacy of smoking cessation intervention using hypnotherapy showed higher rates of abstinence than the controls (Green & Lynn, 2000).

Meditation

This is a simple technique that is practiced twice a day for 20 min while sitting comfortably with the eyes closed. During this time the ordinary thinking processes settle down, and a distinctive psychophysiological state of restful alertness is realized. There are two types of meditation. *Concentration technique* focuses on an object or certain focus that is unchanging, or on a repetitive focal point, such as the heart rate or depth control breathing. *Nonconcentration technique* focuses attention in a nonjudgmental way toward any sensation, emotion, perception, or cognition as it comes forward into the meditator's awareness (Astin et al., 2000).

Meditation is a wakeful, hypometabolic state that has been reported to reduce health care costs, strengthen the immune response, alter anxiety and depression, lower blood pressure, reduce the frequency and prolongation of epileptic seizures, assist with reduction of chronic pain syndrome, lower rates of substance abuse, and countermand some aspects of cardiovascular disease (Freeman, 2004). Meditation can be applied to both mental and physical health problems. Many patients are referred to meditation clinics by their physicians as a complement to traditional medical care in the treatment of chronic illness and stress-related disorders. According to Astin et al. (2000), evidence-based research on the effects of meditation therapy has been observed in studies of cardiovascular disease, chronic pain, anxiety, substance abuse, dermatologic disorders, depressive symptoms, adjuncts to psychotherapy, and other chronic disease states have been observed during meditation therapy.

Many PLWP experience anxiety, depression, insomnia, and tension. These symptoms are meditative-responsive, and therefore meditation may be beneficial to PLWP.

Scientific Evidence. Transcendental meditation as an intervention for cardiovascular disease, chronic pain, posttraumatic stress syndrome, and general health has been proven to be efficacious (Barnes, Treiber, & Davis, 2001; Bishop, 2002; Relman, 2001). Meditation has been shown to produce increases in left-sided brain activity, which is associated with positive emotional states. Also, meditation can increase antibody titers to influenza vaccine and improve immune function (Davidson et al., 2003).

Music Therapy

Listening to music changes metabolism, raises and lowers blood pressure, causes the release of endorphins, reduces fatigue, and promotes relaxation. For PLWP the benefits of music therapy are well documented in clinical literature (Pacchetti et al., 2000; Stern, Lander, & Lees, 1980), demonstrating that music improves rhythmic limb movements, gait, and freezing. Music has a strong contribution to make toward the physical and spiritual well-being of PLWP.

The use and value of music was apparent in ancient and traditional cultures as far back as any records of such activity exist. As the Western world expands its horizons, more people are reevaluating the importance given to music and the therapy it provides. Music therapy has been a Medicare-reimbursable service since 1994 and is considered an active treatment if it is ordered by a physician, is goal directed, and is reasonable and necessary for the illness or injury. Additionally, the patient must exhibit improvement from the therapy (American Music Association, 1999). Many private insurance companies also reimburse for music therapy. Medicaid reimbursement varies from state to state.

The beneficial effect of music was first documented after World War II, when a group of musicians began touring the country, playing their music for the war-wounded veterans in the Veterans Administration hospitals. The nurses and physicians began to document the emotional and physical responses of their patients to the music, which led to hospitals actively hiring musicians to play their music for the patients (Burgner, 2005).

Scientific Evidence. It is a known fact that as we age, our immune systems are often impaired because our natural killer (NK) cells are not as effective as they once were. Music therapy has been found to significantly increase the NK cell count and its activity in older patients with Alzheimer's disease, cerebrovascular disease, and Parkinson's disease. In addition, changes in NK cell counts were independent of neurodegenerative diseases (Hasegawa et al., 2001).

Spiritual Healing and Prayer

The Parkinson's diagnosis can be devastating to patients and families. Prayer and spirituality treatment methods may offer solace against the emotional and psychological ramifications of the disease. The offering of prayers to a higher being for the purpose of healing or arresting the disease may be practiced by the patient or family, or by others as intercessory prayer for the patient. It can be a comfort to the Parkinson's patient that faith is at work on his or her behalf. Literature suggests that patients who are committed to a religious orientation report a better overall satisfaction with life and lower levels of depression and stress (Shafranske & Malony, 1990).

Scientific Evidence. A 2003 NCCAM-funded study on the effect of spiritual well-being on end-of-life despair in terminal cancer patients found that spiritual well-being offers some protection or bumper effect for patients who face imminent death (McClain, Rosenfeld, & Breitbart, 2003).

Yoga

Yoga began in India over 6,000 years ago. The oldest written record of Indian culture is a text, written 3,000 years ago, called the Vedas, which describes the origins of yoga within its hymns and rituals (Quigley & Dean, 2000).

There are many styles of yoga, all of which focus on strict alignment of the body, coordination of breath and movement, and holding the postures or flowing from one posture to another. Control of emotions and mind, meditation, and contemplation are integrated into forms of yoga (Quigley & Dean, 2000). Yoga is a scientific and practical discipline that is not connected to any religion and can be practiced by all denominations and faiths.

PLWP can benefit from yoga because the postures focus on flexibility of the spine through bending, stretching, and twisting movements that work on joints, muscles, internal organs, and glands. These movements increase the flow of blood and oxygen throughout the body and promote balance and strength (Rajendran, Thompson, & Reich, 2001). A small pilot study of yoga for PD patients was done with the patients self-rating their signs before and after 12 weeks of yoga. Amazingly, patients overwhelmingly rated their balance and posture improved, two symptoms resistant to medication treatment. The pilot, funded by the National Parkinson Foundation, ended, and the patients elected to continue yoga on a fee for service basis (G. M. Vernon, personal communication, January 29, 2007). More scientific studies of yoga in PD are warranted.

Scientific Evidence. Five randomized, controlled trials in which yoga was used as an intervention for depression ranging from mild to severe found beneficial effects of yoga intervention on depression. If the depressed patient had reduced or impaired mobility, yoga was not feasible (Pilkington, Kirkwood, Rampes, & Richardson, 2005).

Manual Healing Methods

Alexander Technique

Frederick M. Alexander (1869–1955), with whom the Alexander Technique (AT) originated, was an actor and Shakespearean orator. He developed chronic laryngitis and was determined to restore his voice. He began watching himself in the mirror while speaking and observed unnecessary muscle tension that was responsible for the vocal difficulty. He rediscovered over time a way to speak without tensing the muscles in his neck and discovered the principle that influences health and well-being by changing the way he thought while initiating a body movement. Through work with himself and others, he shared his hands-on teaching method that encourages all the body's processes to work more efficiently (Goldberg, 2004).

AT offers lessons that evaluate the relationship between thought and muscle activity. Many times, the habitual tightening of muscles in our bodies as we walk, sit, stand, lie down, and lift can cause stress and pain.

AT helps the patient see the unconscious movement habits that contribute to the recurring difficulties, then reeducates by focusing on improving awareness of how the patient moves in order to increase the ease of that movement by releasing unnecessary muscle tension (Arnold, 2004).

Multiple colleges and universities, such as the Julliard School of Performing Arts in New York and the Royal Academy of Dramatic Art in London, endorse AT for their performing artists (Goldberg, 2004). AT can be beneficial to PLWP because it helps with the control of balance and movement by showing the relationship between thought and muscle activity through individual lessons. AT teaches the use of an appropriate amount of effort for a particular activity, giving more energy for other activities. AT can be applied to sitting, lying down, standing, walking, lifting, and other activities of daily living.

Scientific Evidence. No well-designed randomized controlled trials exist to test claims by practitioners that AT has beneficial patient effects.

Bowen Technique

The Bowen Technique (BT) is a system of gentle but powerful soft tissue manipulations that affect the body structurally and energetically to restore its self-healing mechanisms (Carter, 2001). The technique was developed in the 1960s by Thomas Bowen, an Australian and self-taught healer who devoted his lifetime to developing the technique. BT uses Bowen *moves,* which are applied over muscles, tendons, nerves, and fascia using the thumbs and fingers in a series of specific sequences of moves called *procedures,* with frequent pauses to allow time for the body to respond.

Thomas Bowen believed that his technique could assist the body's natural ability to repair itself and that dysfunction was the result of disturbance in the tissues. He also believed in the universal life energy called Qi (pronounced "chee") we see in traditional Chinese medicine (Faculty at Harvard Medical School, 2005b).

Scientific Evidence. Evidence suggests that BT is beneficial for frozen shoulder through the use of soft tissue manipulation (Carter, 2001).

Chiropractic Therapy

Chiropractic history dates back to 1895, when David D. Palmer, a grocer from Davenport, Iowa, placed his hands on a janitor who had an irregular protrusion of the spine and, with a vigorous thrust, reduced the irregularity. Afterward, the janitor claimed to hear noises in the street, something he could not hear before the spine adjustment (Hansen & Triano, 2000). Palmer gave credit to a medical physician named Jim Atkinson, who taught him about the use of bone setting in other cultures. Palmer wrote the first chiropractic book in 1910, *The Chiropractic Adjuster,* and Jim Atkinson edited it (Phillips, 2004). In 1906, Palmer became the founder of chiropractic and what is now called the Palmer College of Chiropractic located in Davenport, Iowa. From 1906 to 1963 the Palmer College of Chiropractic published a set of textbooks written by Palmer and his son B. J. Palmer, emphasizing chiropractic technique and philosophy. There are 39 volumes, called the Palmer Green Books, and they are a collector's item today (Library Web Master, 2005).

Chiropractic theory holds that vertebral *subluxations* are the cause of most health problems and are due to blockages of the nerves originating from the spinal column, which connects to organs and other body tissues (Benedetti & MacPhail, 2003). A subluxation can be a vertebral malposition or a mechanical impediment that can affect mobility, posture, blood flow, and muscle tone (Hansen & Triano, 2000). Many manipulative healing methods believe in the principle that the human body can regulate itself and has the ability to heal itself. The chiropractor tailors the therapeutic manipulation to the patient's needs, mostly neck and back pain. There are approximately 100 manipulations or adjustment modalities used, which involve rapid movements by the chiropractor to the spine, joints, or muscles (Benedetti & MacPhail, 2003). Some chiropractors include lifestyle counseling, rehabilitation, nutritional management, and many physiotherapeutic exercises in their patient management.

PLWP may benefit from chiropractic management for degenerative joint disease, mobility, range of motion, and pain relief. However, patients who desire to have chiropractic therapy should inform their physicians before doing so. Chiropractic manipulation is contraindicated in fractures, bone tumors, bone and joint infections, acute cauda equina syndrome, and disc herniation. Those with acute myelopathy, advanced osteoporosis, cancer, deformities, progressive neurological deficits, and vertebral–basilar syndrome should not receive chiropractic therapy in those areas (Hansen & Triano, 2000).

Scientific Evidence. Chiropractic evidence-based research is scant in the literature. In the summer of 2005 the World Federation of Chiropractic's Identity Consultation Assembly declared, "There is little existing research or scientific evidence to support chiropractic's role in overall health improvement" (Jackson, 2005, p. 11). The British Medical Association warned, "There is a lack of sufficient evidence to support many of the claims of efficacy [for chiropractic and CAM]. Without evidence, it is impossible for the public and the medical profession to make informed decisions on the risks and benefits of different therapies" (Jackson, 2005, p. 11). The paucity of clinical trials in chiropractic research where manipulation treatments were performed for low back and neck pain, headache, and neck disorders show mixed results. However, there seems to be some efficacy of chiropractic in treating low back and neck pain for short-term relief (Skargren, 1997). As we can see by the lack of current research, more randomized controlled trials are needed in the chiropractic area.

A study published in 2005 comparing four approaches for low back pain with a cohort of 654 patients whose ratings of disability were similar divided the groups into four different approaches for treatment:

1. medical care by a primary care physician
2. medical care plus physical therapy
3. chiropractic care (spinal manipulation and other adjustments)
4. chiropractic care along with one or more additional treatments: heat, cold, ultrasound, or electrical muscle stimulation.

Information was obtained on the cost of care (except medication costs) and on the outcome of care. Medical care alone was the least expensive treatment, but the costs nearly doubled when physical therapy was added. Chiropractic care and chiropractic plus other methods cost more than medical care alone and did not produce better low back pain outcomes than medical care (NCCAM, 2006).

Feldenkrais Method

Moshe Feldenkrais was a Russian physicist who was disabled from a knee injury. He learned that knee surgery would not guarantee complete use of his knee, and he faced wheelchair confinement. That was unsatisfactory to him. He used his formal training in science and martial arts to become the first non-Japanese native to receive a black belt in judo. He learned about anatomy, kinesiology, and physiology in order to develop an approach that would help his knee.

His therapy restored his knee to almost full function, and afterward, he began to develop the Feldenkrais Method (FM), which he taught around the world during the 1970s and up until his death in 1984 (Wildman, Stephens, & Aum, 2000).

This method is based on the concept that improving patterns of movement may enhance physical and psychological performance and recovery from disabling conditions. The two basic components of FM are *awareness through movement* and *functional integration*. Awareness through movement is a group approach whereby the practitioner leads participants through a series of movements, that is, standing, sitting, reaching, and so on, in order to increase the participants' awareness of what types of movements work best so that flexibility and coordination can be improved. Functional integration involves a hands-on session with the practitioner wherein the participant is taken through a series of passive range of motion patterns that teach the body through more functional patterns of movement so that the participant learns to move in beneficial ways, which results in improvements in activities of daily living (Wildman et al., 2000).

Scientific Evidence. Scientific evidence is lacking at this time.

Massage Therapy

Massage involves the kneading, stroking, and manipulation of the body's soft tissues. It is used to relieve muscle tension and stress and to produce relaxation. There are many different types of massage therapy:

- *Swedish massage.* This is the most common form of massage in the United States. This technique uses long, smooth strokes and kneading movements along the surface of the skin to promote relaxation and improve circulation.
- *Deep massage.* This uses slow, heavy strokes to create pressure and friction in the muscles. This technique seeks deep muscle tissue to relieve muscle strain and tension.
- *Sports massage.* Athletes use a form of massage that focuses on certain muscle groups used in performing their sports. Both Swedish and deep massage could be used.
- *Craniosacral massage.* This massage type focuses on cranial and spinal imbalances that may cause sensory, motor, or intellectual dysfunction. This involves the manipulation of the bones and tissues of the cranium and spine in one continuous massage motion.
- *Neuromuscular massage.* This may be referred to as trigger point therapy, which concentrates on painful areas in the muscles.

Therapists use deep massage techniques to locate and release tender points.

- *Rolfing.* This technique focuses on connective tissues that form a support network. The practitioner uses significant pressure to realign connective tissues they believe are pulled out by stress on the body. The entire technique requires 10 sessions (Dunn, Sleep, & Collett, 1995; Smith & Logan, 2002).

A licensed massage therapist or a physical therapist should perform massage therapy. In some cases, massage therapy is reimbursed by insurance or Medicare if it is part of a physical therapy program ordered by the care provider. PLWP may benefit from massage therapy for muscle aches and stiffness, tension, and sleep disorders.

Scientific Evidence. Several studies exist on the efficacy of massage therapy. The overall results reported that massage therapy reduced blood pressure, heart rate, and pain scores and contributed to improvement in symptom distress among cancer and palliative care patients. The studies reported also used aromatherapy oils as carrier agents applied to the skin during massages, however, it is not known whether aromatic oils are of benefit (Fellowes, Barnes, & Wilkinson, 2004).

Reflexology

Reflexology relieves stress or treats health conditions through the application of pressure to specific points on the feet. Reflexology practitioners believe that certain areas of the feet correspond to certain parts of the body or to certain organs (White et al., 2000).

Forms of reflexology were used over 2,000 years ago in China and Egypt. During the early 20th century a physician named William Fitzgerald determined that the foot could be mapped to other areas of the body to treat medical conditions. He divided the body into 10 zones and mapped the foot to correspond to these zones. He applied pressure to the areas of the foot he believed were connected to the body. This was called *zone therapy* (White et al., 2000).

In the 1930s, Eunice Ingham, a nurse and physiotherapist, further developed Fitzgerald's maps to include reflex points, and afterward, the technique became known as reflexology.

Reflexology charts have pictures of the feet with diagrams corresponding to internal organs or parts of the body. The left foot treats the left side of the body, and the right foot treats the right side of the body. The therapist begins with a foot massage before moving to the reflex points on the foot. The therapist may use many instruments to apply pressure to the reflex points, for example, tongue blades, wire brushes, probes, and so on.

The patient may feel a tingling in the part of the body that corresponds to the reflex point that is being stimulated. This therapy should never be painful (Stephenson & Dalton, 2003).

Scientific Evidence. Theories about how reflexology works have not been proven scientifically. There is a paucity of research in reflexology, however, the Cochrane database reported from a small pilot study that reflexology may offer short-term anxiety relief and relaxation (Sola et al., 2006).

Reiki

Reiki has been practiced for 2,500 years and is documented in the Tibetan sutras and in ancient records of cosmology and philosophy. The name *Reiki* comes from the Japanese words *rei*, meaning "universal spirit," and *ki*, meaning "life energy." Reiki was introduced to the West in the 1930s. Reiki practitioners believe that favorable effects are received from the "universal life energy" that practitioners channel to patients, providing energy, harmony, and balance to the body and mind (Miles & True, 2003). Reiki treats a variety of health problems and is also administered to the dying patient to promote internal peace.

The practitioners place their hands in 12–15 positions over the body, which are held for 5 s each. These hand positions cover all of the body systems within 30–90 min. This technique is called sweeping and allows the practitioner to detect areas of energy disruption, imbalance, or blockage and to cleanse patients of negative feelings, emotions, or physical burdens (Miles & True, 2003). Many patients have reported warmth, invigoration, relaxation, sleepiness, and tingling during Reiki.

Scientific Evidence. A blind pilot study of 45 clinical patients, the objective of which was to test the effects of Reiki on autonomic nervous system function, assigned the participants randomly to three test groups:

1. No treatment (rest only)
2. Reiki treatment by experienced Reiki practitioner.
3. Placebo treatment by a person with no knowledge of Reiki and who mimicked the Reiki treatment.

The results showed a decrease in heart rate and diastolic blood pressure in the Reiki group compared to both the placebo and control groups. The study indicated that Reiki has some effect on the autonomic nervous system (Mackay, Hansen, & McFarlane, 2004).

Trager Approach

The Trager Approach (TA) involves manual therapy and mental exercises known as *mentastics* (from *mental gymnastics*). This approach was developed and practiced by Milton Trager, MD, for over seven decades before his death in 1997. Dr. Trager developed his principles through his own experiences as a beach acrobat, bodybuilder, boxer, and dancer by understanding the importance of how a person's mental state communicates to the musculoskeletal system and patterns of movement (Liskin, 2004). The trained practitioner of TA distinguishes awareness of relaxation and tension of the tissues, and from that point this awareness is taught to the patient so that improvement and skill can alter the patient's own tension patterns. The practitioner seeks to affect the mind of the patient, while working with the body in order to change physical patterns or habits the muscles have developed through unhealthy mental or physical activity. "Physical patterns reflect mental patterns, and such patterns can be changed through special kinds of awareness, movement and skilled touch" (Liskin, 2004, p. 473).

Scientific Evidence. A quantitative research study was undertaken to measure the changes of evoked stretch responses (ESR) in the most rigid arm of PLWP after TA. EMG recordings of the flexor carpi radialis and extensor digitorum passively flexed and extended to an amplitude of 60° and at a frequency of 1 Hz were taken at 1 and 11 min after the treatment was performed. The results from this study showed a reduction in ESR by 36% immediately following the therapy, and ESR remained 32% lower 11 min after the therapy (Duval et al., 2002). TA may be beneficial to PLWP who experience problems with balance, dystonias, and muscle rigidity.

Pharmacological and Biological Treatments

Herbal Medicine

Herbs are the second most common CAM therapy used by the older adult population (Fisher & Morley, 2004). The U.S. Food and Drug Administration (FDA) classifies herbal preparations as dietary supplements. Therefore herbal preparations are not subject to the stringent standards of purity, efficacy, and safety that traditional medications are. Many of us believe that because they are natural, they are safe, however, many times, this is not the case. Currently, there are over 20,000 herbal and natural products available for public use in the United States (Miller et al., 2000). This section will give a brief overview of the most commonly used herbs and the ones that could be used by PLWP.

CoQ_{10}. CoQ_{10} works on the mitochondria of the cell, thereby producing energy. It is used for angina pectoris, Bell's palsy, deafness, diabetes, heart failure, hypertension, immune deficiency, mitral valve prolapse, irregular heart rhythm, and to counter the oncology medication Adriamycin's toxic effects on the heart.

Scientific Evidence. A multicentered clinical trial using 1,200 mg/day of CoQ_{10} showed a 44% improvement in mobility when compared to the placebo group. It is believed that CoQ_{10} can slow the progression of Parkinson's disease through its neuroprotective capabilities (Shults et al., 2002). Further studies by the NET-PD (Neuroprotective exploratory trials in PD group) did not get a robust response using CoQ_{10}. Further studies will undoubtedly be done in PD. Additionally, researchers found that adding CoQ_{10} to other therapies can shorten hospital stays and prevent serious complications in heart failure patients, however, it has not been shown to decrease death rates (Fetrow & Avila, 2000).

Echinacea. Echinacea is a member of the daisy family and is used for treatment of cold or flu symptoms. This herb is also marketed as an immune system stimulator. Echinacea is contraindicated in persons with tuberculosis, multiple sclerosis, HIV, and other autoimmune diseases. The usual dose is 900 mg three times a day.

Scientific Evidence. According to a 1999 study, echinacea is ineffective in treating upper respiratory infections, and persons taking echinacea continuously for long periods of time have more upper respiratory infections than people who do not take the herb (Fetrow & Avila, 2000).

Ginger. Ginger is used as an antiemetic for nausea and vomiting caused by motion sickness or the side effects of medications. One slice of ginger (sold in supermarkets) can be boiled in water for 30 min and consumed as a tea. Capsules are available; the recommended dose for nausea is 500–1,000 mg.

Scientific Evidence. Findings from a meta-analysis suggest that 1 g of ginger is effective in preventing postoperative nausea and vomiting (Reuters Health Information, 2006).

Ginseng. Ginseng is the best selling of all the herbs. It is used for increased concentration, relaxation, vigilance, well-being, and possible antidiabetic effects. The usual dose is 200–600 mg in a single dose or twice daily, and ginseng should be taken with meals because it can cause hypoglycemia. Ginseng is contraindicated in asthma, renal failure, hypertension, infectious diseases, bronchitis, emphysema, heart failure, pregnancy, and gastrointestinal problems (Fisher & Morley, 2004). Medical experts do not recommend taking ginseng daily for more than 3 weeks.

Scientific Evidence. There is no scientific evidence to prove that ginseng improves stamina, boosts energy, or reduces stress (Fetrow & Avila, 2000).

Ginkgo Biloba. Ginkgo biloba is used for intermittent claudication, cerebral insufficiency that displays symptoms of cognitive impairment, memory impairment, and dementia. Persons who are on anticoagulant therapy, such as aspirin, heparin, or warfarin, should not use ginkgo because it has its own antiplatelet qualities. The usual dose for ginkgo is 40 mg three times a day.

Scientific Evidence. A meta-analysis of 40 studies found that ginkgo was more effective than placebo for a variety of patient complaints, including memory and concentration problems, headaches, depression, confusion, dizziness, and tiredness (Freeman, 2004). There are numerous clinical trials on ginkgo, too numerous to mention in this chapter, that prove its benefits scientifically.

Melatonin. Melatonin is a neurohormone produced in the pineal gland that regulates sleep cycles and the hormonal changes that trigger sexual maturity in adolescence. However, melatonin is promoted widely for insomnia. The dosage varies according to the severity of the insomnia, from 5 to 75 mg at bedtime (Fetrow & Avila, 2000). Many stores carry a standard 3 mg tablet.

Scientific Evidence. A meta-analysis of several clinical trials from 1999 to 2003 that used melatonin for the treatment of a number of categories of sleep disorders, including primary sleep disorders, secondary sleep disorders, and sleep restriction, found no clinical significance in treating sleep disorders in all of the populations studied, except for people suffering from delayed sleep phase syndrome. Melatonin promotes sleep in delayed sleep phase syndrome because of its effect on sleep onset latency, but not on sleep efficiency. This analysis could not conclude that melatonin was effective in alleviating sleep disturbances experienced by jet lag or shift work. Evidence does suggest that melatonin is safe for short-term use, has a short half-life, penetrates the blood–brain barrier, and suggests a link between endogenous melatonin and the sleep cycle (Buscemi et al., 2004).

Milk Thistle. Milk thistle is used as a liver protectant from alcohol, drugs, hepatitis, and environmental and industrial toxins and may assist in the regeneration of liver cells through its powerful anti-inflammatory effect. Other uses include treating gallstones, hepatitis, and psoriasis. The recommended dose of milk thistle is based on its silymarin content, the active ingredient in the plant. The usual dose is 70–210 mg three times daily. Milk thistle may increase the clearance of estrogen and decrease the clearance of glucoronidate drugs, such as Ativan, Lamictal, and Comtan. Women with hormone-sensitive conditions, such as breast, uterine, or ovarian cancer and endometriosis or uterine fibroids, should avoid using milk thistle (Freeman, 2004).

Scientific Evidence. In a placebo-controlled study it was found that milk thistle decreased biliary lipid composition in the gallbladder. Milk thistle offers liver protection against harmful toxins, and patients with acute liver disease from alcohol use had a greater decrease in liver enzymes than the placebo group.

Mucuna pruriens. Mucuna pruriens is a climbing legume found in Central and South America and India whose pods contain powder containing a natural form of L-dopa. Mucuna pruriens has long been used in traditional Ayurvedic Indian medicine for diseases, including Parkinson's disease. The seeds are prepared into a powder, which allows for a rapid onset of action of natural L-dopa, which is lacking in PLWP. In India the equivalent of the FDA has approved mucuna pruriens under the brand name Zandopa. It should not be used in people who have glucose 6 phosphate dehydrogenase deficiency due to the risk of hemolytic anemia.

Scientific Evidence. In a randomized, controlled, double-blind crossover trial, Katzenschlager et al. (2004) used 50/200 mg of carbidopa/levodopa and 15–30 g of mucuna preparation in randomized order at weekly intervals. The results showed that mucuna pruriens had a rapid onset of action and a longer on time, without an increase in dyskinesias (Katzenschlager et al., 2004).

St. John's Wort. St. John's wort is used for anxiety, depression, and nervousness. The usual dose is 300 mg three times per day. St. John's wort should not be taken if the person is using tricyclic antidepressants, serotonin reuptake inhibitors, or monoamine oxidase (MAO) inhibitors because of the dopamine, norepinephrine, and serotonin reuptake action of these medications. Photosensitivity is a side effect of using St. John's wort.

Scientific Evidence. In several randomized clinical trials involving thousands of patients, St. John's wort was effective as an antidepressant, superior to placebo, and found to be as effective as tricyclic antidepressants without significant side effects (Freeman, 2004).

S-adenosylmethionine. S-adenosylmethionine (SAMe) is an antioxidant that helps to raise serotonin levels in the brain and may treat depression.

Scientific Evidence. Studies that have compared SAMe and tricyclic antidepressants have found both to be equivalent (Fisher & Morley, 2004). It has also been reported to be effective as a pharmaceutical treatment for pain and inflammation. SAMe is equivalent to nonsteroidal anti-inflammatory agents for the treatment of pain from osteoarthritis and may have other benefits as well (Fisher & Morley, 2004). Studies suggest that it can help normalize liver function in patients with cirrhosis, hepatitis, and cholestasis. It is not recommended for bipolar (manic) depression, and because of its effect on the liver, it may enhance the elimination of various drugs from the body. The usual dose of SAMe is 400–1600 mg two to four times per day (Fisher & Morley, 2004).

Saw Palmetto. Saw palmetto is made from the berries of the American dwarf palm tree that grows in the West Indies and from South Carolina to Florida. It is used to treat benign prostatic hypertrophy (BPH) and was shown to be helpful in reducing nocturia and increasing peak urinary flow (Fisher & Morley, 2004). The usual dose is 160 mg two times per day.

Scientific Evidence. An uncontrolled 3-month trial of 305 men who suffered from BPH showed significant improvement in urinary flow rates, residual urinary volume, and prostate size.

In a double-blind, placebo-controlled trial, 50 patients received saw palmetto, and 44 patients received a placebo. The urinary rate of flow for the saw palmetto group improved by 50%, and the number of nighttime trips to the bathroom decreased significantly compared to the placebo group (Freeman, 2004).

Researchers from the University of California, San Francisco reported that saw palmetto was no better than placebo at relieving urinary symptoms caused by enlarged prostate glands. A study published in the *New England Journal of Medicine* randomized 112 men with benign prostatic hyperplasia to saw palmetto and 113 to sugar pills. After a year, there was no difference between the groups (Bent et al., 2006).

Valerian Root. Valerian root is an herbal sedative. It is used as a sleep aid for insomnia and works by binding benzodiazepine sites in the brain. The usual dose is 400–900 mg taken 30–60 min before bedtime. Valerian root should not be used in patients with liver disease, or in combination with alcohol, other benzodiazepines, or the medication Antabuse.

Scientific Evidence. A few small studies have shown valerian root to be effective in inducing sleep. The German Commission E (similar to the FDA) recommends valerian root for restlessness and sleep disturbances (Fetrow & Avila, 2000).

Energy Medicine and Other Unclassified CAMs

Aromatherapy

Aromatherapy is a form of herbal medicine. Various oils from plants are applied topically to the skin or are nasally inhaled. The action of the antiviral or antibacterial agents is believed to heal the body. The aromatic biochemical structures of certain herbs or flowers are thought to act in areas of the brain related to past experiences and emotions (e.g., the limbic system) of the patient (Buckle, 2004).

Scientific Evidence. Aromatherapy is used for many health conditions. Several small studies suggest that lavender aromatherapy may help relieve anxiety. However, there is no scientific evidence for the effectiveness of any other use or type of aromatherapy (Faculty at Harvard Medical School, 2005a).

Acupuncture

Acupuncture is a traditional Chinese medical technique for unblocking Qi by inserting needles at certain points on the body to balance the opposing forces of yin and yang. Qi is the energy that allegedly permeates all things and is undetectable by methods of empirical science. It is believed to flow through the body along 14 pathways, called meridians. Qi flows freely in the body until illness, which blocks Qi, presents itself (Lee, LaRiccia, & Newberg, 2004). In Chinese medical theory the yin and yang explain polar relationships, patterns, change, and how things function in relation to each other in the universe. Nothing can exist in and of itself, according to the theory. Yin is the shady side and represents cold, rest, responsiveness, passivity, darkness, interiority, downwardness, inwardness, and decrease. Yang is opposite of yin, with qualities of the sunny side, and represents heat, stimulation, movement, activity, excitement, vigor, light, exteriority, upwardness, outwardness, and increase (NCCAM, 2004c). The yang is active when we exercise and heat up. The yin is at work as we sweat and cool down.

Traditional Chinese medicine has identified 500 specific points where needles may be inserted for certain effects. Acupuncture needles range between 24 and 40 gauge and are between 0.5 and 2.0 in. long. It is proposed that acupuncture produces the conduction of electromagnetic signals at a greater than normal rate, thus initiating pain-killing biochemicals, for example, endorphins that may alter brain chemistry by changing the release of neurotransmitters and neurohormones affecting parts of the central nervous system. The exact mechanism of how acupuncture works is unknown (NCCAM, 2004c).

Scientific Evidence. Numerous clinically controlled trials involving acupuncture as a medical intervention for pain performed from 1973 to 1998 demonstrated effectiveness, in varying degrees, in alleviating low back pain, headache pain, pain from osteoarthritis, neck pain, musculoskeletal and myofascial pain, organic pain, and presurgical and postsurgical pain. It has been found effective for postoperative and chemotherapy-induced nausea, neurological dysfunction, gynecologic and obstetric conditions, and as a potential treatment for substance abuse (Barclay & Lie, 2005; Freeman, 2004).

Ayurveda

Ayurveda therapy uses aromatherapy, colors, diet, herbs, massage, sound therapy, and yoga to restore harmony and balance to the spirit–mind–body system. Ayurveda has been used for over 5,000 years and is the ancient traditional medicine of India. The term *Ayurveda* is based on two Sanskrit words: *ayu,* meaning "life," and *veda,* meaning "knowledge" or "science." The fundamental principle of Ayurveda is to treat the disease with the method opposite to it in nature, for example, a warm disease, such as arthritis, which produces warmth in the joints, would be treated with a cold remedy (Halpern, 2000; Hardy, 2001). Aside from knowing disease etiology and the nature of the disease, the Ayurveda practitioner acquires information from the patient and develops an understanding of the patient emotionally, physically, and spiritually. The lifestyle of the patient is considered before the practitioner can prescribe a therapy to treat the opposite (warm vs. cold) qualities of the disease and offer counseling. Ayurveda places a high importance on keeping the body and mind clean and pure to prevent toxins from causing disease. For prevention of disease a regimen called *panchakarma* is used to cleanse and rejuvenate the body, mind, and consciousness. Through this *panchakarma* process of detoxification, cleansing is achieved using all the physiologic systems and orifices of the patient. Before the 15-day process of *panchakarma* can take place, medicated oils are applied externally and internally; this is called *poovakarma*, and it is the initial purging process of detoxifying the body. This process stimulates sweating and facilitates cleansing. Next, *vamana* (emesis) is induced and continues until the patient is vomiting a yellow color (jejunal fluid), which takes about eight bouts of vomiting. This is followed by *paschatkarma*, which basically implies a strict diet regimen. *Virechana* (purgation) is next, eliminating toxic wastes from the intestine. This process takes about 20 purges. From there, *vasti* (enemas) are used to further cleanse the colon with a mixture of honey, rock salt, oils, and medicines. Next is *nasya* (nasal application of herbal medicines, which cleanses the head and sinuses), followed by, finally, *raktamoksha* (blood-letting), often performed by use of a leech to suck out the impure blood from around an infected area. Ayurveda advises undergoing *panchakarma* at seasonal changes to keep the metabolism strong and prevent a buildup of toxins in the body and mind. The *panchakarma* process is meant to make the patient more receptive to the curative process (Life Positive, 2005).

According to Ayurveda, the human being is composed of five elements of nature, three *doshas* (biologic energies), seven *dhatus* (tissues), which maintain and nourish the body, and several *srotas* (channels), which are responsible for transportation of food (blockages cause disease). The five elements found in nature are space, air, fire, water, and earth. The three *doshas,* which are characteristic in all individuals, are space and air, fire, and water and earth. Each type of *doshas* determines the diagnosis and treatment by the physician or practitioner after *nadi vigyan,* which is a detailed technique of pulse diagnosis. A full medical examination of the tongue, voice, eyes, skin, urine, stool, and general appearance is taken in account before prescribing treatment (Halpern, 2000).

Scientific Evidence. Scientific evidence in Parkinson's disease is lacking at this time.

Traditional Chinese Herbal Medicine

Traditional Chinese medicine (TCM) is a system of healing that was developed in China and dates back to 200 B.C. The TCM view believes that the body is a balance between two opposing and inseparable forces called the yin and yang. Yin represents the cold, slow, or passive principle, while yang represents the hot, excited, or lively principle. The yin and yang must remain in a balanced state to prevent disease. When there is an imbalance between the yin and yang, the flow of Qi (vital energy or life force) is blocked along the blood pathways called meridians. TCM is a medical system which believes that the body has the power to heal itself (Bensky & Gamble, 1993; Lee et al., 2004; NCCAM, 2004c). The TCM practitioner may use herbs, acupuncture, or massage to help unblock Qi and bring the body back into a wellness state. Each therapy is individualized according to the area of the imbalance. The practitioner may use any of the following modalities:

1. Massage and manipulation
2. Chinese *Materia Medica* (the encyclopedia of natural products used in TCM)
3. Acupuncture and moxibustion (moxibustion is the use of heat from the burning of the herb moxa for the designed acupuncture site)
4. Diet and exercise.

TCM modalities treat a variety of diseases and symptoms, including movement disorders, depression, and insomnia, often suffered by PLWP.

Homeopathy

Homeopathy is a system of medical theory and practice that dates back to its founder, a German physician named Samuel C. Hahnemann (1755–1843). Hahnemann hypothesized that the selection of a therapy should closely resemble the symptoms of the patient's disease. He called it the "principle of similars." He would give repeated doses of many common remedies to healthy volunteers and record the symptoms the remedies produced. This procedure is called *proving,* or in modern homeopathy, a *human pathogenic trial.* As a result of his experiment, Hahnemann developed treatments for sick patients by matching the symptoms produced by a drug to symptoms in sick patients. At the present time, homeopathy is administered in minuscule or virtually nonexistent dosages. There are some efficacy questions about this practice (Bellavite & Signorini, 1995; Jonas, Kaptchuk, & Linde, 2003).

Homeopathic theory asserts that each individual has a self-healing capacity that homeopathy activates. Homeopathic medicines are extremely dilute and are virtually nontoxic (Bellavite & Signorini, 1995; Jonas et al., 2003).

Scientific Evidence. In a meta-analysis of 110 homeopathy trials and 110 matched conventional medicine trials, the results indicated weak evidence for a specific effect of homeopathic remedies; therefore the benefit is comparable to placebo effect (Shang et al., 2005).

Naturopathy

Naturopathy translates as "nature disease" and is a healing system created in Europe during the 1900s. Naturopathy, or naturopathic medicine, is practiced throughout Europe, Australia, New Zealand, Canada, and the United States. Naturopathy views disease as a manifestation of changes in the processes by which the body naturally heals itself. It not only focuses on disease treatment; it also emphasizes health restoration (Smith & Logan, 2002). Naturopathy does not focus on symptoms, but rather, on underlying disease causes. These causes may occur at many levels, including the physical, mental, emotional, and spiritual levels. The cause of the symptoms must be determined by the practitioner, who must evaluate the root causes of the disease on all levels and choose the treatment for those causes instead of for the symptoms exhibited (Smith & Logan, 2002).

There are six principles that form the foundation of naturopathic practice:

1. The healing power of nature
2. Identification and treatment of the cause of disease
3. The concept of "first do no harm"
4. The doctor as a teacher
5. Treatment of the whole person
6. Prevention

The modalities used in naturopathy include diet modification, nutritional supplements, herbal medicine, acupuncture, Chinese medicine, hydrotherapy, massage, joint manipulation, and lifestyle counseling (Smith & Logan, 2002).

Scientific Evidence. Scientific evidence is lacking at this time.

Tai Chi

Tai chi originated over 1,000 years ago in China. Tai chi uses slow, graceful movements to relax and strengthen muscles and joints. This form of exercise developed from Taoism, an ancient belief system in which movements of the body are coordinated with the mind and breathing to improve physical and psychological well-being. Tai chi places an emphasis on tranquility of the mind and agility of the body. The slow-flowing movements of tai chi maintain flexibility, balance, energy, and relaxation, from which PLWP may benefit.

There are eight *postures* and five *attitudes* in tai chi that drive the movements (Gilchrist, 2005). The eight postures include the following:

1. Ward-off
2. Rollback
3. Press
4. Push
5. Pull
6. Split
7. Elbow strike
8. Shoulder strike

The five attitudes are:
1. Advance
2. Retreat
3. Look left
4. Gaze right
5. Central equilibrium

Tai chi incorporates philosophy, physiology, psychology, geometry, and the laws of dynamics into the postures and attitudes to achieve the slow-flowing body movements. Tai chi has been described as yoga and meditation in motion (Gilchrist, 2005).

Scientific Evidence. In four trials involving 206 participants who were diagnosed with rheumatoid arthritis, evidence showed improvements in range of motion of ankle plantar flexion and lower extremities. A comparison of traditional range of motion exercises with tai chi reported a significantly higher level of participation and enjoyment with tai chi (Han, Judd, Robinson, & Taixiang, 2004).

Diet and Nutrition

Fava Beans

Fava beans are legumes (sometimes referred to as broad or horse beans) that grow in a long pod with large, flat seeds inside. In the Mediterranean region this bean has been eaten for thousands of years and is a good source of iron, magnesium, potassium, zinc, copper, selenium, and vitamin C. Three and a half ounces of fresh cooked fava beans contain 56 calories, 20 g of carbohydrates, 5 g of protein, and 2 g of fiber (1 oz = 2 tbsp; Holden, 2001). Fava beans contain levodopa, which is the same chemical as in carbidopa/levodopa (Sinemet) and other levodopa medications that treat Parkinson's disease. The amount of levodopa in the beans is dependent on soil conditions, rainfall, harvesting season, and other factors. Therefore there can be much variability in the amount of levodopa found in fava beans. Holden (2001) recommends 3 oz of fresh green fava beans, or 3 oz of canned green fava beans, believed to contain 50–100 mg of levodopa. However, too little could result in the undertreatment of bothersome symptoms, while too much could result in overmedication symptoms, such as dyskinesias, nausea, or hypotension. It is not known what the bean's absorption rate is, nor is its duration effect known. People may also have an allergy to fava beans.

PLWP who are depressed and take MAO-A isocarboxazid (Marplan), phenelzine (Nardil), or tranylcypromine (Parnate) should not eat fava beans. Also, PLWP taking MAO-B inhibitors, such as selegiline (Eldepryl) or rasagiline, should not eat fava beans. The combination of fava beans and the above medications can raise the blood pressure dramatically.

These beans can be purchased at specialty food stores or at Middle Eastern grocery stores. They can be cooked, seasoned, and served as a side dish, added to salads, or eaten alone. One serving daily or every other day should be adequate when eaten in conjunction with Parkinson's medications (Holden, 2001).

Scientific Evidence. Multiple reports appear to show that fava bean ingestion can be beneficial as adjunctive therapy in PD. However, clinical research trials are needed to ascertain how to dose fava beans so as to avoid "favism" (i.e., overdosage), or underdosage when used.

IMPORTANCE OF CAM THERAPY
TO NURSING PRACTICE

Nurses frequently see PLWP and their families who, many times, feel hopeless and possibly desperate about their medical condition. In these moments they may turn to CAM therapies, no matter how unrealistic or far-fetched they seem, how much they cost, or whether or not they have relevant scientific justification. Just because the CAM therapy makes perfect sense and seems quite logical or harmless does not mean it works for PLWP.

Patient history and information obtained by the nurse are parts of the patient assessment. The nurse asks medical, surgical, and personal questions regarding the patient's social history, such as alcohol use, religious preference, and so on. PLWP CAM use information should become a part of the patient intake history and can easily be asked with the medication history, that is, use of over-the-counter medications, vitamins, and so on. Health care providers need to know if PLWP are engaged in CAM therapy and may find the need to discuss the risks and benefits of certain therapies with the patient and family. The literature shows that CAM therapy choices selected by the patient are frequently made without consulting a physician (Rajendran et al., 2001).

Currently, and over the past decade, a database with a growing body of evidence about CAM therapy has and is being collected through randomized clinical trials in accordance with sound scientific principles (Spencer & Jacobs, 2003). Nurses may find this information helpful as well as interesting (Table 11.1). This database contains empiric, evidence-based information about the CAM therapies that have scientific proof of their benefits and the ones that have not shown any therapeutic value (Spencer & Jacobs, 2003). The knowledgeable nurse could educate PLWP in the wise use of time and money in relation to CAM therapy. Nurses cognizant of the patient population's growing use of CAM therapies can offer much in the form of CAM education—the CAM therapies available and their purposes—in order to steer PLWP and their families toward health and a feeling of well-being that complements traditional medicine. Always keep in mind that first, we do no harm.

TABLE 11.1 CAM Therapy Resource List

Acupuncture[a]

The American Academy of Medical Acupuncture (AAMA)

5820 Wilshire Boulevard, Suite 500

Los Angeles, CA 90036

(323) 937-5514

Web site: http://www.medicalacupuncture.org

Acupuncture.com

Web site: http://www.acupuncture.com

Acupuncture

Web site: http://nccam.nih.gov/health/acupuncture/index.htm

Alexander Technique

American Society for the Alexander Technique (ASAT)

3010 Hennepin Ave. South Suite 10

Minneapolis, MN 55408

(612) 824-5066

(800) 473-0620

E-mail: ASAT@ix.netcom.com

Web site: http://www.alexandertech.com

American Association of Oriental Medicine (AAOM)

433 Front Street

(303) 449-2265

Catasauque, PA 18032

(888) 555-7999

Web site: http://www.aaom.org

Ayurvedic medicine

National Institute of Ayurvedic Medicine (NIAM)

584 Milltown Road

Brewster, New York 10509

(914) 278-8700

Web site: http://www.niam.com

(continued)

TABLE 11.1 CAM Therapy Resource List *(continued)*

Biofeedback[a]

Biofeedback Certification Institute of America

10200 W. 44th Avenue, Suite 310

Wheatridge, CO 80033

(303) 420-2902

Web site: http://www.bcia.org

Chiropractic[a]

American Chiropractic Association

1701 Clarendon Boulevard

Arlington, VA 22209

(703) 276-8800

Web site: http://www.amerchiro.org

Exercise

The Cooper Institute

12100 Preston Road

Dallas, TX 75230

(972) 233-4832

Web site: http://www.cooperaerobics.com

Guided imagery[a]

The Academy for Guided Imagery

PO Box 2070

Mill Valley, CA 94942

(800) 726-2070

Web site: http://www.healthy.net/agi/index_explorer.html

Herbs[a]

American Herbalists Guild

1931 Gaddis Road

Canton, GA 30115

(770) 751-6021

Web site: http://www.americanherbalist.com

The Herb Research Foundation

4140 15th Street

Boulder, CO 80304

(303) 449-2265

Web site: http://www.herbs.org

(continued)

TABLE 11.1 *(continued)*

Homeopathy[a]

National Center for Homeopathy

801 North Fairfax Street, Suite 306

Alexandria, VA 22314

(703) 548-7790

Web site: http://www.homeopathic.org

Hypnosis[a]

American Society of Clinical Hypnosis

140 N. Bloomingdale Road

Bloomingdale, IL 60108

(630) 980-4740

Web site: http://www.asch.net

International Medical and Dental

Hypnotherapy Association

4110 Edgeland, Suite 800

Royal Oak, MI 48073

(800) 257-5467

Web site: http://www.infinityinst.com/imdha.html

Massage[a]

American Massage Therapy Association

820 Davis Street, Suite 100

Evanston, IL 60201

(847) 864-0123

*Web site:*http:// www.amtamassage.org

Meditation

Center for Mindfulness in Medicine, Health Care, and Society

University of Massachusetts Medical Center

419 Belmond Avenue, 2nd Floor

Worcester, MA 01604

Web site: http://www.mindfulnesstapes.com

(continued)

TABLE 11.1 CAM Therapy Resource List (continued)

Music therapy

American Music Therapy Association, Inc.

8455 Colewsville Road, Suite 1000

Silver Spring, MD 20910

(301) 589-3300

Web site: http://www.musictherapy.org

Spiritual medicine[a]

Institute for Medicine and Prayer

St. Vincent Hospital

455 St. Michael's Drive

Santa Fe, NM 87505

(505) 820-5479

Therapeutic touch

Nurse Healers Professional Associates, Inc.

3760 South Highland Drive, Suite 429

Salt Lake City, UT 84106

(801) 273-3399

Web site: http://www.therapeutic-touch.org

Trager Approach

The Trager Institute

21 Locust Ave.

Mill Valley, CA 94941

(415) 388-2688

E-mail: admin@trager.com

Web site: http://www.trager.com

Other resources

American Holistic Nurses' Association

PO Box 2130

Flagstaff, AZ 86003-2130

(800) 278-2462

Web site: http://www.ahna.org

CAM on Pubmed

Web site: http://www.nlm.nih.gov/nccam/camonpubmed.html

Food and Drug Administration

Web site: http://www.fda.gov

(continued)

TABLE 11.1 *(continued)*

Medline Plus

Web site: http://www.nlm.nih.gov/medlineplus/alternativemedicine.html

National Center for Complementary and

Alternative Medicine (NCCAM)

PO Box 7923

Gaithersburg, MD 20898

(888) 644-6226

Fax: (866) 464-3616

E-mail: info@nccam.nih.gov

Web site: http://nccam.nih.gov/health/advice/index/html

Quackwatch

Web site: http://quackwatch.com

The Integrative Medicine Consult

Newsletter for Health Professionals

Integrative Medicine Communications

43 Bowdoin Street

Boston, MA 02114

(800) 217-1938

White House Commission on Complementary and Alternative Medicine Policy

Web site: http://www.whccamp.hhs.gov

SUMMARY

The biopsychosocial-spiritual patient concept (Astin et al., 2000) appears to be the desired patient model of the present, and the patient seems to be seeking therapies available without consulting the care provider. As more patients seek care alongside and outside of the biomedical model, we need to listen to and look at the actions of our patients. The patient is learning more and more about diseases, symptoms, and treatment options through Internet resources and other media. These resources discuss traditional Western medicine and CAM therapy. The patient is calling on those resources in an effort to broaden health care choices in order to improve quality of life. Health care professionals must become knowledgeable about the CAM therapies the patient is learning about and using so that nurses can guide the patient and be able to recognize any contraindications to patient care.

Nurses should also advise PLWP to consult their physicians before taking so-called natural herbal medicines to ensure that there are no contraindications to their herbal and traditional medication regimens. Also, remind the PLWP to monitor their progress with herbal or CAM therapies and decide whether the improvement, if any, is worth the monetary investment and time commitment.

The National Institutes of Health–sponsored National Center for Complementary and Alternative Medicine is a huge step forward in answering the many questions on the value of the multitude of CAMs our patients are using. With adequate research funding and scientifically based studies to develop evidence-based outcomes, nurses will be in a much better place to guide patients on the use of the myriad of products available to them.

REFERENCES

American Music Association. (1999). Frequently asked questions about music therapy. Retrieved August 5, 2005, from http://www.musictherapy.org/faqs. html

Andrasik, F., & Lords, A. (2004). Biofeedback. In L. Freeman (Ed.), *Mosby's complementary and alternative medicine: A research-based approach* (2nd rev. ed., pp. 207–235). St. Louis, MO: Mosby.

Arnold, J. (2004). *Alexander Technique*. Retrieved August 5, 2005, from http://www.alexandertechnique.com/at/

Astin, J., Shapiro, S., & Schwartz, G. (2000). Meditation. In D. W. Novey (Ed.), *Clinician's complete reference to complementary/alternative medicine* (pp. 73–85). St. Louis, MO: Mosby.

Barclay, L., & Lie, D. (2005, October 24). *Acupuncture may be helpful for chronic daily headache*. Retrieved November 22, 2005, from http://www.medscape.com/viewarticle/515298_print

Barnes, V., Treiber, F., & Davis, H. (2001). Impact of transcendental meditation on cardiovascular function at rest and during acute stress in adolescents with high normal blood pressure. *Journal of Psychosomatic Research, 51,* 597–605.

Bellavite, P., & Signorini, A. (1995). *Homeopathy: A frontier in medical science*. Berkeley, CA: North Atlantic.

Benedetti, P., & MacPhail, W. (2003). *Spin doctors: The chiropractic industry under examination*. New York: Dundurn Press.

Bensky, D., & Gamble, A. (1993). *Chinese herbal medicine: Materia medica* (Rev. ed.). Seattle, WA: Eastland Press.

Bent, S., Kane, C., Shinohara, K., Neuhaus, J., Hudes, E. S., Goldberg, H., et al. (2006). Saw palmetto for benign prostatic hyperplasia. *New England Journal of Medicine, 354,* 557–566.

Bishop, S. (2002). What do we really know about mindfulness-based stress reduction? *Psychosomatic Medicine, 64,* 71–83.

Buckle, J. (2004). Aromatherapy. In L. Freeman (Ed.), *Mosby's complementary and alternative medicine: A research-based approach* (2nd rev. ed., pp. 417–435). St. Louis, MO: Mosby.

Burgner, K. (2005, June 20). Musical intervention. *Advance for Nurses,* 15–18.

Buscemi, N., Vandermeer, B., Pandya, R., Hooton, N., Tjosvold, L., Hartling, L., et al. (2004, November). *Melatonin for treatment of sleep disorders*. Retrieved December 28, 2005, from http://www.ahrq.gov/clinic/epcsums/melatsum.htm

Carter, B. (2001). A pilot study to evaluate the effectiveness of Bowen Technique in the management of clients with frozen shoulder. *Complementary Therapy Medicine, 4,* 208–215.

Davidson, R., Kabat-Zinn, J., Schumacher, J., Rosenkranz, M., Muller, D., Santorelli, S. F., et al. (2003). Alterations in brain and immune function produced by mindfulness meditation. *Psychosomatic Medicine, 65,* 564–570.

Decker, G. M. (2000). An overview of complementary and alternative therapies. *Clinical Journal of Oncology Nursing, 4,* 49–53.

Donaldson, V. (2000). A clinical study of visualization on depressed white blood cell count in medical patients. *Applied Psychophysiology of Biofeedback, 25,* 117–121.

Dunn, C., Sleep, J., & Collett, D. (1995). Sensing an improvement: An experimental study to evaluate the use of aromatherapy, massage and periods of rest in an intensive care unit. *Journal of Advanced Nursing, 21,* 34–40.

Duval, C., Lafontaine, D., Herbert, J., Leroux, A., Panisset, M., & Boucher, J. P. (2002). The effect of Trager therapy on the level of evoked stretch responses in patients with Parkinson's disease and rigidity. *Journal of Manipulative Physiological Therapy, 25,* 455–464.

Faculty at Harvard Medical School. (2005a, July 5). *Aromatherapy.* Retrieved August 5, 2005, from http://www.intelihealth.com/IH/ihtPrint/ WSIHW000/8513/34968/360050.html

Faculty at Harvard Medical School. (2005b). *Complementary and alternative medicine—Bowen Technique.* Retrieved August 5, 2005, from http://www.intelihealth.com/IH/ihtIH?d=dmtContent&c=358741&p=~ br,IHW|~st,8513|~r,WSIHW000|~b,*|

Fellowes, D., Barnes, K., & Wilkinson, S. (2004). *Aromatherapy and massage for symptom relief in patients with cancer.* Retrieved February 9, 2006, from the Cochrane database, http://www.cochrane.org/reviews/ en/ab002287.html

Fetrow, C. W., & Avila, J. R. (2000). Herbal medicines A to Z. In M. Andrews, K. Dodds, C. Harold, & P. Johnson (Eds.), *The complete guide to herbal medicines* (pp. 1–568). Springhouse, PA: Springhouse.

Fisher, A., & Morley, J. (2004). Anti-aging and complementary therapies. In C. Johnson & P. Boyle (Eds.), *Current geriatric diagnosis and treatment* (pp. 468–481). New York: McGraw-Hill.

Freeman, L. (2004). *Mosby's complementary and alternative medicine: A research-based approach* (2nd rev. ed.). St. Louis, MO: Mosby.

Gilchrist, L. (2005, April 13). *Parkinson's disease meeting its match in tai chi.* Retrieved June 15, 2005, from http://www.worldtaichiday.org/ PARKINSONSTC.html

Goldberg, M. (2004). *The F. M. Alexander Technique.* Retrieved March 7, 2006, from http://www.alexandercenter.com/#Anchor6

Green, J., & Lynn, S. (2000). Hypnosis and suggestion-based approaches to smoking cessation: An examination of the evidence. *International Journal of Clinical and Experimental Hypnosis, 48,* 191–211.

Halpern, M. (2000). Ayurveda. In D. W. Novey (Ed.), *Clinician's complete reference to complementary/alternative medicine* (pp. 246–257). St. Louis, MO: Mosby.

Han, A., Judd, M., Robinson, V., & Taixiang, W. (2004). *Tai chi for treating rheumatoid arthritis (1).* Retrieved January 19, 2007 from the Cochrane database, http://www.cochrane.org/reviews/en/ab004849.html

Hansen, D., & Triano, J. (2000). Chiropractic. In D. W. Novey (Ed.), *Clinician's complete reference to complementary/alternative medicine* (pp. 310–324). St. Louis, MO: Mosby.

Hardy, M. (2001). Ayurveda: Where do we go from here? *Alternative Therapies in Health Medicine, 2,* 32–35.

Harvard Medical School Office of Public Affairs (2005, January 12). *Complementary and alternative medicine used widely by one third of US adults—Remains unchanged from 1997.* Boston, MA: Author.

Hasegawa, Y., Kubota, N., Inagki, T., & Shinagawa, N. (2001). Music therapy induced alterations in natural killer cell count and function. *Nippon Ronen Igakkai Zasshi, 38,* 201–206.

Holden, K. (2001). *Fava beans, levodopa, and Parkinson's disease.* Retrieved January 19, 2007, from http://www.parkinson.org/site/apps/s/content.asp?c=9dJFJLPwB&b=108269&ct=89694

Jackson, D. A. (2005). The next step in becoming evidence-based. *Chiropractic Journal, 12,* 11–15.

Jonas, W., Kaptchuk, T., & Linde, K. (2003). A critical overview of homeopathy. *Annals of Internal Medicine, 138,* 393–399.

Katzenschlager, R., Evans, A., Manson, A., Patsalos, P., Ratnaraj, N., Watt, H., et al. (2004). Mucuna pruriens in Parkinson's disease: A double blind clinical and pharmacological study. *Journal of Neurology, Neurosurgery, and Psychiatry, 75,* 1672–1677.

Lee, B., LaRiccia, P., & Newberg, A. (2004). Acupuncture in theory and practice. *Hospital Physician, 40,* 11–14.

Library Web Master. (2005, October). *Palmer College of Chiropractic special collections and archives.* Retrieved December 28, 2005, from http://www.palmer.edu/PCC_Library/Special_Services/special.htm

Life Positive. (2005). *Panchakarma and other Ayurvedic remedies.* Retrieved January 20, 2006, from http://www.lifepositive.com/Body/ayurvedic-remedies.asp

Liskin, J. (2004). Aromatherapy. In L. Freeman (Ed.), *Mosby's complementary and alternative medicine: A research-based approach* (2nd rev. ed., pp. 472–482). St. Louis, MO: Mosby.

Lynn, S., Kirsch, I., Barabasz, A., Cardena, E., & Patterson, D. (2000). Hypnosis as an empirically supported clinical intervention: The state of the evidence and a look to the future. *International Journal of Clinical and Experimental Hypnosis, 48,* 239–259.

Mackay, N., Hansen, S., & McFarlane, O. (2004). Autonomic nervous system changes during Reiki treatment: A preliminary study. *Journal of Alternative and Complementary Medicine, 10,* 1077–1081.

Mayo Clinic. (2004, January). *Biofeedback: Using the power of your mind to improve your health.* Retrieved August 5, 2005, from http://www.mayoclinic.com/health/biofeedback/SA00083

McClain, C., Rosenfeld, B., & Breitbart, W. (2003). Effect of spiritual well-being on end-of-life despair in terminally-ill cancer patients. *Lancet, 361,* 1603–1607.

Miles, P., & True, G. (2003). Reiki—review of biofield therapy history, theory, practice and research. *Alternative Therapy in Health and Medicine, 2,* 62–72.

Miller, L. G., Hume, A., Harris, M., Jackson, E., Kanmer, T., Cauffield, J., et al. (2000). White paper on herbal products. *Pharmacotherapy, 20,* 877–891.

Montgomery, G., Weltz, C. R., Seltz, M., & Bovbjerg, D. H. (2000). Brief presurgery hypnosis reduces distress and pain in excisional breast biopsy patients. *International Journal of Clinical Experimental Hypnosis, 50,* 17–32.

National Center for Complementary and Alternative Medicine. (2004a, October). *Energy medicine: An overview.* Retrieved August 2, 2005, from http://nccam.nih.gov/health/backgrounds/energymed.htm

National Center for Complementary and Alternative Medicine. (2004b, September). *Selecting a complementary and alternative medicine (CAM) practitioner* (NCCAM Publication No. D168). Retrieved December 28, 2005, from http://nccam.nih.gov/health/practitioner/index.htm

National Center for Complementary and Alternative Medicine. (2004c). *Whole medical systems: An overview.* Retrieved August 2, 2005, from http://nccam.nih.gov/health/backgrounds/wholemed.htm

National Center for Complementary and Alternative Medicine. (2006, November). *NCCAM facts-at-a-glance.* Retrieved January 4, 2006, from http://nccam.nih.gov/about/ataglance/index.htm

NurseScribe. (2005). *Nursing theory.* Retrieved March 15, 2006, from http://www.enursescribe.com/nurse_theorists.htm

Pacchetti, C., Mancini, F., Aglieri, R., Fundaro, C., Martignoni, E., & Nappi, G. (2000). Active music therapy in Parkinson's disease: An integrative method for motor and emotional rehabilitation. *Psychosomatic Medicine, 62,* 386–393.

Page, S. J., Levine, P., Sisto, S., & Johnston, M. V. (2001). A randomized efficacy and feasibility study of imagery in acute stroke. *Clinical Rehabilitation, 15,* 233–240.

Phillips, R. B. (2004, May). *A brief history of chiropractic.* Retrieved December 28, 2005, from http://www.chiroweb.com/archives/ahcpr/chapter1.htm

Pilkington, K., Kirkwood, G., Rampes, H., & Richardson, J. (2005). Yoga for depression: The research evidence. *Journal of Affective Disorders, 89,* 13–24.

Quigley, D., & Dean, C. (2000). Yoga. In D. W. Novey (Ed.), *Clinician's complete reference to complementary/alternative medicine* (pp. 141–151). St. Louis, MO: Mosby.

Rajendran, P., Thompson, R., & Reich, S. (2001). The use of alternative therapies by patients with Parkinson's disease. *Neurology, 57,* 790–794.

Relman, A. (2001). A critical view. *Advances in Mind-Body Medicine, 17,* 68.

Reuters Health Information. (2006). *Ginger prevents postoperative nausea and vomiting.* Retrieved January 25, 2006, from http://www.medscape.com/viewarticle/521620_print

Rossman, M. L., & Bresler, D. E. (2000). Interactive guided imagery. In D.W. Novey (Ed.), *Clinician's complete reference to complementary/alternative medicine* (pp. 64–72). St. Louis, MO: Mosby.

Schwartz, M., & Olson, P. (2003). *A historical perspective on the field of biofeedback and applied psychophysiology* (3rd rev. ed.). New York: Guilford Press.

Shafranske, E., & Malony, H. (1990). Clinical psychologists' religious and spiritual orientations and their practice of psychotherapy. *Psychotherapy, 27,* 72–78.

Shang, A., Huwiler-Muntener, K., Nartey, L., Juni, P., Dorig, S., Sterne, J., et al. (2005). Are the clinical effects of homeopathy placebo effects? A comparative study of placebo-controlled trials of homeopathy and allopathy. *Lancet, 366,* 2083–2086.

Shults, C., Oakes, D., Kieburtz, K., Beal, F., Haas, R., Plumb, S., et al. (2002). Effects of coenzyme Q_{10} in early Parkinson disease: Evidence of slowing of the functional decline. *Archives of Neurology, 59,* 1541–1550.

Skargren, E. (1997). Cost and effectiveness analysis of chiropractic and physiotherapy treatment for low back pain: Six month follow-up. *Spine, 22,* 2167–2176.

Smith, M., & Logan, A. (2002). Naturopathy. *Medical Clinics of North America, 1,* 173–184.

Sola, I., Thompson, E., Subirana, M., Lopez, C., Pascual, A. (2006). *Non-invasive interventions for improving well-being and quality of life in patients with lung cancer.* Retrieved February 9, 2006, from the Cochrane database, http://www.cochrane.org/reviews/en/ab004282.html

Spencer, J., & Jacobs, J. (2003). *Complementary and alternative medicine: An evidence-based approach* (2nd rev. ed.). St. Louis, MO: Mosby.

Stephenson, N., & Dalton, J. (2003). Using reflexology for pain management: A review. *Journal of Holistic Nursing, 2,* 179–191.

Stern, G., Lander, C., & Lees, A. (1980). Akinetic freezing and trick movements in Parkinson's disease. *Journal of Neural Transmission Supplement, 16,* 137–141.

White, A., Williamson, J., Hart, A., & Ernst, E. (2000). A blinded investigation into the accuracy of reflexology charts. *Complementary Therapeutic Medicine, 3,* 166–172.

Wikipedia, (2006). Hypnosis. Retrieved February 2, 2007 from www.http:/en.wikipedia.org/wiki/Hypnosis

Wildman, F., Stephens, J., & Aum, L. (2000). Feldenkrais Method. In D. W. Novey (Ed.), *Clinician's complete reference to complementary/ alternative medicine* (pp. 3931–406). St. Louis, MO: Mosby.

Index

Page numbers followed by a t indicate a table on that page; page numbers followed by an f indicate a figure on that page

SPRINGER / PUBLISHING COMPANY

Essentials of Clinical Genetics in Nursing Practice

Felissa R. Lashley, PhD, RN, ACRN, FAAN, FACMG

Refresh your genetic knowledge and enhance your patient care...

We now know that genetic factors can cause disease or affect an individual's susceptibility or resistance to disorders and even to treatment. To provide the best nursing care, it is therefore essential that practitioners and students have a basic knowledge of the science of genetics and how it affects the major areas of nursing expertise.

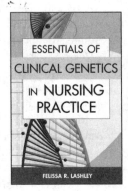

ESSENTIALS OF
CLINICAL GENETICS
IN NURSING
PRACTICE

FELISSA R. LASHLEY

To address this need, Dr. Felissa Lashley has created this "essentials" guide specifically for nurses. From genetic factors and trends affecting health care today, to the more complex discussions of human variation, every genetic topic critical to the practice of nursing and nursing education is covered, including:

- Prevention of Genetic Disease
- Genetic Testing and Treatment
- Genetic Counseling
- Maternal-Child Nursing
- Psychiatric/Mental Health Nursing
- Community/Public Health Nursing
- Trends, Policies, and Social and Ethical Issues

Each chapter examines how genetic information influences treatment and management and is intended to further the development of a nurse's "genetic eye" in the daily care of patients.

2006 · 352pp · softcover · 978-0-8261-0222-5

11 West 42nd Street, New York, NY 10036-8002 • Fax: 212-941-7842
Order Toll-Free: 877-687-7476 • Order Online: www.springerpub.com